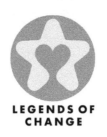

LEGENDS OF CHANGE

A REVOLUTION POWERED BY WOMAN-KIND

REBECCA FRITH

INSPIRATIONAL REAL LIFE STORIES
FROM A GROWING MOVEMENT
OF BRAVE WOMEN WHO ARE
CHANGING THE WORLD...

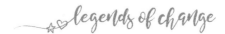

ISBN 978-0-6486720-0-5

FIRST EDITION

www.legendsofchange.com

Publisher's and Author's disclaimer:

Legends of Change book represents a wide range of women's opinions about a variety of topics mostly related to health, well-being, veganism, and a plant-based lifestyle. Certain ideas, procedures, advice, and treatments may be hazardous if undertaken without proper medical clearance or supervision.
We recommend that everyone does their own research and seek further advice. These opinions reflect the research and ideas of the writer and author but are not intended to substitute for the services of a trained practitioner. The author, publisher, and writers disclaim responsibility for any adverse effects resulting directly or indirectly from the information contained in this book.

Design, copy and layout:

Front cover image: Sammy Frith
Lead editor: Sara Hansen
Creative Director: Sammy Frith
Designer: Sammy Frith

Illustrations and art credits:

Single arrow (pg 5) - By Freepik
Boho Hand (pg 10) - By macrovector / Freepik
Big Butterfly (pg 16) - By Visnezh / Freepik
Wind blow (pg 110)- By macrovector_official / Freepik
Indian Hat (pg 191) - By macrovector / Freepik
Big arrows (pg 242) - By Omelapics / Freepik
Mum (pg 312) - By visnezh / Freepik
Big Sun (pg 356) - By macrovector_official / Freepik
Plant plate (pg 410) - By rawpixel.com / Freepik

In loving memory of my beautiful
Aunty Lyn Blake,
who lost her hard fought battle with
breast cancer in 2009.
For inspiring me in life and on this
journey to seek the truth...

CONTENTS

Legends of Change

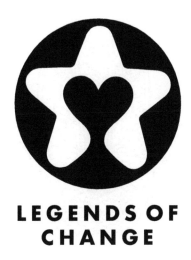

LEGENDS OF CHANGE

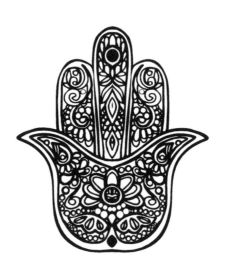

A LETTER FROM THE AUTHOR
REBECCA FRITH

From doctors, nutrition experts and Olympic athletes, to mums, daughters and women struggling with chronic illness, Legends of Change is the ultimate compilation of 85+ first-hand stories, helpful habits, and life-changing tips from women who have transitioned into a vegan lifestyle of plant-based eating. Empower yourself through the stories of people who are just like you, or someone you know, who has suffered through disease, disorders and despair. Passionate about this information and excited to speak out on the incredible benefits plant-based eating has had on their lives, the women featured in these short profiles detail their most personal life experiences in order to inspire you, the reader, to live the life that you're truly meant to live; healthier, happier and more fully alive.

No book can give you all of the answers to your questions, but this book may just be able to answer a few. Each chapter offers suggestions, advice, and simple tips about how to create daily habits that could truly change your life. Some ideas might work for you, while others may not. There are plenty of gems in here for each reader to discover and make their own.

Hi, I'm Bec, "compiler" of these incredible stories and founder of *Legends of Change*, a passionately driven mission to spread the message about the all-encompassing benefits of living a plant-based vegan lifestyle.

I lost my aunt to cancer in 2009, and this great loss to our family impacted me profoundly. After witnessing her long-suffering from this dreadful disease, I vowed that I would never suffer the same fate. The fear that this nasty destroyer of so many lives might be 'genetic' frightened me into finding out all that I could.

So I embarked on a quest to find out how I could prevent this from happening to me or any of my loved ones. After weeks, months, years of research, I believe I am on the right path, and at age 40, I have never looked or felt better.

But what started as a journey into health and nutrition became so much more. As I opened my eyes and mind to what I was putting on my plate and in my body, the inescapable truth as to why veganism is kinder to animals, to people and our planet's future began to shine bright.

In the last four years, I have influenced many of my family members and friends to change their eating habits and lifestyle, along with my husband and two boys Archie and Kik (ages 8 & 6), who are now three years vegan.

This has been a wonderful period of change in all our lives, but I knew it was more than that for me.

I wanted to do more; I couldn't just sit on all that I knew. I needed to find a way to share, inspire, and reach more people.

And that's when the seed for this book was born.

Women account for almost 80% of the Plant-Based/Vegan community, and we're on the front line of this movement.

If you're trying to go vegan, you're a pioneer.

After connecting on social media with so many women around the globe in the past few years, one thing stood out for me. It's the truth of each individual's story that has the biggest impact and influence on others. Real people with real-life stories.

Stories boost our feelings of trust, compassion and empathy. They motivate us to work with others, and they positively influence our social behavior. Because of this, stories have the unique ability to build lasting connections.

When we hear facts, it ignites the data processing centers in our brains, but when we listen to stories our sensory centers are moved.

With a growing ocean of truly moving and inspiring stories out there regarding the endless positives of taking up a vegan lifestyle, I felt like these stories needed to be told and shared. Not only to celebrate the love and power embodied in each of these real-life accounts but more importantly, to serve as a tool and inspiration to influence and help others.

All the brave women contained within these pages have been willing to share their stories, some very personal, and at times very difficult to tell, but they have done it to empower you, encourage and inspire you to help make a change. As human beings, we change through study, habits and real-life, relatable stories. The hope is that each time you pick up this book, you will find some new inspiration from women who you can empathize with and relate too.

As you go through this book, take your time to read the words, and feel the message with your heart as well as your mind. Some stories will speak more loudly to you than others. Some of the women will be familiar to you and will need little or no introduction, but others will be new voices, ones that I think will leave a lasting impression.

Legends of Change is a book you can share with your non-vegan friends, your sister, your grandma, your work colleague, your mom, or even the men in your life. It's a book that you should give to someone close to you for encouragement and inspiration because many of these stories will be relatable to so many people.

We have separated this book into seven different categories, and we have ten or so different questions for each genre. It doesn't have to be to a book that is read from cover to cover, but instead, a source of inspiration and revelation that you can pick up and open at any place or point. Some ideas might work for you; others may pass you by. This is perfectly fine but you might also find that the story you really need to hear may just be the one that you flip to at random.

13

I have laughed and I have cried. Reading these stories has changed my life for the better, I certainly hope the same for you.

I am so proud to be a part of this community of brave and compassionate legends, and to help do my bit to pave the way for a brighter, healthier and more compassionate future on planet Earth.

Finally, I'd like to thank you, the reader, from the bottom of my heart for supporting this book and sharing it with your family and friends.

It's truly been a labor of love.

xx,

With Love - Rebecca

legends of change

" "

I AM THRILLED TO BE A PART OF
THE AMAZING COMMUNITY OF
VEGAN WOMEN WHO ARE TRULY
CHANGING THE WORLD. OUR
ACTIONS TO CREATE A MORE
LOVING AND PEACEFUL WORLD
CARRY GREAT POWER, AND IT
IS NO SURPRISE TO ME THAT
ALMOST 80% OF ALL VEGANS IN
THE UNITED STATES ARE WOMEN.
I KNOW THAT THE STORIES IN
THIS BOOK WILL INSPIRE MANY
AROUND THE GLOBE TO CELEBRATE
THE MOST BEAUTIFUL GIFTS WE
HAVE TO GIVE TO OTHERS... OUR
SENSITIVITY, KINDNESS, LOVE
AND COMPASSION.

DR. JOANNE KONG

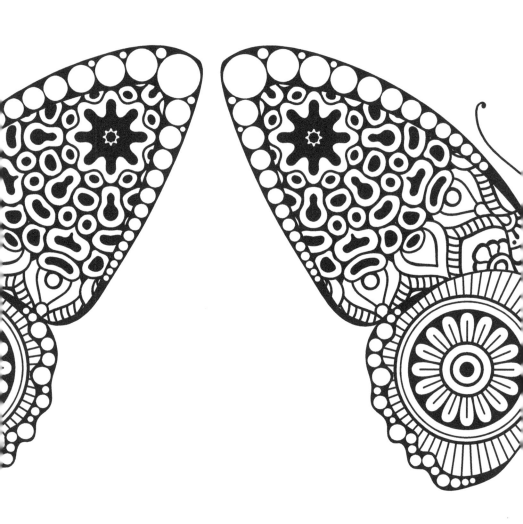

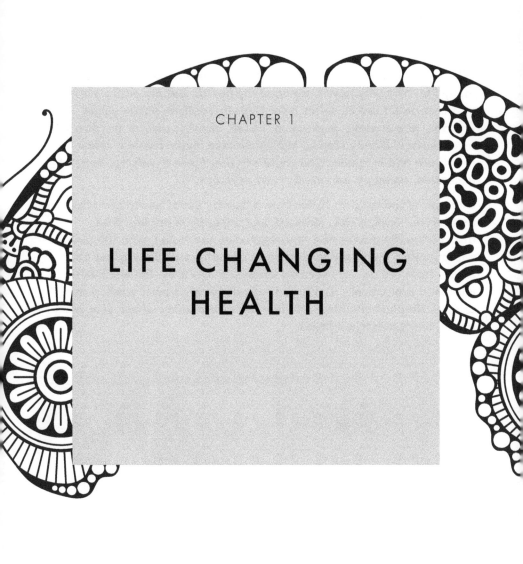

CHAPTER 1

LIFE CHANGING HEALTH

DEBORAH WOOD

CONNECT WITH DEBORAH:
FACEBOOK: DEBORAH.WOOD.1675

REVERSED MULTIPLE CHRONIC ILLNESSES AND DROPPED 100 POUNDS

"Going raw vegan was by FAR the best decision I have ever made in my life. Not only have I regained my health, but my entire life has also changed. I use to suffer from Hypothyroidism, fibromyalgia, arthritis, IBS, anxiety, depression, PCOS, obesity, plantar fasciitis, UTIs, incontinence, kidney stones, kidney disease, hypertension, reflux & heartburn and insomnia. You could say that I was a walking, beyond miserable, unhappy person, but not anymore."

Deborah Wood used to suffer from a laundry list of health complications that left her feeling sick, stressed, and unhappy in her life. After discovering the power of a raw vegan diet and losing over 100 pounds without much physical exercise, years of ineffective dieting and poor advice from her doctors seemed laughable. Once her life and health improved dramatically, Deborah finally discovered what worked was also the simplest and most intuitive path: consuming whole, raw, plant-based, nutrient-packed foods.

18

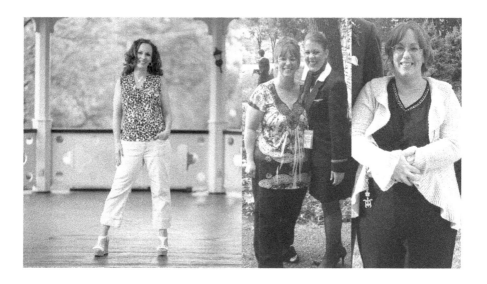

WHAT ARE YOUR DAILY RITUALS/HABITS WHICH YOU BELIEVE HAVE BEEN KEY TO YOUR HEALTH?

I would have to say that I practice positive thinking and gratitude every single day. I believe those two components are essential for success in life in anything and everything you do. I also journal once a week to keep track of the goals I accomplish, failures that happen, food I am currently eating and craving, and all of my health-related problems and improvements. Other daily rituals include food preparation, hygiene, and I try to get some sort of movement in. I don't really exercise as much as I would like to due to an injury, so I strive for movement. I also pray. I pray for guidance, health, strength and peace, as well as many other things.

AT WHAT POINT IN YOUR LIFE DID YOU DECIDE TO CHANGE YOUR DIET? HOW HAS THAT DECISION IMPACTED YOUR LIFE?

I decided on raw vegan. I had tried it in the past but failed. It was too hard for me. It was like trying to relearn everything I knew about cooking and eating, and it seemed so frustrating. But this time I felt I had nothing to lose, and I knew that nutrition was the answer.

In September of 2016, I went raw vegan "cold turkey," as the ironic saying goes. I gave it all up. I gave up holiday dinners and Christmas cookies and birthday cakes and steak and gravy. I gave up pizza and fries and ice-cream and soda. I gave it all up! Was it hard? Sure it was! But I was determined that I was going to do this. I was going to get my life back! I was going to change my attitude and my outlook on life! I was going to heal and inspire others to do the same, and I did.

WHAT THINGS HAVE MADE THE MOST DIFFERENCE IN YOUR ABILITY TO LIVE A GOOD LIFE AFTER LIVING WITH OR CURING YOUR DISEASE?

I think the two things that have made the biggest difference in my life are my attitude and raw vegan food. You have to have the right attitude going into anything you do or try; it's essential. This means that if you go into something with a great attitude, you have more of a chance to succeed at what you're trying to accomplish. A poor attitude is not going to get you anywhere positive, and I am all about the positive!

Food plays an equally essential role, as well. Traditional eating seems normal and fine until it's not working. I always felt that I ate right and that I ate "healthy." I cooked, canned, gardened, preserved food, yet I was still sick, overweight and unhealthy. Why? It was the food! And in all fairness, it was also the doctors and pills that kept me that way. Change the food and change your LIFE. I changed my life!

I never thought my husband or kids would ever go vegan. The difference it makes in your health and even in one's weight is jaw-dropping. I went from a size 22/24 to a size 8, and I am still losing an average of a pound a month with NO exercise other than physical therapy, which isn't all that much. All the different diets I tried and failed at never did anything like this for me. I really feel that the diet industry is taking advantage of desperate people who are trying to find the answer and are STILL being misled. If everyone knew the truth, we could make a huge impact.

It really is insane. This cured nearly every single thing I've ever been doctored for, for my entire life. Through many years of research, I've found that it all stems from nutrition. My mother and her three sisters were starving growing up. So much so that some had to have their teeth removed in their early twenties.

Later in her life, she had my sisters and me. I can remember being sickly all my life. I remember once at age 12 going to the doctors and him diagnosing me with bursitis in both shoulders. I couldn't raise my arms past my rib cage. That makes no sense at that age, and neither did any of the multiple health problems I suffered my entire life. Babies born to malnourished parents are malnourished, it's that simple. If the parent is missing vital vitamins and minerals it makes perfect sense that the offspring are lacking too, yet no one addresses this issue at all. I am just incredibly thankful I've finally figured it out. It took me many years, but I did.

I always thought what we ate was healthy. Growing up, we canned our food and froze it. As an adult, I canned/preserved, froze and grew our own food. I even went so far as raising and processing our own livestock to gain even better health. Don't get me wrong, we did gain better health, but it still wasn't enough. Through even more research, going vegan made sense. And in my case, raw vegan was definitely the best way to complete healing and regaining my health. Plants equal nutrition and nutrition equals health, it really IS that easy, yet no one is willing to talk about it to acknowledge it, especially the healthcare industry. I am very lucky and I just want everyone to know there is hope and plants can return your health and your life. Cleveland Clinic is on board with this they tell me, as is the family doctor it took me years to find. I have definitely raised other doctor's interests as well, so maybe in time and with enough testimony, they will really start to listen.

WHAT WAS YOUR DOCTOR'S REACTION AFTER ANNOUNCING YOUR PLANS TO FOLLOW A PLANT-BASED DIET?

I didn't tell my doctors at first. I just went for it. I didn't tell them because this is not really accepted by people in general. It's considered extreme and certainly not something that my doctor would have recommended.

66 99

IT REALLY IS INSANE. THIS CURED
NEARLY EVERY SINGLE THING
I'VE EVER BEEN DOCTORED FOR,
FOR MY ENTIRE LIFE. THROUGH
MANY YEARS OF RESEARCH,
I'VE FOUND THAT IT ALL STEMS
FROM NUTRITION.

DEBORAH WOOD

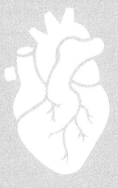

I tried for many years to lose weight. Doctors I used to go to recommend going on diets such as Weight Watchers, low carb and keto. I tried them all, and they all failed. The doctors had no other advice to offer me so I did the research myself. It was probably after a month or two that the doctor I regularly saw for an injury noticed I was steadily losing weight. I finally came clean and told her that I had gone plant-based. I always tell them plant-based because if I use the term vegan, they generally don't know what I mean.

Since then, the doctors that I go to who are very caring are astounded. They have watched me regain my health and lose 103 pounds with no exercise at all, just plant-based eating. I generally don't tell people I am raw vegan because they just don't get it and are way too judgemental about it. The doctors I see are very supportive since they have seen the results that I have achieved first hand. It's hard for them to deny when they have seen and followed my progress the whole time.

AFTER ADOPTING A PLANT-BASED DIET HOW LONG DID IT TAKE BEFORE FIRST, YOU STARTED TO FEEL BETTER, AND SECOND, YOU KNEW YOU WERE NOT GOING TO LET THIS WIN?

I really noticed I felt better after just two weeks. Since I had tried a raw vegan diet years ago, I knew what it could do, and this time I was ready and committed from the start. Honestly, what did I have to lose at this point?

YOU'VE JUST MET A HEARTBROKEN STRANGER WHO HAS JUST BEEN GIVEN A LIFE-THREATENING DIAGNOSIS. WHAT WOULD BE YOUR TOP FIVE TIPS TO HELP THEM?

I have met so many women who are heartbroken and lost like I was. I tell them all the same thing. I tell them that they can heal, they can reverse disease, and to never ever give up. EVER! You don't have to be perfect; you just have to try to eat plants. Loads of plants! As many as you can. Fruits are powerful and healing as well; and eat as many different kinds as you can find. Fresh is always best, but if you do have to cook them or open a can then go for it. Always just try and pick the best option that is available. It's all about choices and doing your research. Find out what food choices you are making and make the best ones available to you at the time. I continue to research every day as I know I would not be where I am with my health today if I had just sat back and listened to my doctors.

DO YOU TAKE ANY SPECIAL SUPPLEMENTS OR POTIONS? MENTION ANY SPECIFIC BRANDS YOU USE AND WHY YOU THINK THESE HAVE BENEFITED YOU AND YOUR HEALTH?

Yes! While doing my research, I came across things that I felt may improve my health and wellness. Each person is different and unique, so that is where research comes into play. I feel years of traditional eating made me deficient in many essential vitamins and minerals, so I am researching and doing my best to replace them. I am also taking cell salts at this time (minerals). Sometimes I take Niacin, and wear a vitamin B12 patch and a vitamin D patch.

WHAT ARE THE TWO OR THREE THINGS YOU HAVE DONE DIFFERENTLY WITH YOUR LIFE AFTER YOUR HEALTH GOT BETTER?

I would have to say that I look at everything differently. I look for the positive in all things. I steer clear of negativity on an epic level. A positive attitude changes everything. I feel the need to inspire people. My physical therapist (whom I see weekly) has even asked me to speak at a local YMCA. I would never have done such a thing before. Being vegan, whether it's raw or regular, really gives you a different perspective on life, which changes many different aspects. I am stronger; I have more energy, I am more positive, more outgoing, and more hopeful. It really is a game-changer.

WHAT ARE SOME OF THE WORST RECOMMENDATIONS THAT YOU WERE GIVEN BY EXPERTS?

Some of the worst recommendations from doctors included bariatric surgery, weight loss pills, more exercise and countless different diets. They focused on my weight and not on my health. I had one doctor who wanted to know who my surgeon was so he could contact him and have him take out my gallbladder without any tests even being done. I tried to tell him that I was a healthy big girl, which he promptly slammed my chart down and yelled BULLSHIT, and went on and on how that was a lie. He took blood work, and I left. I had my daughter drive three hours to the Cleveland Clinic. On our way back from the doctor's clinic, he called with my results from the blood tests and could not understand why my cholesterol was only 164. They could not understand why it was not high since I was so overweight. It goes without saying that I never went back to that doctor again.

ANY INSPIRING STORIES THAT HAVE HAPPENED TO YOU OR PEOPLE CLOSE TO YOU THAT HAVE NOT BEEN COVERED ABOVE. STORIES THAT CAN HELP OTHERS.

Going raw vegan was by FAR the best decision I have ever made in my life. Not only have I regained my health, but my entire life has also changed, and I no longer suffer from the numerous health conditions that I was diagnosed with. I no longer take any pills, and the only doctors that I see are for my Complex regional pain syndrome (CRPS).

I lost 103 pounds with no real exercise, and I am the healthiest and happiest that I have ever been. My health and life in general, have improved so dramatically that my husband went vegan a year after I did. My eldest daughter has also now decided that we looked so good that she too had to go vegan. My two younger children are mostly plant-based, and my physical therapist is also trying to eat more plant-based since seeing the dramatic effects it has had on my life. None of us ever get sick anymore and we all feel the incredible benefits of this amazing and healthy lifestyle.

It can be as easy or as hard as you make it. It can honestly be as easy as eating an apple or making a healthy apple crisp. The benefits are there so just eat more plants! As for those that say it is too expensive, well, it sure is a lot cheaper than the costly doctor's bills I was constantly paying for, the endless prescriptions, and the time it took to attend all of these appointments. I used to suffer from hypothyroidism, fibromyalgia, arthritis, IBS, anxiety, depression, polycystic ovary syndrome, obesity, plantar fasciitis, UTIs, incontinence, kidney stones, kidney disease, hypertension, acid reflux, heartburn and insomnia.

The health improvements I've gained after changing to a raw vegan diet are as follows: my hair grew back, I sleep better, I have softer skin, improved eyesight, no body odor, improved dental visits, I no longer sunburn, no longer have high blood pressure, no more foot pain, no more anxiety, easier time going to the bathroom, better stress management, a general positive feeling of being alive, almost all body pain is gone with the exception of the CRPS/RSD, no more carpal tunnel symptoms, no more shingles (I have had them five times), no more adult cystic acne, no more oily skin, I require less sleep, and I have way more empathy towards others. I am leading a very happy and health-filled life.

CASSANDRA BANKSON

CONNECT WITH CASSANDRA:
INSTAGRAM: @CASSANDRABANKSON
FACEBOOK: CASSANDRA BANKSON
YOUTUBE: CASSANDRA BANKSON
cassandrabankson.com

REVERSED GASTROINTESTINAL ISSUES AND SEVERE ACNE

"After struggling for years to fit into the modeling industry as well as with high school judgment and my own negative self-image, I began developing gastrointestinal issues that doctors couldn't explain. I would have severe swelling, pain, and internal bleeding after I ate. Doctors put me on an elimination diet and a bland diet, but to me, it felt so restrictive that I did not feel nourished, I felt deprived. One day when I was surfing the web, I accidentally came across a YouTube video titled 'The Best Speech Ever.' It's a video about animal rights, and though I only anticipated watching the first five minutes, I was sucked in for the whole hour. The video was a wake-up call to me: I have six cats and I love animals and always try my best not to harm others. So why was I making dietary choices that don't match my morals and values?"

Cassandra Bankson is a model, blogger, and plant-based social media influencer who has over a million followers/subscribers over a variety of social media platforms. Passionate about science-based skincare, cruelty-free makeup, and healthy, plant-based eating, Cassandra shares her story in an honest, relatable way in order to inspire her audience to embrace their unique beauty while focusing on healthy eating and self-love.

WHAT ARE YOUR DAILY RITUALS/HABITS WHICH YOU BELIEVE HAVE BEEN KEY TO YOUR HEALTH?

Throughout my youth, I would always wake up to scarf down breakfast, throw clothes on my body, and pray that my little brother and I weren't late for school. As I got older, I realized that rituals and routines were there to help me – the more I can plan ahead, the more time I would save later stressing, worrying, and forgetting to bring an item or complete a task. I've also realized that if you can't take care of yourself, it's impossible to continue taking care of those around you. For those reasons, I put my mental clarity and health first every single morning.

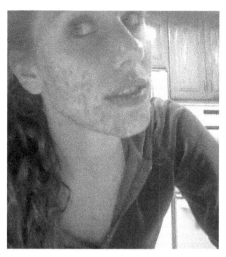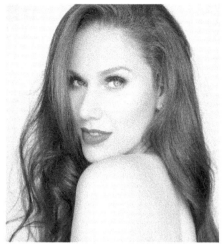

When I first wake up, I turn off my alarm, chuck my phone across the room so that I am not tempted to scroll through Instagram, and tuck in the corners of my bedsheets so that I don't climb back in. I always make myself a healthy breakfast, and usually a warm cup of Matcha green tea. I do my best to read a book and take notes on what I'm learning or thinking. I find that I am the most creative in the morning, which is why I try to allow myself this time. Watching the sunrise is a relaxing and reconnecting moment that I strive for whenever I can. Day after day, it never ceases to blow me away. It is also very humbling – reminding me of what a small yet important part of such a beautiful system each and every one of us are.

When my morning begins on the right foot, usually, the rest of my day goes smoother. I do my best to remind myself of my positive qualities throughout the day. Even if I've failed to understand something or I messed up on a project at work, I remind myself that failure is one step closer to success. Giving myself this kindness has allowed me to take on life with a growth mindset and has helped me to be kinder to others.

Because I live my life trying not to harm others, I made the decision to eat vegan – this also makes healthy choices a bit easier! If donuts or cake show up at an office meeting, I have no problem saying no – not because I am depriving myself, but because I choose to nourish my body while making choices that don't harm others in the process. By the end of the day even if I am tired and exhausted, I try to make a quick note on my calendar of something I achieved that day. Making a note of something as simple as completing a project, or making a difference in someone else's life really does make me feel like I'm contributing positively to society. When I look back at all of the notes (especially on my bad days), it reminds me that life really isn't so negative. Life is a roller coaster and if things are down, it means that soon they will be looking up.

AT WHAT POINT IN YOUR LIFE DID YOU DECIDE TO CHANGE YOUR DIET? HOW HAS THAT DECISION IMPACTED YOUR LIFE?

As much as I try to avoid talking about it, when I was younger I didn't have the healthiest relationship with food. Because I had always thought about food in a negative way, I thought this was normal. It wasn't until those patterns stopped that I realized something had been wrong. After struggling for years to fit into the modeling industry, as well as with high school judgment and my own negative self-image, I began developing gastrointestinal issues that doctors couldn't explain. I would have severe swelling, pain and internal bleeding after I ate. Doctors put me on an elimination diet and a bland diet, but to me it felt so restrictive that I did not feel nourished, I felt deprived.

One day when I was surfing the web, I accidentally came across a YouTube video, titled 'The Best Speech Ever." It's a video about animal rights and, though I only anticipated watching the first five minutes, I was sucked in for the whole hour. The video was a wake-up call to me: I have six cats, I love animals, and I always try my best to not harm others. If this was all true, why was I making dietary choices that didn't match my morals and values?

The speaker said a quote that really hit me in the gut – "if it's not good enough for your eyes, why is it good enough for your stomach?" When I realized that cruelty was so prevalent in the meat and dairy industry and that I couldn't handle watching it, I decided to stop choosing to eat it. For me, this decision happened about four years ago. It also happened overnight, which was extremely difficult. I didn't know what to eat, or how to make healthy choices, I simply knew that I no longer wanted to contribute to someone else's pain and suffering.

It took a few weeks, but I started exploring new options, such as new flavors, new cuisine (such as Thai and Iranian), and even mock meats and cheeses. This choice went completely against what doctors are recommending: beef and vegetables. Wouldn't you know it, something interesting started happening. My stomach swelling and bloating started to clear up. The issues I was having with the stomach bleeding began to cease over a couple of weeks, and after six months, my acne started to clear. That was an ailment I suffered with for over fifteen years. It was amazing to me that a choice based on ethics would have such a profound impact on other areas of my life. Not only did my body feel better, but I also started aligning myself with more everyday kindness towards others and towards myself.

My acne ended up clearing, and I started to feel more confident about my body, understanding that it is a beautiful piece of biology that has carried me through every day, not an object that I should punish or detest. I never expected that switching to plant-based would benefit my life in so many other ways, but making a decision that was aligned with my morals and values ended up bringing everything else into alignment for me.

WHAT THINGS HAVE MADE THE MOST DIFFERENCE IN YOUR ABILITY TO LIVE A GOOD LIFE AFTER LIVING WITH OR CURING YOUR DISEASE?

After going vegan, many things started to change positively. I embraced that life isn't always positive. Sometimes I do make bad decisions.
But reminding myself that this is all part of the process allows me to get up off my knees and continue forward while also extending compassion to others who might make decisions I don't agree with.

WHAT WAS YOUR DOCTOR'S REACTION AFTER ANNOUNCING YOUR PLANS TO FOLLOW A PLANT-BASED DIET?

My doctors were originally very skeptical. They did not seem to understand that I was feeling nourished and choosing to eat well, as opposed to focusing on restriction or deprivation. Specifically, because of my medical condition, they urged me against it. They wanted me to continue eating a bland diet of beef and vegetables. However, even after six months on that diet, my bloating and internal issues were not fixed. When I became plant-based, it seemed to heal quicker (within the span of a few months). Per doctor's recommendations I did decide to do some blood tests, fecal tests, scans and samples, and my doctors were just as surprised as I was when they came back showing that my body's hormone levels were more normalized, my blood panels were healthier, and the internal bleeding and swelling seemed to have stopped completely.

Years later, it became evident that my body was reacting to specific antibiotics that animals were fed as some of those trace compounds ended up in the meat. Having taken antibiotics for acne and reacted negatively years earlier, some of these compounds were disrupting the inside of my stomach and intestinal linings. Upon my own research and speaking to dietitians and research professionals in the medical field, there also seems to be links between dairy and acne which are statistically significant but not always taught or studied. Coming across these professionals and research papers helped me understand from a scientific perspective why cutting out dairy has been so helpful in my own personal journey.

AFTER ADOPTING A PLANT-BASED DIET HOW LONG DID IT TAKE BEFORE FIRST, YOU STARTED TO FEEL BETTER, AND SECOND, YOU KNEW YOU WERE NOT GOING TO LET THIS WIN?

When I first went vegan/plant-based, it took about four to six weeks before my stomach swelling went down. It took about three to six months to completely heal, and that's when I noticed my skin starting to change. It was around the six-month mark that I looked in the mirror and realized that my acne was not as inflamed. Looking back at the video diary that I had been putting on YouTube, it seems that even after three to four months, my skin was already improving. It really is hard to track progress if you gauge success by just looking at yourself in the mirror every day. However, having quantitative and qualitative results, such as blood tests, journal entries, or a video diary, it really does help you see the progress that you might have turned a blind eye to otherwise.

YOU'VE JUST MET A HEARTBROKEN STRANGER WHO HAS JUST BEEN GIVEN A LIFE-THREATENING DIAGNOSIS. WHAT WOULD BE YOUR TOP FIVE TIPS TO HELP THEM?

Number one: your feelings are valid. I don't know how you feel, but I can be sympathetic because I have dealt with elements of my own. Even if somebody else you talk to tries to tell you that it's not a big deal, allow their opinion but remember that you are also allowed to have your own experience.

Number two: I know it might feel debilitating, but ask what you can do. One of the most powerful things that I have ever heard Oprah Winfrey say is, "in life, we can never control our circumstances, but we do get to choose how we react to them." Ask yourself what you can do.

Number three: don't stay quiet. I suffered for so many years with my acne and other issues, feeling ashamed and embarrassed because nobody else seemed to know or understand what I was going through. The truth is that other people were just as hurt and hiding the same way that I was. If you don't speak up, you will never be able to find others who are going through the same thing. I found that connecting with others who understood me was essential in helping myself through the negative parts of the process.

Number four: find the silver lining. As horrible as things can be, there is always a hidden positive. Having acne for over 15 years was something that almost caused me to end my own life multiple times. As horrible as it was and as much as I would never wish the continuous judgment, physical pain, and emotional turmoil on somebody else, I look back, and I am happy that I suffered with acne. Yes, happy. The reason is that I can see now how it taught me to connect to others. It taught me how to find my value as a human instead of what I look like. It gave me my purpose and passion in life to help others feel confident in their own skin and understand their skincare and cosmetic ingredients so that they can make conscious choices about what they are putting on and in their bodies. I am proud of the woman that I am today, and acne was a part of my past. If it weren't for acne, I would not be the strong and empowered person I am today.

Number five: remember that failure is a stepping stone to success. Nobody wakes up and is successful overnight. You didn't learn how to walk, read, or pursue a passion overnight. For every single thing you have achieved, there were failures along the way that got you to this point. I feel that the educational system seems to prioritize perfection and not leave a lot of room for error, but I do feel that error is where most of the growth happens. Remember that any failures are stepping stones to success. Celebrate them in their own unique ways.

DO YOU TAKE ANY SPECIAL SUPPLEMENTS OR POTIONS? MENTION ANY SPECIFIC BRANDS YOU USE AND WHY YOU THINK THESE HAVE BENEFITED YOU AND YOUR HEALTH?

To be honest, the more I decided to seek out knowledge and an understanding of my condition, the more I realized the power of taking action by looking at the details.

Take action - If you don't start, you will never get anywhere. Whether it is a fitness routine, a healthy habit, playing a musical instrument or learning something new, if you don't start it, it won't happen.

Look at the details - Whether it is a food label or cosmetic label, see what's in it first. You might notice that although all of the supplements have different brand names and packaging, most of them only contain a handful of beneficial ingredients. Although there are so many cosmetic products on the market, the few that actually work all have the same active ingredients. Do your research and seek those things out. For me, there are five foods that I eat every single day. From a scientific and research-based perspective, these foods contain essential nutrients that I know my body needs to function best. I really notice after a work trip or vacation where they are not available that my body is not functioning at its best.

Every day I try to have a scoop of protein powder in the morning. I normally despise protein powders – most of them are oxidized and expensive powdered crap. Mostly, I choose to eat the Garden of Life Raw Protein Powder with no Stevia. From a scientific and nutrient perspective, this one is stable and digestible by the body, plus it contains a beautiful array of vegan amino acids that my body can use to turn into proteins.

I also try to drink almond-based milk, especially in my Matcha latte or coffee. Flax milk from Good Karma is one that I personally enjoy, especially because it's omega 3, 6, and 9 ratio is beautifully balanced. Our bodies need omega fatty acids to run well, and I find that this is the perfect way to get mine every day.

Every day, I also try to eat an apple. I find that the sugars, vitamin C, and antioxidants make me feel great, and prevent me from chewing down cookies or other foods that wouldn't serve my body as well. Whether it's for lunch or dinner, I always try to grab some spinach as well. It is high in vitamins and minerals such as vitamin A, C, K, calcium, iron, folic acid, and of course a good source of protein and even some trace omega fatty acids.

I also always try to have lentils or chickpeas. Beans digest in the body in a very interesting way, regardless of what form they are served in. They break down beautifully in the intestines and feed the beneficial bacteria in our guts. I usually go for lentils or beans, but sometimes enjoy Banza pasta – a pasta made from chickpeas. Sometimes hummus with carrots or some other kind of vegetable. They have amazing amounts of fiber, protein, and minerals such as iron, magnesium, and calcium.

WHAT ARE THE TWO OR THREE THINGS YOU HAVE DONE DIFFERENTLY WITH YOUR LIFE AFTER YOUR HEALTH GOT BETTER?

Since my health got better, I feel so much stronger, both emotionally and physically. Although I have always enjoyed exercising, I never truly loved to be outdoors. Now I thoroughly enjoy running through the hills, scaling mountains, and even rock climbing. After changing my diet, I realized how beautiful my body is because now, having it in working ability, it'd be a shame not to use it! I choose now to use and celebrate my body, and who knew that I might actually someday be able to do a pull-up?!

I also judge others less. When I would judge myself harshly, I would often point fingers at others, scrutinizing their image, dietary, or lifestyle choices. Once I switched things in my physical diet, as well as in my own psyche, I realize that everybody is on their own journey. I want to be compassionate with others because I know that growth happens at a different pace for all of us. If I can lead by a kindhearted and vibrant example, others are more willing to listen to me. If I yell about their insecurities, they are more likely not to listen to the advice I may have to offer.

ANY INSPIRING STORIES THAT HAVE HAPPENED TO YOU OR PEOPLE CLOSE TO YOU THAT HAVE NOT BEEN COVERED ABOVE. STORIES THAT CAN HELP OTHERS.

Growing up as a model with acne, judging myself for my skin, my body, and for who I was intrinsically, was a miserable existence. People often look at a model in a magazine and wish to be her. Most of the time, however, she is so photoshopped and manipulated that she doesn't even look like that. I struggled silently for so many years with my issues and concerns, not once thinking that others were struggling in silence as well. It wasn't until I started opening up online, choosing to free the pain within myself by allowing it to console others, that I realized I wasn't truly alone.

Whatever it is that you are struggling with or going through, please remember that in a strange way, it is shaping you into who you are meant to be. You are not alone, and there are other people who are going through it too – people who've done it before and people who somebody in the future will do it after. If you choose to open up, you might be able to help some of them as well. As you get through this, I know it's hard, and I know that words may hurt. Anyone who says otherwise is a liar. But at the same time, we can choose to try our best to remember to be compassionate in our words and actions. Remember that you must grow out of who you currently are in order to grow into who you are meant to be. You are beautiful and worthy in your own way. Even on the darker days, please do not ever forget that.

32

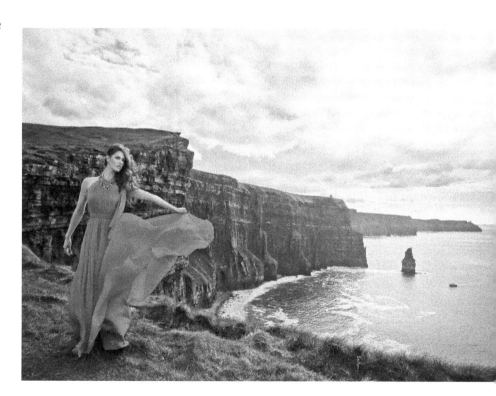

JANETTE MURRY WAKELIN

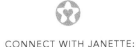

CONNECT WITH JANETTE:
rawveganpath.com

REVERSED AGGRESSIVE BREAST CANCER 18 YEARS AGO, WAS "GIVEN" SIX MONTHS TO LIVE

When Janette Murray-Wakelin was diagnosed with highly aggressive carcinoma breast cancer over 18 years ago, she was "given" six months to live. The tumor was three centimeters, and cancer had spread into her chest wall and her lymph nodes. It was recommended that she undergo conventional chemotherapy and radiation treatment to "possibly" extend her life a further six months. At 52 years old, a mother of two, and grandmother of one, she was not willing to accept this prognosis.

"12 years after my cancer diagnosis, I ran together with my partner Alan Murray around Australia to show by example what is physically possible with a plant-based diet and to inspire and promote kindness and compassion for all living beings, and to raise environmental awareness for a sustainable future. In total we ran 15,782 kilometers, running 366 marathons each in 366 days, with no days off."

WHAT ARE YOUR DAILY RITUALS/HABITS WHICH YOU BELIEVE HAVE BEEN KEY TO YOUR HEALTH?

The daily rituals and habits that I believe have been key to my health are exercise, consuming a raw-vegan-plant-based diet, taking time for myself in natural surroundings and sleeping. Exercise includes going for a run or walk, and a river swim early in the morning, doing an hour of yoga and strength exercises with weights, and using the core pump machine.

I have been consuming a raw vegan, nutrient-rich, and plant-based diet since my cancer diagnosis in 2001. On a daily basis I generally have two meals per day; one after my exercise routine about mid-morning that consists of fresh fruit and fruit juice or smoothie, and the other is usually mid to late afternoon and may include fresh veggie juice, a salad with fresh ingredients from the garden, or a large seasonal fruit meal such as melons, oranges, mandarins, or any tropical fruit.

Wherever I am, I try to take time for myself in nature. It may be a walk in the forest or on the beach, sitting quietly in the garden, or meditating on my deck overlooking the river. Sleeping is also an important key to health, and I try to get at least 8-9 hours of sleep per night.

AT WHAT POINT IN YOUR LIFE DID YOU DECIDE TO CHANGE YOUR DIET? HOW HAS THAT DECISION IMPACTED YOUR LIFE?

When I was diagnosed with terminal cancer in 2001, I rejected the allopathic treatment that was offered (as it didn't make sense to me to compromise the body further) and decided to do everything I could to help my body heal and rejuvenate.

The first consideration was to start a holistic therapy to kickstart the healing process. At the same time, I changed my diet to 100% raw vegan and plant-based, as it was clear to me that giving the body the most nutrient-laden food would help with healing and rejuvenation. I had already been eating vegetarian for most of my life, so making the change to raw vegan was an obvious choice. I knew that environmentally my body had been compromised, so I also became more conscious of the lifestyle choices I could make that would make a difference. This was not only for my health but for the health and well-being of all living beings and for the health of the planet. In making these conscious lifestyle choices, I was also, in effect, taking control of my own destiny. In doing so, I had overcome any fears that I may have had when first diagnosed. It really was, and is, all about making the connection.

WHAT THINGS HAVE MADE THE MOST DIFFERENCE IN YOUR ABILITY TO LIVE A GOOD LIFE AFTER LIVING WITH OR CURING YOUR DISEASE?

After living with and curing my cancer, I have found that the difference in my ability to live a good life is phenomenal! Because I continue to live a conscious, raw vegan lifestyle since my diagnosis and healing of cancer, I have increased the clarity of my mind, improved my physical fitness, unlocked unlimited energy, and overall enjoy optimal health. I have not had any ill health nor had the need to see a doctor since. I have sustained some (accidental) injuries, including broken ribs but found that I was able to heal quickly without any medication nor medical protocol.

Due to living a conscious, raw vegan lifestyle, I continue to get stronger and more physically fit as I get older (in years), so the good life continues.

WHAT WAS YOUR DOCTOR'S REACTION AFTER ANNOUNCING YOUR PLANS TO FOLLOW A PLANT-BASED DIET?

After announcing my plans to follow a plant-based diet, my doctors had mixed reactions. My general doctor was supportive of my choices, but the cancer specialists, oncologists, and radiotherapists were not. Mostly, they told me that I was making a big mistake by not having their recommended treatment, but they also expressed concern that I would not "get enough protein" with a plant-based diet. Apart from finding that rather amusing, I was able to enlighten them to the benefits of a raw vegan diet in the healing process, especially once I was completely clear of cancer within the time (six months) that they predicted I would die.

WHAT WAS THE CRAZIEST THING YOU DID TO TRY AND FIGHT YOUR DISEASE? DID IT WORK OR MAKE ANY DIFFERENCE TO YOU?

After I was diagnosed with terminal cancer, in my opinion, the only crazy thing I could have done was to follow the recommended cancer treatments of chemotherapy and radiation. Instead, I decided to do everything I could that made sense to help with the healing process.

I did try several different holistic protocols (all-natural), but I wouldn't consider any of them to be crazy. And, of course, it worked. I was cleared of cancer. So, the difference it made to me is that I am not only alive, but optimally healthy, vibrant, and thriving.

AFTER ADOPTING A PLANT-BASED DIET HOW LONG DID IT TAKE BEFORE FIRST, YOU STARTED TO FEEL BETTER, AND SECOND, YOU KNEW YOU WERE NOT GOING TO LET THIS WIN?

After adopting a plant-based diet, it only took five days before I started to feel better, particularly with increased clarity of mind. This was helpful in my circumstances, as I was able to make crucial decisions and choices almost instantly and know that they were the right choices for me. During the first few months of being on a raw vegan, plant-based diet, my body was going through many changes; from detoxing to healing. However, after only six months (the time given for the prognosis of death), I was completely clear of cancer. From the moment of my diagnosis of cancer, I considered it a challenge that I was going to overcome, and there was no doubt in my mind that I would win.

YOU'VE JUST MET A HEARTBROKEN STRANGER WHO HAS JUST BEEN GIVEN A LIFE-THREATENING DIAGNOSIS. WHAT WOULD BE YOUR TOP FIVE TIPS TO HELP THEM?

My top five tips to anyone receiving a life-threatening diagnosis would be;

1. Get a second or third opinion. If you believe the prognosis is the same, then take time to find your truth before making any decisions regarding treatment or therapy. Decide what is right for you and not necessarily what is generally considered "normal." Whatever decisions or choices you make, be sure that you are happy with them.

2. Everything in your life is a choice that is yours to make. Start making (more) conscious lifestyle choices that will make a difference in your health immediately. Start with food choices and make plant-based food a priority. Consuming a raw plant-based diet ensures 100% nutrient-laden food that will assist with faster healing. Include exercise, meditation, and/or yoga, visualization, and gratitude in your daily regime.

3. Ask your family and friends to unconditionally support you with the choices you make, even if they may not agree with them. This will help to eliminate added emotional stress, which is not beneficial to your healing.

4. Find a reputable holistic practitioner who can advise you on the benefits of fasting and juicing. During healing, it is essential not to place too much of a burden on the body, so with making a change to a plant-based diet, juice and/or blend for simpler digestion and to consume more nutrients from the food than if you were to eat it.

5. Make sure you get at least eight or nine hours of tranquil sleep each night. This is the time when the body can prioritize healing. Believe in yourself, smile, laugh and breathe. Place the highest value on yourself - you are worth it.

DO YOU TAKE ANY SPECIAL SUPPLEMENTS OR POTIONS? MENTION ANY SPECIFIC BRANDS YOU USE AND WHY YOU THINK THESE HAVE BENEFITED YOU AND YOUR HEALTH?

I do not take any special supplements (processed vitamins, minerals, superfoods, etc) or potions (processed, herbal, or otherwise), no processed "pain-killers," and no drugs of any kind (including caffeine, alcohol, nicotine, etc). I get all the nutrients I need in their natural form from fresh, ripe, organic, and preferably locally-grown fruit and vegetables.

WHAT ARE SOME OF THE WORST RECOMMENDATIONS THAT YOU HAVE BEEN GIVEN BY "EXPERTS."?

Some of the worst recommendations that I have been given by "experts" include: treating cancer with chemotherapy and radiation, taking chemotherapy drugs, having a mastectomy (surgery to remove the breast), having surgery to remove tumors and cancerous lymph nodes, wearing restrictive stockings, restricting exercise, restricting the consumption of fruit, and increasing the consumption of animal products such as milk and yogurt.

HOW DO YOU HANDLE THE UPS AND DOWNS OF GOOD AND BAD DAYS? WHAT STRATEGIES DO YOU USE?

During the initial six months of holistic therapy, I experienced some uncomfortable detox symptoms, which may have been considered down

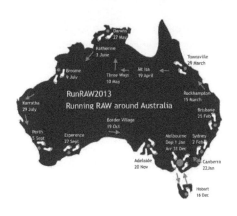

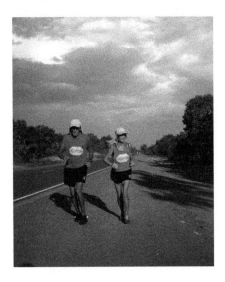

days, but I recognized them as healing symptoms, so they became good days. While I was having daily therapy, I had a lot of time to think about my situation, which sometimes made me feel emotional. I used meditation and visualization to help me through those times. Once I was clear of cancer and have continued living a conscious vegan lifestyle, I have only good days.

WHAT ARE THE TWO OR THREE THINGS YOU HAVE DONE DIFFERENTLY WITH YOUR LIFE AFTER YOUR HEALTH GOT BETTER?

The most important thing that I have done differently with my life after my health got better is to live every moment with gratitude, kindness and compassion. I also became passionate about sharing what I learned from my experience so that others may also make more informed choices. My partner and I moved to a cleaner, more natural environment, and endeavor to live a self-sustainable lifestyle in an area where we can grow our own food or obtain it locally, and where there is also a large community of like-minded people.

ANY INSPIRING STORIES THAT HAVE HAPPENED TO YOU OR PEOPLE CLOSE TO YOU THAT HAVE NOT BEEN COVERED ABOVE. STORIES THAT CAN HELP OTHERS.

After my six month journey with cancer, my partner and I founded a Centre for Optimum Health in Canada, encouraging healthy conscious lifestyles through living nutrition and exercise for the mind, body and spirit. We established a highly successful Living Food & Conscious Lifestyle Program and shared our knowledge of attaining optimal health through a series of inspirational presentations. We did this internationally during the ten years following my cancer recovery. The response was overwhelming with hundreds of people being encouraged to make their own informed choices with regard to diet, exercise and maintaining a healthy and conscious lifestyle.

We moved to Australia in 2009 and continue to offer personalized conscious lifestyle programs and retreats in our home, as well as giving inspirational talks worldwide.

We have both participated in many international marathons, and ultra runs, and to celebrate my 50th year, we ran the length of our home country, New Zealand. We covered 2,182 kilometers, running 50 marathons in 50 consecutive days.

13 years after our New Zealand run and 12 years after my cancer diagnosis, we ran together around Australia in order to inspire conscious lifestyle choices, promote kindness and compassion for all living beings, and to raise environmental awareness for a sustainable future. In total we ran 15,782 kilometers, running 366 marathons each in 366 days, with no days off. On January 1, 2014, we acquired world acclaim by setting a new World Record as the only couple over the age of 60 fuelled entirely on a raw vegan, plant-based diet, wearing barefoot shoes, to run 366 consecutive marathons while Running Raw Around Australia, thus proving beyond any doubt that living a raw, vegan conscious lifestyle results in optimal health where physically, mentally and emotionally, anything is achievable.

In March 2014, we were approached by a filmmaker to make a cinematically produced film based on our Run Around Australia and the positive message that it conveys with the intention of showing the documentary in cinemas worldwide. A short version of the film, RAW the documentary, was selected and screened at the prestigious Cannes Film Festival in France in May 2015. The finished film was released in February 2017. It was officially selected and screened with The Australian Transitions Film Festival throughout Australia and premiered in Australia, New Zealand, USA, Hong Kong, China, and Indonesia. In 2018 the film was officially selected to screen with the American Documentary Film Festival in the USA and screened in Paris, France in conjunction with our running the Paris International Marathon with the France Vegan Marathon Team.

RAW the documentary is now available on DVD internationally through my website. I am also the author of the best selling book, Raw Can Cure Cancer (now in its 6th edition), and my second book, Running Out of Time, based on the Run around Australia. Both are available through my website: rawveganpath.com

LAUREN NOWELL

CONNECT WITH LAUREN:
INSTAGRAM: @ACTIVATEYOURSHINE
FACEBOOK: LAUREN NOWELL

> **SUFFERED WITH CROHN'S DISEASE FOR NEARLY HER ENTIRE LIFE**

Having suffered from Crohn's disease for nearly her entire life, Lauren Nowell is a blogger and plant-based eating advocate who is passionate about finding peace, wellness and harmony in life. She attributes much of her current health to switching to a plant-based diet and is interested in sharing her success story with as many sufferers of chronic illness as possible to teach others the important, life-changing link between health and nutrition.

WHAT ARE YOUR DAILY RITUALS/HABITS WHICH YOU BELIEVE HAVE BEEN KEY TO YOUR HEALTH?

The key to health is keeping a clean internal environment, a diet full of nutrition and hydration, incorporating movement and flexibility, and enhancing your mind to be a powerful force that propels you into the greatest version of yourself. To master incorporating all of these into my daily life, I begin each morning with hydrating my cells with fruit.

Whether it's starting with lemon water, fresh raw juice, a smoothie, or a bowl of fruit. I follow with stretching my body, regulating my energy, and then set my intentions for the day with gratitude journaling, meditation, reading, or listening to inspiring audiobooks. Remaining in this flow state where I'm staying on top of hydration, nutrition, and elimination (through periodic detoxes) and feeding my mind empowering thoughts, I'm able to maintain amazing vitality. Keeping my physical, mental and spiritual body plugged into nature, and source energy has radically changed my health and outlook on life.

AT WHAT POINT IN YOUR LIFE DID YOU DECIDE TO CHANGE YOUR DIET? HOW HAS THAT DECISION IMPACTED YOUR LIFE?

At age two, I started to display symptoms, and at age six, I was diagnosed with Crohn's. For 20 years, I suffered from debilitating intestinal pain, chronic headaches/migraines, and arthritis. I was treated with antibiotics, toxic immuno-suppressants, steroids and surgeries. I later suffered from Lyme,

Candida, infections, chronic inflammation, skin cancers and chronic pain.

Doctors told me for years that there was no cure, that food had nothing to do with how I was feeling nor could it help, and that I'd have to remain on medication my whole life and get surgery every ten years to remove sections of my inflamed intestine. I accepted this fate. I only knew of pain, and I learned to get comfortable with the future my doctors had laid out for me. That was until things got much worse, and the suffering was starting to be too much for me.

I remember laying in bed not being able to walk because I was recovering from surgery where they removed a large chunk of skin cancer that was in my knee. These melanomas and abnormal moles were appearing all over my body, and it was from a side effect of a drug I took for my Crohns.

I was at my rock bottom, and I made the decision in that moment that I didn't want to live like this anymore. I knew there was more to life, and I finally felt the desire to discover life outside of the pain I was living in. That's when I started researching, and I kept coming across Dr. Robert Morse. His raw food diet, juicing and detoxification teachings resonated with me immediately. I started watching more of his YouTube videos day in and day out and started taking notes and implementing what I was learning. I started to feel positive changes within weeks, and that's what made me a believer. That was the start of my new life and the beginning of hope for me.

40

WHAT THINGS HAVE MADE THE MOST DIFFERENCE IN YOUR ABILITY TO LIVE A GOOD LIFE AFTER LIVING WITH OR CURING YOUR DISEASE?

The things that led me to be able to live a good life after healing was changing my relationship with food, connecting more to nature, as well as detoxing my body, my home and my mind. I am a firm believer in raw foods and fresh raw juice cleanses, simple mono-meals, fasting, colonics/enemas, herbs, liver cleansing, saunas, chiropractic care, Epsom salt baths, castor oil packs, massages, hemp oil, bio-electric-magnetic-energy-regulation, journaling, yoga, meditation, and lots of self-love, gratitude, and a positive mindset.

WHAT WAS YOUR DOCTOR'S REACTION AFTER ANNOUNCING YOUR PLANS TO FOLLOW A PLANT-BASED DIET?

Throughout my life, my doctors were never truly supportive of my decisions to seek alternative natural care. I started to see doctors for my Crohns at a very young age and sought advice and treatment from many specialists up through my mid-20's. None of them understood or supported natural medicine. They all told me that diet and food had nothing to do with my debilitating digestive condition.

" "

WHEN A DOCTOR DECLARES
YOU HAVE SOMETHING WRONG,
THEY IMMEDIATELY LABEL YOU
WITH A TITLE AND FEAR YOU
INTO OWNING IT AND INTO
TAKING ACTION WITH WHAT THEY
ARE TAUGHT TO TREAT WITH:
PHARMACEUTICALS, *RADIATION*,
OR *SURGERY*. ONE MUST NEVER
ALLOW A TITLE TO DEFINE THEM.
THIS CONDITION WAS CREATED
AND IT CAN BE DISMANTLED WITH
THE RIGHT TOOLS AND MINDSET.

LAUREN NOWELL

When I was young, I decided I wanted to no longer eat meat or take my medications, and my doctors made my parents bring me to a psychologist because they thought I was unfit to make such a crazy decision since I suffered so much with deficiencies. During that appointment, I remember sitting in the corner with my back turned towards the doctor the whole time. I was a smart little girl and intuitively knew what was right for me all along but unfortunately was never able to make those changes due to the pressure and fear instilled by my doctors.

AFTER ADOPTING A PLANT-BASED DIET HOW LONG DID IT TAKE BEFORE FIRST, YOU STARTED TO FEEL BETTER, AND SECOND, YOU KNEW YOU WERE NOT GOING TO LET THIS WIN?

When I reached my rock bottom, I was in a debilitating, desperate state. I wanted to feel better so badly, and I was willing to go into territory I'd never wanted to go to, which was giving up the one thing I was so addicted and attached to: animal products. As I embarked on a journey to heal myself, and the more I researched natural healing, the more I saw a correlation and common factor. No one was healing or regenerating on animal products. These are the very things that cause disorder, deficiencies, and disease within us.

I slowly started to incorporate more fruits and more raw, living foods. These were the very things that my doctors always told me to stay away from because they said my body couldn't handle fiber. I started decreasing my animal consumption dramatically and saw results almost immediately.

When I finally eliminated all animal products from my diet and started cleansing out the acidic ash and debris left behind from eating all that wrong chemistry my whole life, my symptoms started to fade and lessen one by one. Some of the major ailments I had been dealing with for almost 20 years improved within weeks. Some took a lot longer to heal through years of dedicated cleansing and detoxification, but it didn't take long for me to become a believer and never look back. I embrace this vegan detox lifestyle to its full capacity because I know it is the very thing that saved my life!

YOU'VE JUST MET A HEARTBROKEN STRANGER WHO HAS JUST BEEN GIVEN A LIFE-THREATENING DIAGNOSIS. WHAT WOULD BE YOUR TOP FIVE TIPS TO HELP THEM?

I would tell them immediately to never accept a theory or fate given by another person. When a doctor declares you have something wrong, they immediately label you with a title and fear you into owning it and into taking action with what they are taught to treat with: pharmaceuticals, radiation, or surgery. One must never allow a title to define them. This condition was created, and it can be dismantled with the right tools and mindset.

Which brings me to my second tip. We must first and foremost make a decision that we want to heal. Decide that you have the power to reclaim your life. Don't worry about the how just make a definitive decision that you will heal yourself and break down the paradigms in the mind that tell us we cannot. An amazing person to listen to for this is Bob Proctor. Our paradigms (patterns and conditions) are what hold us back from believing we can do, be, or have anything it is that we want. Our thoughts are energy and very powerful in creating our reality. Another person to research is Dr. Joe Dispenza, who teaches how to rewire neural pathways and the subconscious. Watch the documentary Heal as well, where they discuss the body's ability to self-heal. Our minds are a huge factor, just as much as addressing the physical body is.

Another very big decision we need to make if we want to heal is to understand why the physical body gets sick and out of balance, how the body truly functions, and how to optimize the functioning of our elimination, circulation and utilization. This is why I am so passionate about regenerative detoxification. When we learn to eliminate the things that are toxic to our bodies, clean up the residue and waste inside that has built up, take in the things that provide our body with proper fuel, hydration and nutrition, and encourage life-force energy to return, our bodies can heal and regenerate. Once I learned how important it is to keep our inside terrain clean, I found the golden keys to what it means to heal. I encourage people to start learning about regenerative detoxification by watching "The Great Lymphatic System" series by Dr. Robert Morse on YouTube.

Another tip I need to emphasize is to live in the present moment. Don't get too far ahead of the now. Each day you wake up, look at it as a way you can enhance and improve your health and only worry about what act(s) of self-love you will be giving yourself that day. You can plan ahead in your mind by visualizing yourself healthy and full of life. Move towards the steps that need to be taken to heal with ease, with grace, with gusto, but never with urgency.

My last tip is to surround yourself with community. It is so important to have support from others who have healed naturally and from those who are currently on the path of healing naturally just as you are. I love Instagram so much because there is a huge community of conscious people to connect with, get inspired by and learn from. Find your high vibe tribe and allow them to support you on your journey.

DO YOU TAKE ANY SPECIAL SUPPLEMENTS OR POTIONS? MENTION ANY SPECIFIC BRANDS YOU USE AND WHY YOU THINK THESE HAVE

43

BENEFITED YOU AND YOUR HEALTH?

Outside of sunshine, deep breathing, meditating, gratitude journaling, and stretching, there are a few other things I supplement with on a day to day basis to boost and maintain my health. I prefer getting most of my nutrients from real food sources and herbal botanical formulas from Dr.Robert Morse. I also take a CBG enriched sonicated liposomal hemp extract every day by Prime My Body. After discovering what an important role the endocannabinoid system (ECS) plays in homeostatically regulating our body and how it assists our body in healing itself, it is a very important tool I use in my arsenal. After trying many brands, I have found Prime My Body to be the highest quality, most effective and the best for my body. It helps me stay calm, creative, balanced and in a flow-state. I also take a liposomal B12 and vitamin D by Quicksilver Scientifics as needed in winter, and I love powdered mushroom blends by SuperFeast for boosting my immunity. I also love Markus Rothkranz Wild Green Force powder and vitamin C powder when I need a boost of alkalinity, energy, and Puradyme enzymes/probiotics if I need some extra gut support.

Another very important part of my daily health regimen is not necessarily a supplement, but is my magic weapon in keeping my river of life flowing and circulating. I have discovered an advanced technology called BEMER, which uses a special signal to enhance general blood flow & circulation within the 74,000-mile span of microvessels that make up 74% of our vascular system. Being that poor circulation stands behind many of people's health issues, I am so excited to have found this! It is a German technology being used by over a million people worldwide that have been used in Europe for 20+ years, and it has been the most researched mat with data and studies proving its effects. For just eight minutes, twice a day, I lie on the BEMER mat, which stands for Bio-Electro-Magnetic-Energy-Regulation. When blood flow is enhanced, our tissues and organs are supplied with oxygen, nutrients, and energy, and metabolic waste & carbon dioxide is disposed of. It has been a total game-changer for me and has brought my health to all-new levels. I am so passionate about sharing this exciting technology with others who are looking for a better quality of life! You are going to see more and more of these being used because just as Thomas Edison, Nicola Tesla, Albert Einstein and many more spoke about...we are energetic beings and the future of medicine will be that of energy & frequency.

WHAT ARE THE TWO OR THREE THINGS YOU HAVE DONE DIFFERENTLY WITH YOUR LIFE AFTER YOUR HEALTH GOT BETTER?

Since I have healed, I have finally eliminated fear out of my realm. I used to avoid making plans and leaving the house, and continually cancelled plans with friends and family because I had a fear of getting unexpectedly sick. Now that I feel amazing I never worry, but live in the present moment and try to enjoy life to the fullest, no matter what comes my way! I have replaced fear with trust and I do not worry about the "what ifs" anymore.

Another thing I can do now is to eat in abundance and eat beautiful, colorful, raw, living foods! My inflamed intestines used to always be raw, swollen, and restricted, so I dealt with a lot of pain every time I ate. Sometimes I couldn't eat anything but liquids. I was afraid to eat any roughage or fiber so I avoided fruits and vegetables. Now that my digestive system is stronger, I get to eat!

Another thing I've discovered is how much more energy and vitality I have, so I'm doing more and loving it! I now get to live life to the fullest, whereas before healing, I was very restricted. My mind is in such a better place too, I'm more positive and incredibly empowered knowing that I have control over my health.

ANY INSPIRING STORIES THAT HAVE HAPPENED TO YOU OR PEOPLE CLOSE TO YOU THAT HAVE NOT BEEN COVERED ABOVE. STORIES THAT CAN HELP OTHERS.

I suffered for the majority of my life. In the moments of pain and chronic illness, it is so hard to see that it is not the luck of the draw or a bad card given. You feel as if everything is against you, but as you find your power and step into the greatest version of yourself, you will look back upon the suffering and see it as a total blessing. There are lessons and blessings in everything we encounter, and we have the choice to grow and expand. I made the decision that I no longer wanted to suffer, and from that time on, I was guided to the information that was meant to help me.

Pain and suffering can be a catalyst for great change. As you set your mind to believe you can heal, doors will start opening for you, and it will turn into this organic unfolding of opportunities to help you grow. After I regained my health, I found a great passion for wanting to help others attain vibrant health. I now see my pain as such a blessing because if I didn't go through all of it, I wouldn't know what so many on Earth are going through right now. I know how people feel, and I want to help end that suffering. I found my purpose in my pain, and I am forever grateful for all the adversities I've been put through because they have empowered me to be the person I am today. It is my mission to end the suffering in our world and re-ignite the Light within each and every one of us so that we can live a bright life full of purpose, passion and joy, and experience what it is like to be physically and mentally free with nothing to weigh us down.

JAYNE LOGHRY

ANOREXIA, GASTROINTESTINAL PROBLEMS, INFLAMMATION, AND PAIN.

"There came a point when nothing I was doing was working. I was simply struggling through health issues and digging through research, trying to find the truth I knew existed. I knew there had to be a natural way to heal what was going on inside of me. After suffering from an eating disorder, it is finally nice to be in control and LOVE what food can do for my body and not worry about restricting myself."

Jayne Loghry struggled with multiple health issues, including anorexia, gastrointestinal problems, inflammation and pain. Her chronic conditions are what led her on the path towards a plant-based lifestyle, and she hasn't looked back since.

AT WHAT POINT IN YOUR LIFE DID YOU DECIDE TO CHANGE YOUR DIET? HOW HAS THAT DECISION IMPACTED YOUR LIFE?

There came a point when nothing I was doing was working. I was simply struggling through health issues and digging through research, trying to find the truth that I knew existed. I knew there had to be a natural way to heal what was going on inside of me, but I was at a loss for how to do that.

That's when I watched a documentary called Forks Over Knives, and realized that I had examples living right in front of me: my in-laws. They had already switched to a whole-food, plant-based diet, and their energy and zest for life that was renewed through their diet had really inspired me.

WHAT THINGS HAVE MADE THE MOST DIFFERENCE IN YOUR ABILITY TO LIVE A GOOD LIFE AFTER LIVING WITH OR CURING YOUR DISEASE?

I have battled with undiagnosed gastrointestinal issues for quite a while, as well as fatigue and inflammation in joints. This has caused me a decent amount of pain throughout the majority of my life. Currently, I'm in a place where I am feeling more energy, more alive, and honestly, less afraid of eating than ever before in my life. The food I choose now on a daily basis fills me up in a good way and gives me the energy to live my days fully present in all that I do. This is what I love most about having adopted this diet.

AFTER ADOPTING A PLANT-BASED DIET HOW LONG DID IT TAKE BEFORE FIRST, YOU STARTED TO FEEL BETTER, AND SECOND, YOU KNEW YOU WERE NOT GOING TO LET THIS WIN?

I started feeling better around the second or third week. After a month, I was on track with my gastrointestinal issues, which are mostly cleared up. My energy levels rose as well, I lost some fat percentage in my body, and I am overall happier.

YOU'VE JUST MET A HEARTBROKEN STRANGER WHO HAS JUST BEEN GIVEN A LIFE-THREATENING DIAGNOSIS. WHAT WOULD BE YOUR TOP TIPS TO HELP THEM?

My top tips are:

1. Start small. You're not solving this issue today, but slowly and surely you can start to change your diet.

2. Believe in yourself and find someone else who does too. We are all human and have weak points. Your weak points will come, so prepare for this. Find someone to be on your team and help you through when things get tough.

3. There are so many vegetables and fruits out there. Don't limit yourself and also, check what's in season. In-season fruits and veggies have been a lifesaver for us. Try to have fun trying new things and experimenting.

4. Switching your diet may seem like a small thing, but it can have huge benefits. You really help yourself by giving yourself a chance.

DO YOU TAKE ANY SPECIAL SUPPLEMENTS OR POTIONS? MENTION ANY SPECIFIC BRANDS YOU USE AND WHY YOU THINK THESE HAVE BENEFITED YOU AND YOUR HEALTH.

Generally, since I have begun eating a whole-food, plant-based diet, I don't take anything. I simply try to "supplement" through a variety of vegetables and fruits throughout my day.

WHAT ARE THE TWO OR THREE THINGS YOU HAVE DONE DIFFERENTLY WITH YOUR LIFE AFTER YOUR HEALTH GOT BETTER?

1. Food freedom. End of story. Eating real, whole, food - gives me complete food freedom.

2. I embraced cooking and eating meals with my husband. I was always so worried about portion sizing for the both of us, but now we both help out in the cooking process, and we're always full by the end of our meals. Before, I

always had to add more fat or meat to my husband's meals. Now, we both fill up on the same exact meal; he just usually has more on his plate!

ANY INSPIRING STORIES THAT HAVE HAPPENED TO YOU OR PEOPLE CLOSE TO YOU THAT HAVE NOT BEEN COVERED ABOVE. STORIES THAT CAN HELP OTHERS.

I used to be obsessed with the next nutrition or diet craze, constantly going from one thing to the next. I was over-exerting myself and anorexic. I was also stressed, anxious, and honestly felt a lack of control in most areas of my life, which is why I took control of my eating...or lack thereof. It's something I've always struggled with.

My husband and I journeyed through several ways of eating, and our journey led us to many documentaries. I'm not sure what thing finally got our attention, but I'm so happy it did. We decided to try the whole-food, plant-based diet and honestly, it's changing both of our lives.

As I said, I've struggled with an obsession of food, numerous gastrointestinal issues, as well as inflammation in my joints. These physical symptoms have cleared up and, on top of that, this way of enjoying life has changed my perspective on food entirely.

We eat what was made and created on this earth for consumption.

It's hard when you've had an eating disorder and have become confused as to what is right. But it's simple really. Michael Pollan says it best when he says, "Eat food. Mostly plants. Not too much," and I couldn't agree more. You'll know it's food by its name and something that isn't made of a list of things that you can't pronounce.

I've found a new identity now that I am no longer consumed by what is going into my body. Rather, for the first time in my life, I'm looking up and around at those sitting at the table with me.

You can do this too.

The people sitting at the table with you deserve your best you.

LORNA McCORMACK

CONNECT WITH LORNA:
INSTAGRAM: @ESSENTIALLYPLANTBASED
lornamccormack.com

SUFFERING FROM LIFELONG CHRONIC ECZEMA & ASTHMA

"When it comes to food, no one wants to be told what to eat. But very often we don't realize that we are trapped by our food choices. It is only when we have enough information on how food can help us live a better quality life and how to do it that we can break free from the old habits to truly enjoy our food and live better."

Lorna McCormack is a nutritionist & medical herbalist, who helps her patients understand the benefits of a plant-based lifestyle for creating and sustaining a healthy body and mind. She now offers classes and various educational programs on food, essential oils and healthy habits with the simple goal of creating a healthier, happier and more balanced life.

49

WHAT ARE YOUR DAILY RITUALS/HABITS WHICH YOU BELIEVE HAVE BEEN KEY TO YOUR HEALTH?

My daily rituals are a constant work in progress. I'm a particularly strong believer in morning rituals. This is the part of the day that I have the most control. My morning rituals set me up for the day with a feeling of accomplishment before I even get started on my "to do's."

My long-term habits have been;

Drinking one liter of water upon waking. I usually bring a water bottle with me to bed so when I wake up it's beside me and I'll drink it while I'm getting ready.

When I get down to the kitchen, I'll take a shot of apple cider vinegar. Again I leave the bottle at the sink as a reminder every morning. I believe if you want to create new habits, you need to set yourself up for success by having visual reminders and making it convenient.

Then, I'll take my daily supplements, which are always whole-food, plant-based supplements. Then, I'll refill my water bottle and add two drops of peppermint and lemon essential oil.

Next, I make myself a green drink. Depending on how much time I have, I'll either make a green smoothie or a green juice containing cucumber, celery, kale, spinach and only a small piece of fruit for the taste. I'll also add some superfood powders. Some of my favorites are spirulina, chlorella, cinnamon and slippery elm.

I've always had a strong interest in food as nourishment for my body, so when I began my own health journey, most of my rituals focused on food. However, over the years of training in holistic health (herbal medicine, essential oils and lifestyle) I've become more aware of the need to build on my diet with other practices to nourish my mind and soul.

This year I've been building on my morning routine with the following rituals;

Ten minutes morning meditation
Five minutes morning affirmations
Five minutes gratitude journaling

My week also includes yoga. I love yin yoga. I'll practice at home two times weekly and also attend a class once a week.

I also use an infrared sauna one or two times weekly, mostly just during the winter months.

My exercise routine is very sporadic and random. It's anything from bouncing on the trampoline with the kids after school and daily walks in the fields surrounding my house, to short runs with a local running group.

AT WHAT POINT IN YOUR LIFE DID YOU DECIDE TO CHANGE YOUR DIET? HOW HAS THAT DECISION IMPACTED YOUR LIFE?

My journey to a plant-based diet was not a straight line from A to Z. It started when I was 23 and suffering from lifelong chronic eczema, asthma, and with an impending wedding that motivated me to lose weight. It was around this time that I picked up a book called, The Easy Way to Lose Weight. It's not a vegan book, but for the very first time, I was introduced to the idea that dairy and meat might not be the best thing for me.

I was intrigued and started to find myself reading book after book about juicing, detox and cancer survival stories. Very quickly, I eliminated almost all dairy and meat from my diet. I lost 28 pounds in a few months, my eczema vanished, and my asthma symptoms significantly reduced. I went from using a brown inhaler daily and a blue inhaler up to 30/40 times daily, to eliminating the brown inhaler and only using the blue inhaler occasionally.

The weight loss was amazing to me because I'd been "trying" to diet since I was 15. There honestly probably wasn't a day in my life until that point that I didn't think about what life would be like if I lost weight. But it felt impossible for me to diet. It felt like punishment, so my dieting attempts never usually got past noon!

At this point, it had never occurred to me to call myself vegan; I was just keeping my intake of animal foods very low, which was a big mistake. As life got busier, I still had a taste for these foods, so it became very easy for me to slip back into the standard Irish diet. And I did. My weight started to creep up again, and my asthma symptoms returned.

My awakening came in 2012 when my father was diagnosed with prostate cancer. We had very little knowledge of what this meant in terms of survival rates compared to other types of cancer. We just heard the C-word, and everyone got scared.

Although I had reverted to old habits at this point, I had read enough cancer survival stories to know that we needed to look at diet. So, instead of hiding from the C-word and wallowing in despair, we got to work with researching and experimenting. With his positive mindset and tendency to be proactive, my Dad was the ideal 'first client.' He embraced these changes and began juicing greens every day, growing wheatgrass, and much more. This is when my real journey began.

Soon after, I watched a documentary called Eating. I looked in my fridge the next morning at what I had originally planned for dinner. I had planned to cook a "ham joint," but now all I could see was a lump of dead, decaying, flesh in my fridge, and I definitely didn't want it decaying inside my body! That was the end of meat and milk for me.

Cheese was a different story. I had a strong attachment to it and, though I'd stopped buying it and eating it at home, I couldn't resist the fancy melted cheeses when we went out to eat. It took me about two years to break that addiction.

At this point, I had no fears and was fully in control of where I was going. I was quite happy to experiment with new dishes, and I wasn't disheartened when I got it wrong! I just keep at it. Today, most people look into my food cupboard and fridge and ask, "what do you do with all that stuff?"

Following Dad's diagnosis, I began the process of educating him about what I was learning. Reading the book, The China Study was a pivotal moment for me. Up until this point, I had only read about how animal foods are not the best foods for me with my skin and respiratory conditions. It was easy to think that it was just me who couldn't eat these foods. To say I was shocked about what I was learning about cancer would be an understatement.

I recall attending a doctor's appointment with my father where we shared some of the information we had learned about survival rates for men who receive treatment versus men who don't. Fortunately for us, this doctor had just returned from a conference where they had talked about this.

My Dad left this meeting feeling relieved that he wasn't going to be stuck in the middle of a tug of war between his doctor and me. I left feeling sad and worried about what might have happened if the timing was different. Could my Dad have been railroaded into treatment that would be aggressive and complicated? Why was I the one teaching my Dad how to make lifestyle changes to support his health? Why was no one in the medical profession talking to him about lifestyle and diet?

This sparked a whole new life and career change. I now practice as a nutritionist and essential oils educator, and at the time of writing this, I am a few months away from receiving my license to practice medical herbalism.

WHAT THINGS HAVE MADE THE MOST DIFFERENCE IN YOUR ABILITY TO LIVE A GOOD LIFE AFTER LIVING WITH OR CURING YOUR DISEASE?

Mindset is really important. I didn't overwhelm or restrict myself with labelling myself vegan or vegetarian. Whenever I did, it quickly threw me into a "diet mentality," and I'd begin to focus on what I couldn't eat. And, to be honest, veganism wasn't even my goal. My goal was and remains to be a focus on eating a whole-food, plant-based diet, which just so happens to be vegan.

Through continued education, my eyes were eventually opened. Watching the film, Earthlings, was another pivotal moment. Today, eating plant-based means a lot more to me than personal health. It's about doing the very best I can to protect our animal friends and our planet.

I don't believe in shaming myself or anyone else, but if I did, I'd say that I am ashamed that I didn't do it for the animals sooner. I cannot fathom how I was blinded for so long about the cruelty of animal production. I live in the countryside in Ireland and most days I am a firsthand witness to the reality of animal cruelty. While these scenes bring me great sadness today, I grew up believing there was nothing wrong with that.

This makes me acutely aware of where most people are at.

Therefore, rather than try to guilt or scare people into veganism, my mission has become to inspire and help people to change in a way that is supportive and non-judgmental. It's inclusive and meets people where they are at. I take them step by step towards a lifestyle that's healthier for their body and our planet.

WHAT WAS YOUR DOCTOR'S REACTION AFTER ANNOUNCING YOUR PLANS TO FOLLOW A PLANT-BASED DIET?

With my asthma, I never needed to return to the doctor. I became my own doctor! However, it shocks me that every doctor and "specialist" I visited in relation to my eczema and asthma never even asked my Mum or me (when I was an adult) to consider dietary changes.

My Dad's doctor, on the other hand, expresses an interest in the lifestyle changes Dad has made, but he remains fully focused on the numbers. While this information is important, I find this frustrating because it's not the full picture; it's only a piece of information at a single point in time. We need a health service that treats the whole person and not just one body part.

WHAT WAS THE CRAZIEST THING YOU DID TO TRY AND FIGHT YOUR DISEASE? DID IT WORK OR MAKE ANY DIFFERENCE TO YOU?

It depends on what you call crazy. Some people think that eating only plants is crazy!

When it comes to taking care of your body, there are no big secrets or wacky potions. It's simple…

Move your body
Get lots of good sleep
Rest well – stress management, for example
Eat plants
Limit your exposure to toxins

That's what I do. Some people think it's crazy. Some people think it's unrealistic. Some people think it's expensive. However, I know that living this lifestyle is easier, more practical, and more cost-effective than the so-called standard Western diet and lifestyle.

It's a continuous journey for me. I don't seek a "final destination." It's a case of continuous improvement every day. #progressnotperfection

AFTER ADOPTING A PLANT-BASED DIET HOW LONG DID IT TAKE BEFORE FIRST, YOU STARTED TO FEEL BETTER, AND SECOND, YOU KNEW YOU WERE NOT GOING TO LET THIS WIN?

Within weeks my eczema went away, and I had significantly cut back on inhaler use. With regards to my weight, I wasn't on the scales every week (in fact I abandoned the scales completely), but I do recall around that six-month mark I had to go shopping because my clothes were literally hanging off me. By the time I reached my wedding day, I was the slimmest I had ever been. It's 13 years later, and my wedding dress still fits me!

YOU'VE JUST MET A HEARTBROKEN STRANGER WHO HAS JUST BEEN GIVEN A LIFE-THREATENING DIAGNOSIS. WHAT WOULD BE YOUR TOP FIVE TIPS TO HELP THEM?

The short answer would be (in no particular order);

- Nourish your body by eating lots of plants and drinking lots of water
- Move your body
- Get lots of good sleep
- Rest well – ie. Stress management
- Limit your exposure to toxins

And, as a bonus: to find a network of like-minded people that will support, inspire, and encourage you

The reality of change is very different though. In my day-to-day role, people come to me, asking for help. There are two types of people:

Those that seek the cure: a diet, a herb, a potion, a drug, etc.

Those that seek to learn about a lifestyle that supports their body's ability to heal itself.

With the first person, I must put significant effort into inspiring and educating that person to take charge of their own body and to know that everything they need to heal their body is inside them. Everything else is just a "tool."

With the second sort of person, I can get into the details of teaching them how to create a lifestyle that supports and helps to heal their body, which is really exciting.

DO YOU TAKE ANY SPECIAL SUPPLEMENTS OR POTIONS? MENTION ANY SPECIFIC BRANDS YOU USE AND WHY YOU THINK THESE HAVE BENEFITED YOU AND YOUR HEALTH?

My daily regime includes:

doTERRA's Lifelong Vegan Lifelong Vitality Kit – a whole-food, vegan multivitamin, along with antioxidants, and omega supplements

doTERRA's Terrazyme - digestive enzymes

I vary the superfood powders that I put into my green drinks – my favorites are spirulina, chlorella, cinnamon, turmeric, slippery elm, moringa.

I use doTERRA essential oils in many many ways throughout the day to support the health of everyone in our home & keep toxin exposure to a minimum.

As a herbalist in training, I am fortunate that I can also take individually-made herbal remedies when I feel the need for additional support.

HOW DO YOU HANDLE THE UPS AND DOWNS OF GOOD AND BAD DAYS? WHAT STRATEGIES DO YOU USE?

My strategy is to avoid bad days by managing my need for perfectionism. I don't have bad days when I don't beat myself up over it not being perfect. I focus on progress, not perfection.

However, I do feel that having a strong morning ritual/routine is my secret sauce when it comes to having "my ideal day."

WHAT ARE THE TWO OR THREE THINGS YOU HAVE DONE DIFFERENTLY WITH YOUR LIFE AFTER YOUR HEALTH GOT BETTER?

Suffering from asthma was very debilitating. I had two young kids at this time. I can recall the days when I would avoid bringing them outside for a walk or bouncing on the trampoline because I couldn't breathe. At one point I couldn't walk up a set of stairs without using the inhaler.

Not being able to breathe is a horrible and scary feeling. There were so many restrictions on what I could or couldn't do. While exercise is known to help asthma sufferers, I personally couldn't exercise because I couldn't breathe! It felt like a very cruel, vicious cycle. Changing my diet was the catalyst for change in all areas of my life.

ANY INSPIRING STORIES THAT HAVE HAPPENED TO YOU OR PEOPLE CLOSE TO YOU THAT HAVE NOT BEEN COVERED ABOVE. STORIES THAT CAN HELP OTHERS.

There is so much information out there, and so much of it is conflicting, with one "expert" as convincing as the next. I feel sorry for people who genuinely make an attempt at creating a healthier lifestyle, but often end up confused and disempowered.

I attend a lot of events where I talk to the public, and it shocks me how confused people are about nutrition. They make it sound so complicated. The reality is that it's so simple: eat plants; fruits, vegetables, whole grains, legumes, nuts and seeds. Eat a variety from each of those plant-based food groups in a minimally processed state. That's it.

The public has been duped into believing that the solution to the healthcare crisis is complicated. Maybe they need to believe that it's complicated to justify their bad habits. People don't believe that the solution to some of the largest problems our society is facing is to just eat more plants!

"

ANY FRUIT OR VEGETABLE SHOULD BE CONSIDERED A SUPERFOOD

NARA SCHULER

MINDY MYLREA

CONNECT WITH MINDY:
INSTAGRAM: @MINDYMYLREAFITNESS
FACEBOOK: MINDY MYLREA
bruceandmindy.com

HUSBAND SURVIVED CANCER AND LOWERED HIS CHOLESTEROL BY 100 POINTS IN SIX WEEKS

Mindy Mylrea is no stranger to the fitness scene and has starred in over 400 fitness videos, created cutting edge education for the fitness industry, including the award-winning Tabata Bootcamp program. She has won almost every major award the industry has to offer including IDEA Fitness Instructor of the Year, PFP Trainer of the Year, and International Presenter of the Year. In 2011, in an attempt to treat her husband, Bruce's, high cholesterol numbers, both Bruce and Mindy transitioned to a whole-food, plant-based diet. An unexpected cancer diagnosis for Bruce threw the couple for a loop and opened their eyes to the truth about wellness. For the past three years, Bruce and Mindy have been touring the country in a large RV, lecturing at fitness conferences on the truth about nutrition in order to spread the word about the importance of whole, plant foods.

WHAT ARE YOUR DAILY RITUALS/HABITS WHICH YOU BELIEVE HAVE BEEN KEY TO YOUR HEALTH?

I am thankful for every gift every day, and I let those around me know. I acknowledge and appreciate the simplest of actions and I never take those for granted. Every day I take time to live in the moment and create memories from those moments that might pass me by otherwise.

AT WHAT POINT IN YOUR LIFE DID YOU DECIDE TO CHANGE YOUR DIET? HOW HAS THAT DECISION IMPACTED YOUR LIFE?

Nine years ago, Bruce and I read, The China Study, by T. Colin Campbell. That was the catalyst we needed to make the shift. From there, we dove into the research, and Bruce went on to lecture on plant-based nutrition. Because of Bruce's cancer diagnosis eight years ago, we have become wellness missionaries, passionate about spreading the truth about evidence-based nutrition and how to live an optimal life even when one is dealing with a debilitating disease. This has now become a mission we dedicate our lives to.

We have rented out our house in Santa Cruz, CA for at least two or three years and are traveling around in the Wellness Wagon (a 32-foot RV wrapped in our logo with fruits and veggies) speaking about evidence-based nutrition and wellness. We are a non-profit and do not accept any money from industry influence, because when you do your message can become compromised

WHAT THINGS HAVE MADE THE MOST DIFFERENCE IN YOUR ABILITY TO LIVE A GOOD LIFE AFTER LIVING WITH OR CURING YOUR DISEASE?

Living every day with a purpose and having meaning to the message. We do not believe the saying "things happen for a reason." This is a shallow and empty statement. What we do believe in is that everyone has turbulent times and tragedy. It is what you do with the mud that counts. Do you create something worthwhile? Or, do you dwell in your sorrow?
We choose to be an open book and reach out to as many people as we can who are open to our message.

WHAT WAS YOUR DOCTOR'S REACTION AFTER ANNOUNCING YOUR PLANS TO FOLLOW A PLANT-BASED DIET? WAS HE/SHE SUPPORTIVE?

Yes, very supportive, but not very educated on plant-based eating. They are all blown away by Bruce's lack of side effects and his energy and gusto. Many doctors ask lots of questions and want to be more informed, but their medical training has been limited and lacking nutritional education.

AFTER ADOPTING A PLANT-BASED DIET HOW LONG DID IT TAKE BEFORE FIRST, YOU STARTED TO FEEL BETTER, AND SECOND, YOU KNEW YOU WERE NOT GOING TO LET THIS WIN?

After adopting a WFPBD, the transformation was immediate. Bruce lowered his cholesterol by one hundred points in just six weeks, and I lost ten pounds right away. Our energy was through the roof with no more dip in the day from lack of energy. Plus, now that we don't eat any oil, our taste buds have completely shifted to loving all foods from the earth.
We are never going back.

YOU'VE JUST MET A HEARTBROKEN STRANGER WHO HAS JUST BEEN GIVEN A LIFE-THREATENING DIAGNOSIS. WHAT WOULD BE YOUR TOP FIVE TIPS TO HELP THEM?

- Start shifting to a WFPBD
- Meditate
- Come to our program, "One Day to Wellness"

DO YOU TAKE ANY SPECIAL SUPPLEMENTS OR POTIONS? MENTION ANY SPECIFIC BRANDS YOU USE AND WHY YOU THINK THESE HAVE BENEFITED YOU AND YOUR HEALTH.

Bruce and I take B12, vitamin D, and Dr.Furman's EPA DHA. Bruce also takes citric pectin and wild raspberry extract.

WHAT ARE SOME OF THE WORST RECOMMENDATIONS THAT YOU HAVE BEEN GIVEN BY "EXPERTS."?

There have been a lot of them including: Eliminate soy, drink milk, eat meat. Don't fast because you need the protein. The list goes on...

HOW DO YOU HANDLE THE UPS AND DOWNS OF GOOD AND BAD DAYS? WHAT STRATEGIES DO YOU USE?

Meditation and being mindful. The good news is that Bruce and I are so fine-tuned that when one of us is down, the other is there to lift that person up. It is very rare that we both have a down day at the same time. One of us always comes to the rescue.

WHAT ARE THE TWO OR THREE THINGS YOU HAVE DONE DIFFERENTLY WITH YOUR LIFE AFTER YOUR HEALTH GOT BETTER?

We live in the moment. We live in an RV currently and travel all across North America spreading this message.

ANY INSPIRING STORIES THAT HAVE HAPPENED TO YOU OR PEOPLE CLOSE TO YOU THAT HAVE NOT BEEN COVERED ABOVE. STORIES THAT CAN HELP OTHERS.

Cancer sucks, and it changes everything. Bruce and I will most likely live with cancer for the rest of our lives. It certainly is not a gift we wanted, but it has allowed us to truly live the life we were meant to live. Cancer has allowed us to acknowledge that life is finite and precious. Having the purpose of helping others has opened our hearts to the beauty and grace that an optimal life has to offer. We live every day by what Gandhi preached, "You must be the change you wish to see in the world."

NARA SCHULER

CONNECT WITH NARA:
INSTAGRAM: @NARASCHULER
FACEBOOK: SECRETS OF MY VEGAN KITCHEN
secretsofmyvegankitchen.com

REVERSED DIABETES WITHOUT MEDICATION

Nara Schuler is a graduate of the Durham College Culinary Skills Program, a graduate from the Plant-Based Nutrition Certificate at T. Colin Campbell Center for Nutrition Studies (Cornell University), and a graduate of the Professional Coach Certification, SLAC/SP. Nara has chronicled her journey towards healing her body in her book, Secrets of My Vegan Kitchen - Reversing My Diabetes without Medication, where she shares how she reversed her diabetes through healthful eating habits and whole-food, plant-based recipes.

WHAT ARE YOUR DAILY RITUALS/HABITS WHICH YOU BELIEVE HAVE BEEN KEY TO YOUR HEALTH?

I don't really have any rituals or daily habits. I only changed my diet, cutting all animal products from it, and at the beginning of my new lifestyle, I had to reinvent my recipes. For the first three months, I ate a very strict vegan diet focusing on foods that are nutrient-dense. I ate exclusively; greens and cruciferous vegetables, beans, non-starchy vegetables, fruits, mushrooms, seeds, and nuts. My breakfasts were mostly smoothies, followed by a salad and beans and vegetable soup with fruit for lunch. For dinner, I would eat a modified version of what was left from lunch. I never ate grains or starchy vegetables during the healing period. Before bed, I would drink a cup of freshly made vegetable juice.

In the beginning, I felt quite sorry for myself, as I thought I would never again feel pleasure in eating. I now know that this thought couldn't be further from the truth.

Within a few months after my healing, I started to reintroduce grains into my diet. This addition has impacted my weight loss because I stalled a little before reaching my ideal weight goal.

At this moment, I consider my lifestyle very close to a conventional one, with the difference that I eat a vegan diet (absolutely no animals) and give more importance to eating salads, vegetables, soups, and beans over grains and sweets. My first meal is usually at lunchtime. I avoid coffee but occasionally drink a black decaf to start the day. Lunch normally consists of a salad, rice, beans, or potatoes and a dessert which may be a fruit or low fat and low sugar cake or another dessert. My next meal is the last one of the day. I try to eat before 6 pm to give my digestive system a rest and time to detoxify. Sometimes it can be a wrap or sandwich with vegetables. Sometimes a smoothie or a vegetable juice.

The most important change in my diet, beyond becoming vegan, is the variety of ingredients I choose for my meals. I find it extremely important to have a large variety of greens, vegetables, fruits, seeds and nuts in my salads, day after day. I never eat exactly the same recipe as I am convinced that our body needs numerous nutrients that can only be found when we eat a variety of different types of fruits, legumes, and vegetables.

AT WHAT POINT IN YOUR LIFE DID YOU DECIDE TO CHANGE YOUR DIET? WHY DID YOU DECIDE TO CHANGE TO A VEGAN/PLANT-BASED DIET AND HOW DID YOU OVERCOME YOUR FEARS AND TAKE CONTROL OF YOUR OWN DESTINY?

From my 40's to my 50's, my weight escalated enormously. I went from 180 pounds to 245 pounds and I did not really worry about it, because most women get heavier as they grow older. I was under the impression that the increase in body fat was a normal part of life.

I had headaches and hip pain. I also struggled with sleep apnea, depression and constipation. I was developing high blood pressure and losing my sight. With all of these symptoms, I still believed I was healthy since my blood tests only showed some abnormal results. These were considered acceptable by my family doctor.

My doctor used to assure me that I did not really need to lose weight since I was not obese, just overweight. As time passed my sight was getting worse and I was required to use a CPAP machine to sleep. Still, I was not too worried about my health since it seemed normal to have to breathe through a machine. Little by little though, things got worse. My vision kept weakening, and I was having to rely on painkillers to sleep almost daily. At some point, I got a urinary tract infection that did not subside for a few weeks. This is what prompted me to go to my family doctor to get antibiotics.

Once I was at the doctor's, he measured my glucose and told me I was diabetic. He said I would have to start taking some pills right away since my glucose level was seventeen when a normal level is below seven. I asked him how long I would have to take the medication, and he told me that now that I had developed diabetes, I would never again be able to stop the medications. I was in shock! I did not want to have diabetes. He told me that it was not my choice; it was in my genes since two of my older sisters were already diabetic. I did not accept that; I was furious with him and went home to research about diabetes.

The internet was my best friend those days. I read all the articles I could find. Some were scary, but most of them confirmed my doctor's point of view. Finally, I came across Dr. Joel Fuhrman's book, Eat to Live, where he explains how chronic diseases are created and what to do to reverse them. I downloaded the book and spent the whole night reading it. It made sense. I decided to experiment with his diet.

It was the fear of becoming dependent on medications for the rest of my life that finally spurred my change; the fear of allowing someone else to be in control of my health. After understanding what I had to do and that I was the only one that had the power to heal myself, I went back to my doctor's office and told him I wanted a probation period before starting to take any medication. I told him I needed three months, and if nothing changed, I would submit to his orders and follow his recommendation. He agreed with me, certain that I would return sicker and in need of medications.

WHAT THINGS HAVE MADE THE MOST DIFFERENCE IN YOUR ABILITY TO LIVE A GOOD LIFE AFTER LIVING WITH OR CURING YOUR DISEASE?

Curing my disease has completely changed the way I eat. It changed the way my family eats as well. At the time, I was in charge of making our family meals. In the beginning, my family did not want to eat the same way as I did. I did not want to eat that way either, but it was clear to me that my choices were to change my diet and have a shot of recovering my health or to stay sick and only get sicker over the years. I was 52, and I thought it was too early to have a miserable diseased life.

At some point after the cold turkey diet change and feeling sorry for myself, I started to perceive a large number of options I had when choosing food. I thought to myself that with so many variations of salads I was having every day, I could easily broaden my menu. I have always been a good cook, and this moment gave me the opportunity to experiment with unfamiliar ingredients, so I reinvented my recipes. I got more and more excited about creating new dishes. I started to make interesting meals that not only looked good but smelled and tasted fantastic. My family's interest started to grow.

Meanwhile, my weight was dropping, even though I was not exercising. My blood sugar had decreased to below seven, and I was feeling more and more energized. My family members were more and more interested, and within a couple of months succumbed to eating what I was preparing for myself. First at home only, and within a few extra months, they concluded that my choice was the right one and joined me in my new lifestyle.

WHAT WAS YOUR DOCTOR'S REACTION?

My doctor was sure I would come back again for medication. Three months later, after my diagnosis, when I went back for my blood tests, I was obviously slimmer. My looks and energy did not impress him, and a blood test was requested to check my condition. The results came back in a few days, and he was appalled by them. All my blood parameters were back to normal. Not only normal but in the healthiest range of normal. He was looking at both results. The one from three months before and the one from two days before and he told me it looked like results from two different people. My A1c went from 0.10 (10%) to 0.5 (5%), and he told me he could confidently say that I was not diabetic.

I was very proud of my achievements and was so eager to tell him everything I had done, but to my surprise, he told me he could not recommend this to his other patients as I was the only one he knew who would have the strength to endure such drastic changes in a diet. Unfortunately, his point of view didn't change, despite my continued excellent blood test results over the past nine years.

WHAT WAS THE CRAZIEST THING YOU DID TO TRY AND FIGHT YOUR DISEASE? DID IT WORK OR MAKE ANY DIFFERENCE TO YOU?

I didn't really do anything crazy to fight my disease; I just addressed it right from the start with a diet change. Some might think that a diet change is a crazy thing though.

Feeling sorry for myself was a big feeling at the time. I had never really been sick before, and it feels very strange to be in that position.

The healing process was very interesting. After a few weeks, I could feel that my body's discomfort was not coming back. That is the most amazing feeling one can have. I was so used to taking painkillers on a regular basis, and day after day, I started needing less and less of those over the counter medications. At a certain point, I felt my pain and discomfort disappear completely, and I got my energy back.

AFTER ADOPTING A PLANT-BASED DIET HOW LONG DID IT TAKE BEFORE FIRST, YOU STARTED TO FEEL BETTER, AND SECOND, YOU KNEW YOU WERE NOT GOING TO LET THIS WIN?

The first three weeks were the hardest since I did not really like anything I was eating. My diet used to be mostly composed of grains and animal products high in salt, oil, and sugar.

Fortunately, my blood sugar started to go down from the very first days of my diet change, and that was stimulating. Seeing that I was reversing my diabetes was a great incentive to continue to eat the new foods.
I introduced a lot of vegetable juices during that period, and I believe that it has increased the number of vitamins and antioxidants in my body.
It gave my organs and cells the power to detoxify.

YOU'VE JUST MET A HEARTBROKEN STRANGER WHO HAS BEEN GIVEN A LIFE-THREATENING DIAGNOSIS. WHAT WOULD BE YOUR TOP FIVE TIPS TO HELP THEM?

Every day when I go grocery shopping, I see so many people with obvious painful diseases buying the products that contribute the most to their suffering. I have to tell myself to ignore them because I do not have the right to intrude in their lives. I would love, however, to share my experience and knowledge with them, and that is why I am participating in this amazing project.

There were some situations where I have had the opportunity to talk to people who are battling a life-threatening chronic disease. I normally start by sharing my story and wait for them to ask me questions about the food I eat. Once we get into it, I can slowly tell them that I eat now a fairly normal diet, but it is totally absent of animal products and mostly based on whole-foods that are minimally processed. These words are so unusual to them, yet it is so simple, basic and affordable.

- In order to change someone's perspective on their health, people must have an interest and desire to address their disease. I believe it is impossible to change someone who is not open to trying a different approach.

- One should always ask the doctor how many of their patients have successfully recovered from their diseases under the same treatment you are being suggested to follow.

- Remove from your life, home or pantry all highly processed ingredients and foods, all animal-based products. Throw these things in the garbage with the understanding that when you do, you are freeing your body from getting sicker.

- Fill your kitchen with a variety of non-starchy vegetables, mushrooms, beans, fruits, seeds and nuts. Start eating them in abundance.

- Do a blood test before you begin this journey and keep records of the improvement you feel in your body.

DO YOU TAKE ANY SPECIAL SUPPLEMENTS OR POTIONS? WHY DO

YOU THINK THESE HAVE BENEFITED YOU AND YOUR HEALTH?

In my opinion, any fruit or vegetable should be considered a superfood, as each plant has numerous health benefits. If we use only plants in our diet, we can achieve the best possible health. However, to achieve such benefits, we need to eat an abundance and a large variety of them to be able to absorb the most diversity of vitamins, minerals, and micronutrients from nature as possible.

I only supplement with B12 as our foods are too sterile and we can no longer yield the necessary number of bacteria from soil. My skin is moisturized with coconut oil to keep it smooth and protected from sun burning. That is as far as I go in supplementing on a regular basis.

WHAT ARE SOME OF THE WORST RECOMMENDATIONS THAT YOU HAVE BEEN GIVEN BY "EXPERTS."?

When I was diagnosed with type two diabetes, and I decided to change my diet as my only form of treatment, my doctor suggested that I should contact the Diabetes Association. Fortunately, I followed my instincts and changed my diet according to the literature I found in my research about diabetes reversal. Had I followed the directions of the Diabetes Association, I would still be diabetic and taking medications, maybe even insulin shots. I feel very sorry that people are told to follow a modified diet and continue to be sicker and in need of increasing medications.

WHAT ARE TWO OR THREE THINGS YOU HAVE DONE DIFFERENTLY WITH YOUR LIFE AFTER YOUR HEALTH GOT BETTER?

After I regained my health, I became extremely interested in nutrition. I dove into nutrition literature and read almost anything I could get my hands on. I translated my favorite book from English to Portuguese, with the aim of sharing with a world full of people that suffer from chronic diseases, why their troubles are rooted in misinformation about diet choices.

I wrote my own story and self-published it, to help people learn what I have experienced and how amazing my health recovery was. I really wanted to open people's eyes to such a simple and satisfying experience.

Since 2011, I have been a volunteer for the Vegetarian Association, for which I am the current leader, and where I created the DurhamVeg Fest to promote veganism in my region. I went back to school, graduated with a Culinary Skills Certificate from Durham College, and graduated with a Plant-Based Nutrition Certificate from the T. Colin Campbell Centre for Nutrition Studies at eCornell.

I created videos for online TV in Brazil where I talk to people about diet change, how to do it and give as much information as I possibly can.

Within a few years of becoming vegan, I finally understood the horrible treatment of animals in general, which opened up another area of interest in my life. I understood that animals should never be our food. They have their own lives and feelings. We don't take any of this into consideration when killing them for food or other practices.

A little bit later, I became aware of the impact our diet has on the environment as well, and all of this knowledge has improved my commitment to this lifestyle.

ANY INSPIRING STORIES THAT HAVE HAPPENED TO YOU OR PEOPLE CLOSE TO YOU THAT HAVE NOT BEEN COVERED ABOVE. STORIES THAT CAN INSPIRE AND HELP OTHERS

When I attended Culinary School, I realized how biased our chefs and culinary schools are. This industry runs what we eat and what we choose to have on our table. I made a huge effort to educate not only my colleagues but also my professors and other staff at the school about a vegan diet. I veganized all the dishes we had to prepare in school. Our curriculum was based on traditional French cuisine. Everyone was very impressed with my dedication; however, none of them were interested in cooking vegan meals. Occasionally, they ventured to try my dishes, but the resistance to modifying the way we eat is very high in this area.

I was fortunate enough to have found this amazing way of eating and also being able to influence most of the people I love. My husband of almost 40 years embraced the vegan diet three months after me. He has lost about 30 pounds, and he is in his 60's with intense energy physically and mentally. My two sons and daughters in law are vegan and their families were also exposed to the benefits and the information about a plant-based diet. Many of them have introduced more plants into their diets even if they have not become vegan yet.

In the last few years, there has been a huge growth in vegan interest, and hopefully, we will attract more and more people to modify their way of thinking. Three years after my graduation at cooking school, I finally had the opportunity to open my own vegan restaurant. It is located downtown in a small conservative city in Canada. All 33 items on the menu are 100% plant-based and imitate the traditional foods we are used to. It is one more attempt to guide the general public into changing their view on their diet.

BARBARA TAYLOR
(AUTHORS MUM)

TAKEN OFF HIGH BLOOD PRESSURE MEDS AFTER 25 YEARS

"I have had high blood pressure and had been on medication for the past 25 years. I was told that once I went on it, I would need to be on it for the rest of my life. At the time, I didn't know any better. I needed to get it under control, so I followed my doctor's advice. Over the past three years, my cholesterol was also a little on the high side, according to my doctor, and she was keen to start me on an anti-statin. I believed I could lower this myself but had not yet been able to do so. Once I made the switch to a plant-based diet, I quickly lowered my cholesterol, lost 4kg and within six months was off my blood pressure medication, and my blood pressure was at an optimal level. It's such a wonderful feeling to have taken back my health and not need to take any prescription medication."

Barbara's story is an extra special one because she is my mum and the sister of my loving aunt that we lost to cancer.

Mum pays us a visit every year in Thailand (where we live). On this particular trip (over three years ago now) I had just decided that I was going vegan. I remember Sam ringing mum and warning her about the changes she was about to embark upon. Mum was a little concerned as she was worried about what she was going to be eating while staying with us.

On her first night with us, rather than field all of the usual questions, I decided to sit down with mum and watch What The Health on Netflix. This gave her the confidence that this change could in fact be good for her health. Spending this time with us and immersing herself in plant-based eating was a great way for her to give it a go and see how she felt after the month was up.

After the 30 days mum was feeling amazing. She had lost 4kg without even trying and she had more energy. She had actually just been and had blood tests done before coming to visit us, so as soon as she returned home she was excited to go and get re-tested, to see if her blood results concluded the way she was feeling and they absolutely did.

Her cholesterol was back down to a normal level and she was no longer a candidate for medication. Mum was feeling so great that she also felt as though she may no longer need to be taking blood pressure medication. Something she had been doing for as long as I can remember.

She spoke with her doctor about this, who was not so enthusiastic about getting her off this medication. Well, my mum is a strong and determined women so insisted that she would reduce her medication and she would monitor the results herself and that is exactly what she did.

WHAT ARE YOUR DAILY RITUALS/HABITS WHICH YOU BELIEVE HAVE BEEN KEY TO YOUR HEALTH?

Awareness, knowing my body and what it requires to keep it healthy and energized every day. Breakfast is a must as well as variety in my weekly choices. Having yummy snacks for when I'm feeling hungry is important and also when I need that mid-morning cuppa. Some form of exercise as well, like walking, yoga or going to the gym. I like to move my body every day and yoga is what I have been doing for the past year. I am seeing such great results with my flexibility and I feel much calmer.

AT WHAT POINT IN YOUR LIFE DID YOU DECIDE TO CHANGE YOUR DIET? HOW HAS THAT DECISION IMPACTED YOUR LIFE?

My beautiful daughter (Rebecca Frith) was the catalyst for me deciding to change my diet. Three years ago, I went for my regular visit with her and her family. She told me that they were now following a plant-based diet. At first, I was not sure what that meant for us. I used to be a big salmon eater and when I say big I mean I would probably eat salmon three to four times per week. I was sure I was going to miss this. I was also unsure about how healthy we were going to be as we would be missing a lot of protein, calcium, and omegas! My first question to her was, "so what does that mean for me? What can I eat or, more importantly, what can I not eat?"

When she went through what it all meant, I was not too fazed. I was not a big meat eater anyway, and I actually thought this could be a good change for me. I was interested to see if it could make a change to my health and change my mind about the few concerns that I had.

I am a healthy person; however, I did have high blood pressure and had been on medication for the past 25 years, which I was not happy about. However, I was told that once I went on it, I would need to be on it for the rest of my life. At the time, I didn't know any better. I needed to get it under control, so I followed my doctor's advice. My cholesterol was also a little on the high side according to my doctor, and she was keen to start me on an anti-statin. I believed I could lower this myself, but had not yet been able to do so. This was my chance to see if this really was diet-related as we had some family history of high cholesterol.

On the first night of staying at my daughter's while on that visit, we watched a documentary called *What the Health*. This was a real eye-opener for me. After seeing this documentary, I truly believed that I could not only lower my cholesterol, but perhaps I could even get off this blood pressure medication. So I did.

WHAT THINGS HAVE MADE THE MOST DIFFERENCE IN YOUR ABILITY TO LIVE A GOOD LIFE AFTER LIVING WITH OR CURING YOUR DISEASE?

I have so much more energy now, and I just love that. I have always been an active and vibrant person, but I feel the best I have ever felt.

It is so amazing that I don't have to take medication every day. It is something I truly hated and was never really comfortable with, but believed I needed to do it. It's such a wonderful feeling to have taken back my health and not need to take any prescription medication.

I am a much happier person; I feel like my hormones are stable and no longer have mood fluctuations, which I now believe were a side effect of the chemicals and hormones that are in the animal products I was consuming.

My body and organs feel clean. I know that may sound a little strange, but they feel like they are working the way they should be.

WHAT WAS YOUR DOCTOR'S REACTION AFTER ANNOUNCING YOUR PLANS TO FOLLOW A PLANT-BASED DIET?

At first, my doctor was very skeptical about me wanting to cut out my blood pressure medication and suggested that perhaps this was not a good idea. But, after knowing what I knew from watching What the Health and doing my research, I was going to give this a try, no matter what my doctor had said.

For the first six months of following my plant-based diet, I monitored my blood pressure twice a day. Then, when I was due to have my prescription for medication renewed, I decided it was time to make the change. I no longer was going to take my medication.

At first, it was a little all over the place. I continued to monitor it, and it did take a few months to completely stabilize. Now it is stable and an almost perfect reading every time. I am so pleased that I made this change and I could never go back.

My doctor also commented that she could see that I had lost weight (about four kilograms). I am not a very big person and did not have much to lose, but I have to say I was happy to see that little roll around my midsection disappear, especially because I didn't even have to try to lose it. I explained to the doctor that it was due to my plant-based diet.

WHAT WAS THE CRAZIEST THING YOU DID TO TRY AND FIGHT YOUR DISEASE? DID IT WORK OR MAKE ANY DIFFERENCE TO YOU?

Nothing crazy! I always believed that I was put on blood pressure medication due to a stressful time in my life. I was told that I needed to take it to stabilize my blood pressure and that once I started it that I would always need to take it. Finding out that this was not the case and that there was a way that I could come off them was a moment in my life, I will always remember and be grateful for. I hated the fact that I had to take this pill every single day, and I felt like it had control over me. It felt like if I did not take it or if I forgot to take them, I could possibly have a heart attack. Now, I feel like I have taken back the control!

AFTER ADOPTING A PLANT-BASED DIET HOW LONG DID IT TAKE BEFORE FIRST, YOU STARTED TO FEEL BETTER, AND SECOND, YOU KNEW YOU WERE NOT GOING TO LET THIS WIN?

I guess it took about six months. I continued to keep up my exercise, gym work, walking and yoga. Nothing changed other than my diet, so I knew that this was the underlying cause of the issues that I faced. Once I was able to go off my medication and I felt so amazing, I knew that I had made the right decision to change my diet and that I would never look back.

ANY INSPIRING STORIES THAT HAVE HAPPENED TO YOU OR PEOPLE CLOSE TO YOU THAT HAVE NOT BEEN COVERED ABOVE. STORIES THAT CAN HELP OTHERS.

I am so happy with myself for having made the change to a plant-based diet. I live in an area where people would not even know what a vegan or plant-based diet means. Eating out is a challenge because there are generally no options for me on the menu. I know to either phone in advance and ask for a plant-based option or, if it is a place that won't cater for me or a party we are going to, I generally eat before I go or take my own. I find this lifestyle incredibly easy, and I can always make something with the things I have in the fridge or cupboards.

Seeing the changes in my health, I know that I could never live any other way now. I just wish more people could get past their, "I can't live without meat or cheese" belief, to see just how amazing you can feel once you have given it up. I don't look at it as what I can't eat, I look at it and think, "look at all this AMAZING food that I can eat and eat as much of it as I like because it will nourish my body."

I lost a sister to cancer, and that is not going to happen to me! I just wish I knew then what I know now.

" "

LOOK AT ALL THIS AMAZING FOOD THAT I CAN EAT, AND EAT AS MUCH OF IT AS I LIKE BECAUSE IT WILL NOURISH MY BODY

BABARA TAYLOR

STELLA

CONNECT WITH STELLA:
INSTAGRAM: @STELLATHELIGHT
FACEBOOK: STELLA THE LIGHT
YOUTUBE: STELLA THE LIGHT
StellaTheLight.com

CONTROLLED DEPRESSION, EATING DISORDERS, ANXIETY, OCD, AND DRUG ADDICTION

"Be kind, for everyone you meet is fighting a hard battle you know nothing about." - Wendy Mass

This was Stella's eighth-grade yearbook quote - when her father had stage 4 cancer. She hit her rock bottom at 18-years-old, struggling with depression, anxiety, OCD, and drug addiction. After two stays and six months in rehab, Stella began the process of healing herself and her previous poor lifestyle choices. From a life of disordered eating, restriction, and gimmick diets, to one based around eating plant foods and finally feeling the healing powers of simple, whole-foods, Stella turned her life around.

WHAT ARE YOUR DAILY RITUALS/HABITS WHICH YOU BELIEVE HAVE BEEN KEY TO YOUR HEALTH?

A plant-based lifestyle / education! Allowing myself to dive into this lifestyle 100% with no holding back. Opening my mind to the idea of not eating animals anymore. I wish I would have done it sooner!

Also, my Vitamix. I use it literally three or four times daily! Whether it's for soups, smoothies, ice cream, or flours, it can blend just about anything up with ease! They are strong machines with amazing warranties.

AT WHAT POINT IN YOUR LIFE DID YOU DECIDE TO CHANGE YOUR DIET? HOW HAS THAT DECISION IMPACTED YOUR LIFE?

I happened upon the lifestyle via another crazy search on social media for yet another diet to help me "become healthy."

I had developed an eating disorder due to heavy animal-based dieting over the years. I tried all the normal trendy diets: low carb, low fat, carb cycling, insane cleanses, fasting, paleo, IIFYM etc. I felt worse and worse as time went on and continued to fluctuate in weight like crazy. My mental health was also the lowest it had ever been. I eventually developed a binge eating disorder along with other disordered patterns.

I found a few women who were all about five to ten years in the plant-based vegan movement and knew I had to give it a go! Within the first week, I fell in love, and I have never turned back. Life only gets better, and I only want to share this movement more and more!

I have high energy, compassion for myself, and every living being, my digestion is healed, I am the "fittest" I have ever been, and I don't restrict or limit my food. I would honestly say that every aspect of my life has been positively amplified - mental, physical, emotional, and spiritual!

WHO HAS BEEN THE BIGGEST PLANT-BASED DIET INFLUENCER IN YOUR LIFE AND HOW HAVE THEY HELPED YOU?

I found Ellen Fisher, EarthyAndy, and Loni Jane (via Instagram and YouTube) and just fell in love with how content they seemed to be. They seemed content with themselves, their families, their health, and their confidence... it almost seemed too good to be true!

But also, they were the first group of women who weren't lying to me. They weren't trying to sell me a restrictive diet that I would fail at, and that would bring me more harm than good. They were promoting abundance, self-love, doing no harm to animals, and just 100% honest, wholesome living!

HOW DO YOU THINK WE CAN ALL HAVE A BIGGER IMPACT ON INFLUENCING PEOPLE AND HELPING THEM MAKE THE CONNECTION TO HEALTH AND EATING A PLANT-BASED DIET?

Show them!!

I always tell people who struggle with trying to convince others that plant-based is the way to go, to cut those conversations off and never feed an argument over veganism or plant-based living.

Focus on the people who have an open mind and focus on just being the prime example! Post your yummy meals, talk about how amazing you feel, discuss the benefits, and SHINE THAT LIGHT!!

I love the quote: "First, they ask you WHY?! Then they ask you HOW?!"

When people first see you living this way they will make rude comments, ask why you would ever want to not eat junk food/meat/dairy, and it will feel hurtful! But, as time goes on and they see your delicious food, amazing health, happiness, and well being, they will want to know HOW! They'll want to try your recipes, get your advice on how to start, and learn more about the movement. Never lead by force, lead by example!

WHAT WAS THE REACTION YOU RECEIVED FROM PEOPLE WHEN YOU ANNOUNCED THAT YOU WERE GOING VEGAN? WHO WAS YOUR BEST AND WORST SUPPORTER?

My close friends and family thought, "Oh, she's doing another diet..."

But, within six months, a majority of those people wanted in!! Now most of my friends and family are plant-based vegans, including both of my 50-year-old parents and my partner (who went plant-based when he was just 19!!)

It is easy to think this is a restrictive diet. No meat?! No eggs?! No junk food?! But, it simply takes a shift in the mind to realize that those foods are not treats for the body. In reality, they are harming us in such detrimental ways that are both short term AND long term. Digestive upset, weight gain, mental health issues, heart disease, autoimmune diseases...the list goes on and on and on.

THERE ARE SOME PEOPLE THAT DON'T LIKE TO USE THE WORD "VEGAN." DO YOU USE BOTH "VEGAN" AND "PLANT-BASED," OR ARE YOU STRICTLY ONE OR THE OTHER AND WHY?

I use both. I know the word "vegan" can definitely turn some people off but I am 100% a vegan! I do it not only for my own health, but for the environment and the animals.

Initially, I didn't go plant-based for those reasons. I went entirely for my own health. Then, later on, I learned exactly what veganism was (that is where my passion really started!!) I learned about the craziness that goes on behind closed doors with the meat and dairy industries. This tipped the scale for me, big time.

I think that it truly is an individual choice whatever you want to label yourself, or if you want to label yourself at all. At the end of the day it doesn't matter to me! All I want is for folks to realize that more plant foods and less junk is the way to go. We each have our own journey and we all are doing the best we can.

IF YOU COULD DO ONE THING DIFFERENTLY FROM YOUR PAST FIVE YEARS, WHAT WOULD IT BE?

I don't usually like to think this way. Right now, in this moment, I am HAPPY, healthy, and living my best life! I don't enjoy thinking about my past too in-depth, and I have been plant-based for four of those five years. I have been healing for most of those years anyway.

WHAT BOOK/INFLUENCER COULD YOU NOT LIVE WITHOUT AND WHY?

Can I say Google? I am always Googling and researching on the daily!! Not just about veganism, but about so many other things. This lifestyle has opened up a craving for MORE information, more education, more knowledge and more sharing. I love learning new things.

WHAT ADVICE WOULD YOU GIVE A SMART AND DRIVEN 18-YEAR-OLD TODAY? WHAT ADVICE SHOULD THEY IGNORE?

1. Take care of your mental health - that is so important. Get to know yourself and heal!

2. DON'T DO DRUGS! Don't drink alcohol, don't smoke cigarettes, don't try drugs. Bad news all around.

3. GO VEGAN!

Things to ignore:

1. Your own ego and the egos around you. Ten years from now nobody is going to give a hoot about any of it!

2. Ignore anyone who tells you your dreams are silly or not "right."

3. Don't feel obligated to do what everyone else is doing - be different from the rest. Take care of your body, mind, health, and happiness, and you will thrive for the rest of your life!

ANY INSPIRING STORIES THAT HAVE HAPPENED TO YOU OR PEOPLE CLOSE TO YOU THAT HAVE NOT BEEN COVERED ABOVE. STORIES THAT CAN HELP OTHERS.

It is NEVER too late to begin again.

I was a drug addict. I had a heavy eating disorder. I treated myself so poorly and lost everything and everyone in my life. Lost my job, dropped out of college, lost my family's trust...

Begin again, begin now, talk to new people, travel, eat wholesome foods, go vegan, dive into mental health healing, find yourself, your passions, and what drives you. Bring you back to YOU. The whole, healthy, happy you that is underneath. If I can come out of the fog - you most definitely can. This lifestyle will spur more than just a new way of eating; it is an entire shift back into our true selves!

REMY PARK

CONNECT WITH REMY:
INSTAGRAM: @VEGGIEKINS
FACEBOOK: VEGGIEKINS
YOUTUBE: VEGGIEKINS
veggiekinsblog.com

SUFFERED FROM MENTAL ILLNESS, ANOREXIA, OCD, SELF-HARMING, AND SUBSTANCE ABUSE

"I discovered my love for health and wellness through my journey to recovery from mental illness. At age seven, I developed anorexia. Coupled with my OCD, I took to a variety of consequential destructive behaviors including self-harming and substance/alcohol abuse. By age seventeen, I had reached what was probably the lowest low, with my graduation from high school in jeopardy.

In college, I was exposed to the vegan lifestyle, and after trying vegan for about a week, I noticed significant improvements in chronic stomach issues I had been experiencing prior. In addition to physically feeling better, I felt a stronger connection to food and discovered a passion for veganizing recipes, cooking and eating once again. After cleaning up my nutrition, permanently removing substances and alcohol from my life became much easier because feeling so energetic and actually good was far more appealing than the feeling of hangovers and withdrawal symptoms.

My approach to wellness is a holistic approach because to be well is not only to have a healthy body, but also a healthy mind and spirit. Having come from the opposite end of that spectrum, my purpose is to spread love and light in the form of delicious and nourishing vegan recipes, health tips, and positivity."

Remy Park is a full-time recipe developer, food photographer, blogger, and creator of Veggiekins, a social media platform dedicated to promoting health and wellness. Her recipes have been featured on Mind Body Green, Well + Good, whole-foods Market and Thoughtfully Magazine and partnered with brands like Nike, Sephora, and Samsung. Offline, Remy is a certified yoga and meditation teacher, mindfulness coach, and holistic nutritionist, all which aid in her mission to make holistic health accessible for all.

WHAT ARE YOUR DAILY RITUALS/HABITS WHICH YOU BELIEVE HAVE BEEN KEY TO YOUR HEALTH?

I believe that the way you start your morning sets the tone for how the rest of your day will go. I am definitely a natural early bird, so I like to start every morning watching the sunrise. This is a routine for me that really helps me appreciate the day and have a moment to myself before the rest of my day continues.

Another daily for me is movement of some sort. This could be yoga, a walk in the park, a weight session at the gym, or a gentle stretch before bed. It always improves my mood and has been something that helps me feel physically healthy but also mentally strong and clear. As simple as it sounds, staying hydrated is also a must for me. I drink lots of water (sometimes with lemon!).

Finally, sleep! I struggled a lot with sleep in the past, but nailing a solid sleep routine has really helped me balance my energy levels and improve productivity during the day.

AT WHAT POINT IN YOUR LIFE DID YOU DECIDE TO CHANGE YOUR DIET? HOW HAS THAT DECISION IMPACTED YOUR LIFE?

I used to tell people that I was vegan when I was still struggling with anorexia. At the time, I had no idea what it meant, but I knew that it meant there were a lot of ingredients I couldn't eat, so I used it as an excuse to refuse food. Fortunately, at that time (about 13 or so years ago), the average person did not know what veganism was either, so my excuse really held up.

It wasn't until I was in college that I realized that dairy really made my stomach upset. I cut out dairy, and in search of dairy-free recipes, ended up testing out a lot of vegan recipes. I felt incredible after cutting dairy out of my diet, so I decided on a whim to go vegan for a week. Afterward, I couldn't go back because I had never felt so energized and healthy before.

I didn't go vegan to heal my eating disorder intentionally, but I did notice that my relationship with food has improved significantly because I was no longer able to obsess over labels as much. This was because fruits and vegetables don't come with nutrition fact labels, and I felt more connected to my food choices as I became more aware of the ethical and environmental aspects of veganism. It made me feel GOOD about eating for once and really allowed me to heal that disordered relationship.

WHAT THINGS HAVE MADE THE MOST DIFFERENCE IN YOUR ABILITY TO LIVE A GOOD LIFE AFTER LIVING WITH OR CURING YOUR DISEASE?

Gratitude and perspective always shift my life significantly. Having been in

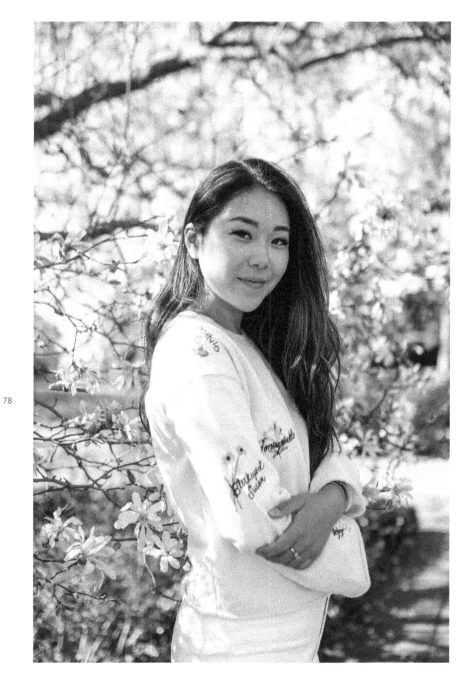

Chapter 1 | LIFE CHANGING HEALTH

a negative situation and having dealt with disorders, I have been able to appreciate life and just being okay. Each day is truly a gift.

WHAT WAS YOUR DOCTOR'S REACTION AFTER ANNOUNCING YOUR PLANS TO FOLLOW A PLANT-BASED DIET?

Initially, my doctor was worried that my choice to go vegan was a means of further restricting food. It is common, but once my doctors began to see improvements in my relationship with food and genuine excitement to cook/learn new recipes, they were very supportive. I actually created my Instagram account with the intention of using it as a private account to share photos of my food intake. It used to serve as a log for my doctor to keep tabs on me.

DO YOU TAKE ANY SPECIAL SUPPLEMENTS OR POTIONS? MENTION ANY SPECIFIC BRANDS YOU USE AND WHY YOU THINK THESE HAVE BENEFITED YOU AND YOUR HEALTH.

The first is simple and very common: lemon water. Every single morning I start my day with hot water plus fresh lemon juice, and it wakes up my system, improves my digestion, and has done wonders for my skin as well.

Amazing Grass greens powder is another part of my routine. I like to add this to smoothies or a drink during my day to get extra greens in. It contains a blend of a variety of super greens and is especially great for travel.

79

I also take a vegan B12 (everyone should, too!), and I like to supplement vitamin D as well.

WHAT ARE THE TWO OR THREE THINGS YOU HAVE DONE DIFFERENTLY WITH YOUR LIFE AFTER YOUR HEALTH GOT BETTER?

I have really learned the value of health and investing in it. There are times when "healthier" options are more costly, but small investments in your health will save you long term costs.

ANY INSPIRING STORIES THAT HAVE HAPPENED TO YOU OR PEOPLE CLOSE TO YOU THAT HAVE NOT BEEN COVERED ABOVE. STORIES THAT CAN HELP OTHERS.

When I created my social media platforms, I was in a dark place both mentally and physically. I would go so far as to call it one of the lowest points in my life, but I am also incredibly grateful for that moment because, without it, I would not have the platform that I do now. I believe that we can move towards the light no matter how dark it is where you start.
My favorite reminder is to let your past make you better, not bitter.

MARY JANE MENKE

CONNECT WITH MARY:
FACEBOOK: MARY JANE MENKE

TWO-TIME CANCER SURVIVOR AT AGED 77

At 77 years old and a two-time cancer survivor, Dr. Mary Jane Menke attributes her health turnaround to plant-based eating. Once she decided to make the switch, she marveled at her cholesterol levels that went from the 280s to the 150s, her improved blood sugar, and that she no longer needs to use a walker!

WHAT THINGS HAVE MADE THE MOST DIFFERENCE IN YOUR ABILITY TO LIVE A GOOD LIFE AFTER LIVING WITH OR CURING YOUR DISEASE?

My cholesterol has reduced from to 280s to 150s, and I suspect it is lower now. My blood sugar has improved, and I've gone from a walker to a cane. Some days I even go without a cane. I'm 77 years old and am a two-time cancer survivor.

YOU'VE JUST MET A HEARTBROKEN STRANGER WHO HAS JUST BEEN GIVEN A LIFE-THREATENING DIAGNOSIS. WHAT WOULD BE YOUR TOP FIVE TIPS TO HELP THEM?

1. Stop eating meat and animal products.
2. Find a plant-based believing physician. It's hard to find them but totally worth it.
3. Increase your movement. Exercise everything that moves on your body.
4. Be positive, find like-minded people, and surround yourself with good thoughts and actions.
5. Help others and do so by being a good example and feeding good information in a positive way. Don't preach or condemn, just share what good has come to you.

DO YOU TAKE ANY SPECIAL SUPPLEMENTS OR POTIONS? MENTION ANY SPECIFIC BRANDS YOU USE AND WHY YOU THINK THESE HAVE BENEFITED YOU AND YOUR HEALTH?

I was severely anemic when I started eating vegan. My oncologist wanted to do IV iron and B12 injections. I said "no" and did sublingual Vitamin B12 and currently take an iron pill every day along with an orange or vitamin C for absorption. I also take vitamin D. I was told by my oncology team that LOTS of their patients are low in Vitamin D and high in copper. I keep a record of my blood tests and am aware of myself and changes to the different readings.

WHAT ARE THE TWO OR THREE THINGS YOU HAVE DONE DIFFERENTLY WITH YOUR LIFE AFTER YOUR HEALTH GOT BETTER?

I now travel more and walk/exercise more. I also make it a fun project to find restaurants that have the kinds of food I can eat and enjoy. I'm discovering more of them all the time. It seems more people are waking up to eating healthier foods

ANY INSPIRING STORIES THAT HAVE HAPPENED TO YOU OR PEOPLE CLOSE TO YOU THAT HAVE NOT BEEN COVERED ABOVE. STORIES THAT CAN HELP OTHERS.

My son, my nephew, and a few of my friends have started eating veggie burgers, and when we eat out, they are ordering more salads and healthy foods than before. I've tried to teach by example and tell them what benefits I've experienced. I wear a Happy Cow t-shirt, and people often ask what that is all about. If they seem to be jovial people I sometimes tell them I don't eat anything that poops. I saw that comment on a t-shirt and find it fun to use at appropriate times.

I love exploring in the produce section of stores and finding foods I've never eaten before. My doctor has classes in her office, where she lectures about nutrition and cooks for us. We get in on the food prep sometimes and we get to actually see and taste things. I like funny comments (when appropriate) like not eating eggs because they come out of a chicken's butt. My doctor commented that eggs are part of a chicken's menstrual cycle - that was pretty attention-getting as well.

I like the energy in a vegan or vegetarian restaurant where I'm not inundated with the smell of burning flesh, like in a steakhouse. However, I have been able to find something to eat anywhere I go. One of my friends insists on a BBQ restaurant, and I just do the salad bar and a baked sweet potato, which works for me. I have been shocked in a couple of nice restaurants where they didn't have the bottles of vinegar and oil. In those cases, I just use a squeeze of lemon or ask for extra tomatoes or something on my salad.

Living with plant-based foods is an adventure, but it's a fun one, and it's for a good cause; a healthier and longer life.

EMILY SKAMLA

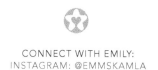

CONNECT WITH EMILY:
INSTAGRAM: @EMMSKAMLA

SUFFERING WITH TYPE 2 REFLEX SYMPATHETIC DYSTROPHY

"Living with complex regional pain syndrome (CRPS) has been my longest and most life-altering health condition that will be a disorder my body will have for the rest of my life. CPRS is a chronic pain condition and is believed to be caused by damage to or malfunction of the peripheral and central nervous systems. CRPS is characterized by prolonged or excessive pain and changes in skin color, temperature, and/or swelling in the affected area. Unfortunately, I was diagnosed long after my initial injury, making the damage irreversible and much more painful. I have never-ending pain on the left side of my upper body, especially in my left arm. The pain worsens when I use it or partake in any repetitive motion. Even running is extremely painful, and often I cannot complete runs due to the severity of the pain. However, despite the worsening symptoms and fear of it spreading, I have learned to turn my situation around and use my pain to push me to achieve my goals. My pain is unbearable, but eating whole-foods has allowed me to use the pain to make me stronger and mentally capable of living every day with it."

Emily has been suffering since the age of seven with Type 2 Reflex Sympathetic Dystrophy (RSD; now known in medical circles as Complex Regional Pain Syndrome.) She suffered fourteen years of a childhood with an invisible disorder that her doctors didn't recognize or understand what caused her severe pain that wasn't solved by surgeries, prescriptions, or other traditional treatments. Eventually, Emily took matters into her own hands, beginning with a whole-food, plant-based diet. Her lifestyle and nutritional makeover led her to an increase in energy and a newfound passion for physical fitness and exercise, turning her into a formidable athlete. Though not "cured," this plant-based diet has allowed Emily the mental and emotional stability to better her life and keep her as healthy as possible through the pain.

WHAT ARE YOUR DAILY RITUALS/HABITS WHICH YOU BELIEVE HAVE BEEN KEY TO YOUR HEALTH?

I practice the belief that you should own the day and own your life.
I begin and end every day by writing in my journal and planner. Before bed, I outline my day ahead. I am someone who needs structure and doing this sets my day up for success.

In the morning, I write a gratitude list as well as remind myself of recent personal victories. This starts my day in a beautiful light and exercises my mind in a positive and powerful way.

When I can, I try to include meditation into my mornings. Another rule that I live by is to drink 32 ounces of water or more within the first half-hour of waking. This simple habit sets your body up for optimal digestion.

AT WHAT POINT IN YOUR LIFE DID YOU DECIDE TO CHANGE YOUR DIET? HOW HAS THAT DECISION IMPACTED YOUR LIFE?

I first went vegan for ethical reasons in my first year of college. However, as a college athlete, I became interested in how my diet could be affecting my athletic ability. In addition, I had been experiencing ongoing general health problems for many years. I became increasingly interested in how a plant-based diet might play a role in changing how I was living my life.

My first major influence in my journey came from Dr. Gregor's book, How Not to Die. After reading his book, I soon found my passion for researching a plant-based lifestyle. Changing my diet lead to increased athletic performance and proper digestion. Equally exciting was that I found my health problems dissipated, and my mood increased substantially. These major life changes allowed me to be confident with my new way of living.

During the first year that I was plant-based, I suffered from depression due to tough personal setbacks in my life. I found myself relying on a lot of convenience vegan foods. I became caught in a pleasure trap with the processed foods and my own inability to regulate my satiation mechanisms.

After discovering a whole-plant-foods diet, I was able to heal myself physically and emotionally. These foods are still in the process of healing me, but I am much more aware of my body and take care of my mental health, which is a necessity.

A whole-foods plant-based diet provides us with the nutrients we need to thrive in a modern food world congested with oils, high-fat processed foods and dangerous disease-causing meat. I have never felt more compassionate about animals, the planet and people. I also take responsibility to research and understand the science behind a plant-based diet so that I can inform others. Empowerment and strength are what this diet fuels me with daily, along with sufficient calories.

WHAT THINGS HAVE MADE THE MOST DIFFERENCE IN YOUR ABILITY TO LIVE A GOOD LIFE AFTER LIVING WITH OR CURING YOUR DISEASE?

Living with complex regional pain syndrome (CRPS) has been my longest and most life-altering health condition that will be a disorder my body will have for the rest of my life. CPRS is a chronic pain condition and is believed to be caused by damage to or malfunction of the peripheral and central nervous systems. CRPS is characterized by prolonged or excessive pain and changes in skin color, temperature, and swelling in the affected area. Unfortunately, I was diagnosed long after my initial injury, making the damage irreversible and much more painful. I have never-ending pain on the left side of my upper body, especially in my left arm. The pain worsens when I use it or partake in any repetitive motion. Even running is extremely painful, and often I cannot complete runs due to the severity of the pain.

However, despite the worsening symptoms and fear of it spreading, I have learned to turn my situation around and use my pain to push me to achieve my goals. My pain is unbearable, but eating whole-foods has allowed me to use the pain to make me stronger and mentally capable of living every day with it.

Like everyone, I have my bad days. Nevertheless, I design my life to be a picture of someone who is healthy, and that is how I wake up every morning. The biggest difference for me is that a plant-based diet alleviates a lot of inflammation in my body and keeps me healthy so I can focus on other aspects of my life. Also, a plant-based diet has been extremely beneficial for my mental health, which can be easily compromised due to the pain and difficulty of completing simple tasks. This way of eating is not just a diet for me; it is a lifestyle.

WHAT WAS YOUR DOCTOR'S REACTION AFTER ANNOUNCING YOUR PLANS TO FOLLOW A PLANT-BASED DIET?

This was not a decision I discussed with my doctor. I had early influences from family members who were also vegan, and I took it upon myself to find the research to back up the major benefit claims. I read many, many books such as The China Study, WHOLE, How Not to Die, The Starch Solution, and The Pleasure Trap. Furthermore, I was active in reading online studies such as work from Dr. Campbell, Dr. Esselstyn, and Dr. McDougall. And of course, nutritionfacts.org, created by the amazing Dr. Greger.

AFTER ADOPTING A PLANT-BASED DIET HOW LONG DID IT TAKE BEFORE FIRST, YOU STARTED TO FEEL BETTER, AND SECOND, YOU KNEW YOU WERE NOT GOING TO LET THIS WIN?

I did not see profound results until I made that switch from a "junk food vegan" to eating a whole-foods diet. In the first couple of months, I had radically improved my digestion and was not as bloated or uncomfortable after eating. I noticed immediate increased energy and was sleeping more deeply throughout the night.

My favorite benefit from the diet is my newfound athletic ability that I discovered by having the energy to begin working out. I went from never being able to run a mile in high school gym class to not needing my inhaler anymore and crushing long runs daily, as well as participating in marathons.

Small benefits came within a year, such as thicker and more vibrant hair, stronger nails, brighter skin, and most importantly, a sense of self-confidence. You can see how such changes can lead to success when it comes to working on mental health. I knew I would never need to question my diet and am constantly reinforcing my passions for the plant-based lifestyle by keeping up with my reading, attending events such as Plant Stock, and humbly being a guest on podcasts such as Plant Yourself.

YOU'VE JUST MET A HEARTBROKEN STRANGER WHO HAS JUST BEEN GIVEN A LIFE-THREATENING DIAGNOSIS. WHAT WOULD BE YOUR TOP FIVE TIPS TO HELP THEM?

The five core elements to optimal health are social support, resilience, movement, mindfulness and optimal diet.

Social support involves having a network of family and friends that you can turn to in times of need. These relationships play a critical role in how you function in your day-to-day life. A sense of belonging, involving emotions in relationships, and participating in social integration, can also be psychologically beneficial. These groups and people can encourage healthy choices and behaviors as well as help you cope with stressors.

Resilience is the ability to bounce back from stress or adversity. How you adjust to the news of your diagnosis determines what your life may be like moving forward. Thriving is living with this adversity, but seeing the light through the darkness. Resilience can be built by reframing your situation, leaning on social supports, practicing positive thinking and even practicing mindfulness and meditation.

Movement is no doubt very important to avoiding anxiety and depression, which is associated with many health diagnoses. Things as simple as taking a walk outside to get the mail and seeing the sun and breathing fresh air can be beneficial.

Mindfulness is a big buzz word in the field of psychology lately. Mindfulness is as easily explained as the statement we all hear at one point, "enjoy every moment. Life is short." Being aware of the present moment and seeing the good and bad without judgment or preconceived notions is a healthy practice. Mindfulness practices help people manage stress, improve coping skills and reduce depression. Mindfulness also cultivates optimism.

An optimal diet is extremely important for not only your physical health but for your mental health as well. Eating healthier leads to heightened self-confidence and value to one's own life. After receiving such news regarding a life-threatening diagnosis, supporting the body through a plant-based diet could improve your healing, address other health concerns that could alleviate certain symptoms (such as inflammation), and provide essential energy and nutrients. Each core element influences the other, and inclusion of all five would lead to an extremely beneficial lifestyle.

DO YOU TAKE ANY SPECIAL SUPPLEMENTS OR POTIONS? MENTION ANY SPECIFIC BRANDS YOU USE AND WHY YOU THINK THESE HAVE BENEFITED YOU AND YOUR HEALTH?

86

A whole-food, plant-based diet can provide the body with all the necessary nutrients for optimal health except B12. This is because B12 is found in soil, but modern-day soil is often depleted, and produce is washed and disinfected extremely well. Not only might vegans be deficient, but those who eat meat may be as well.

WHAT ARE THE TWO OR THREE THINGS YOU HAVE DONE DIFFERENTLY WITH YOUR LIFE AFTER YOUR HEALTH GOT BETTER?

The most impactful change I have made after my health got better (and during the process) was to readdress my priorities. As someone who regularly would partake in the "college party scene," I fully acknowledged without hesitation, that this no longer served me. I took huge leaps to clean up not only my diet, but my social scene as well and how I spent my personal time. I now focus on a healthy, fulfilling lifestyle that incorporates frequent exercise, reading about my passions and spending time with those whom I align.

Recognizing my path did not feel restrictive; it felt liberating. Changing my mindset, diet and lifestyle was huge, and every day since the decision to change these areas of my life, I make choices that recognize and adhere to the importance of those elements.

ANY INSPIRING STORIES THAT HAVE HAPPENED TO YOU OR PEOPLE CLOSE TO YOU THAT HAVE NOT BEEN COVERED ABOVE. STORIES THAT CAN HELP OTHERS.

The number of people who currently report depression or anxiety is astronomically high. You would never know it by looking at all of the happy faces on social media. I was one of these people. It would be unrealistic to offer practical tips on how to "cure" anxiety and depression because even today, I am still working on this myself. I battled with my health and emotional stress for many years. This often leads to detrimental habits. I should have expected to feel this way due to my reliance on an overly processed diet (junk food vegan diet). What you eat matters to your wellbeing. A number of reasons contributed to my depression and stress. I was feeling inadequate, which contributed to self-sabotage. As a society, we are made to feel never good enough. We are terrified of failing and exposing our real selves to the world and being rejected.

I couldn't climb out of my depression until I addressed how these thought patterns made me feel. I began to use diet and lifestyle changes to support my emotional stability. Deciding to be "the real me" in public, changing my diet to support what my body needed, and starting the process of not living for other people's expectations, were the biggest changes I made. I work towards these goals every day.

87

When my depression was at its worst, I did not know the difference between what I wanted and what I thought I was supposed to want. I thought I was supposed to go out drinking with friends, I was supposed to spend all my money on cute clothes, and I was supposed to always be liked by everyone. All along, my true self would say things like, "why are you living a life that you know that isn't working?"

Becoming plant-based wasn't just a significant diet change; it was a lifestyle change and the start of a beautiful personal journey. I started to understand what I really want out of my life by finding true inspiration in myself.

The change did not happen fast, but it was the start of imagining a beautiful future for myself. I now have a sense of hope and productivity and don't run away from my feelings. I have compassion for myself, which came with a lot of resilience. This was my prescription for managing my depression and anxiety. Feelings of sadness and hopelessness are not forever, and by eating healthy foods, and I've found that being in tune with myself, is very healing. Greater contentment came with purposely cultivating a life I wanted to live. I now surround myself with the people that inspire me and disregarding the social judgments I used to put on myself.

EMMA McENEANY

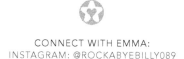

CONNECT WITH EMMA:
INSTAGRAM: @ROCKABYEBILLY089

STRUGGLING WITH ENDOMETRIOSIS, PCOS, AND HIGH CHOLESTEROL

"The biggest difference I have noticed since moving to a whole-food, plant-based diet is that my energy levels have risen. And hormonally I feel more in balance than I have done in a long time...

Most importantly, the way I feel about the future has changed in that I no longer feel like I have the looming presence of illness over me. I am in control of my health and my future. I'm going to be here to not only have kids but to see them grow up!"

Struggling with endometriosis, PCOS, and high cholesterol, Emma McEneany was no stranger to suffering. At age 29 with a long list of health complications and what looked like more on the horizon, she made the change to whole-foods, plant-based diet, and slowly watched her life change for the better.

WHAT ARE YOUR DAILY RITUALS/HABITS WHICH YOU BELIEVE HAVE BEEN KEY TO YOUR HEALTH?

Plenty of water: sometimes I add lemon, lime or cucumber.

I have assorted fruits or overnight oats for breakfast, and I find that this really kick starts my day. I love to snack on assorted veggie sticks or fruit and nut mixes that I make up myself.

I try to minimize my soy intake, and I tend to like to find soy-free alternatives to food, like Burmese tofu! Give me Burmese tofu with lots of vegetables, and I am one happy lady!

AT WHAT POINT IN YOUR LIFE DID YOU DECIDE TO CHANGE YOUR DIET? HOW HAS THAT DECISION IMPACTED YOUR LIFE?

For years I have struggled with my weight, eating habits, cholesterol, PCOS, and endometriosis. I have had numerous procedures to try and help, I've gone on different diets, and tried numerous supplements. You name it; I've tried it!

Two years ago, I decided I wanted to go vegetarian, and though my intentions were great, I found myself back to eating an omnivore diet within eight months. This was due to lack of motivation/inspiration, and quite honestly, I was putting too much pressure on myself. I focused 100% on the ethical animal aspect and put little to no focus on ensuring that I was eating the correct foods to fuel my body.

Then, at the end of 2018, I decided it was time to make some changes and really take control of my health and my weight. Being 29 with a long list of health issues and the risk of more on the horizon was not something that I was comfortable with, so I decided to take the plunge and have gastric surgery. Given that diabetes and cancer are prevalent in my family, I wanted to try and start taking steps to mitigate future risks to my health and give myself a chance to find a happier and healthier me.

After my surgery, I really started to feel that consuming meat and dairy products were not giving me the nutrients that my body wanted or craved. I felt that since I could only eat small portions, it was imperative that I packed as many nutrients into those portions as I could. Both my partner and I decided to get rid of animal products out of our diets and our lives!

I researched and read as much as I could about plant-based diets, the benefits, and how I could transition us both off animal products to living solely on plant-based food and products.

It took time, research and patience. It was a huge learning curve. I could not believe how I had let fear and inaccurate information steer me wrong for so long!

I began to understand the myths around questions like "How will you get your protein?" or comments like, "Being vegan will make you sick!" The list of myths got longer the more I dove into research, and I quickly realized that none of it was true! I decided then and there that this was my path to a healthier, happier me.

WHAT THINGS HAVE MADE THE MOST DIFFERENCE IN YOUR ABILITY TO LIVE A GOOD LIFE AFTER LIVING WITH OR CURING YOUR DISEASE?

The biggest difference I have noticed is my energy levels. I used to always feel tired, cranky and lethargic. Now, even when I have my period, my energy levels are great. I may still be sore and a little grumpy sometimes, but what woman isn't? Another benefit is that my skin has cleared up and is less oily.

Most importantly, the way I feel about the future has changed in that I no longer feel like I have the looming presence of illness over me. I am in control of my health and my future. I'm going to be here to not only have kids but to see them grow up!

WHAT WAS YOUR DOCTOR'S REACTION AFTER ANNOUNCING YOUR PLANS TO FOLLOW A PLANT-BASED DIET?

My regular doctor is actually on maternity leave at the moment, so she doesn't know. I am hoping to surprise her with my progress when she returns to work.

AFTER ADOPTING A PLANT-BASED DIET HOW LONG DID IT TAKE BEFORE FIRST, YOU STARTED TO FEEL BETTER, AND SECOND, YOU KNEW YOU WERE NOT GOING TO LET THIS WIN?

I would say it was around the three-week mark was when I really started to feel better. I realized I was eating better, eating more regularly and had a whole lot more energy.

Hormonally, I felt more in balance than I had done in a long time. Which, as I am sure any woman with PCOS can attest to, it's not often that we feel that way!

I also felt that many other aspects of my life were also starting to improve. It felt like everything was suddenly starting to fall into place. It is moments like these when I knew I had made the right choice for my health, for animals and for the environment.

YOU'VE JUST MET A HEARTBROKEN STRANGER WHO HAS JUST BEEN GIVEN A LIFE-THREATENING DIAGNOSIS. WHAT WOULD BE YOUR TOP FIVE TIPS TO HELP THEM?

Do good and be good to all living beings. I believe it's important to live your dream and make a positive impact on the world because no matter how bad things may seem, there are always those that are worse off.

Fuel your thoughts with positivity, not negativity. Unhealthy minds lead to unhealthy bodies.

Know that you are not alone and lean on those you love for support. Nothing hurts more than someone you love pushing you away.

Do not be afraid of change. Instead, embrace it. Yes, it may be scary, but you don't want to die wondering what could have been.

Be your own moral compass. Find what is important to you and what you are passionate about and fight for it!

DO YOU TAKE ANY SPECIAL SUPPLEMENTS OR POTIONS? MENTION ANY SPECIFIC BRANDS YOU USE AND WHY YOU THINK THESE HAVE BENEFITED YOU AND YOUR HEALTH?

I recently started taking high-absorption magnesium supplements. I have read that these can help immensely with endometriosis pains. I purchased the Doctor's Best brand off eBay, and they are vegan. I also have a Vitamin B12 injection every three months.

WHAT ARE THE TWO OR THREE THINGS YOU HAVE DONE DIFFERENTLY WITH YOUR LIFE AFTER YOUR HEALTH GOT BETTER?

I am a lot more conscious about what food I put into my body.

I now find myself actively looking for new places to go on adventures, whether it's somewhere new to hike or just simply explore.

I've found myself considering going back to school and hopefully learning how to help others on their path to better health and wellness.

ANY INSPIRING STORIES THAT HAVE HAPPENED TO YOU OR PEOPLE CLOSE TO YOU THAT HAVE NOT BEEN COVERED ABOVE. STORIES THAT CAN HELP OTHERS.

When people talk about how a positive mindset can change your path, the reason that this really resonates with me is my mother. Not only is she the strongest woman I know, but she is also the most positive. Eleven years ago, she was diagnosed with terminal cancer. She was told she had six to ten years to live. Instead of curling up in a ball and giving up, I have watched this woman thrive. Though she does not follow a strictly plant-based diet, she has completely overhauled her food choices, her lifestyle and always has a positive mindset. She has had minimal treatment, and she continues to amaze me each and every day. Just by looking at her, you wouldn't know that she has terminal cancer.

My mother is by far, my biggest inspiration. She taught me that we all have our own journey to go on and that we need only have the courage and conviction to follow and stand up for what we believe in.

Everyone's story is different; it's part of what makes the world so amazing and exciting. Sure, there is some bad, but there is also a whole lot of good; we need only open ourselves up to seeing it.

If you are reading this, I wish you all the best on your journey and welcome you to plant-based living. It's so good for the mind, body, and soul.

LILY KOI

CONNECT WITH LILY:
INSTAGRAM: @LILYKOIHAWAII
FACEBOOK: LILYKOI HAWAII
YOUTUBE: LILYKOI HAWAII

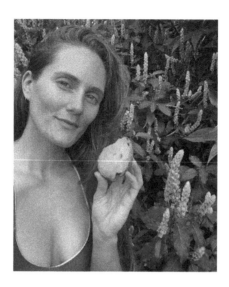

REVERSED HYPOTHYROID - HER DOCTOR SAID SHE'D BE MEDICATED FOR THE REST OF HER LIFE

"I decided to try veganism as a desperate bid to regain thyroid function after a hypothyroid diagnosis. My doctor said I'd be medicated for the rest of my life and I said, "give me six months... It took a week for my blood sugar levels to normalize. After a month, my energy was higher and stable. Within six months, I felt like a new person."

Plant-based eating changed the direction of Lily Koi's life exponentially. After healing her body from a hypothyroid diagnosis and regaining her physical, emotional, and mental strength, she began sharing her knowledge and personal journey across various social media platforms to a far-reaching audience.

WHAT ARE YOUR DAILY RITUALS/HABITS WHICH YOU BELIEVE HAVE BEEN KEY TO YOUR HEALTH?

I believe the habits that have been instrumental in transcending disordered eating and regaining my health is time set aside each day for meal prep, large batch cooking of our staple foods, and my dedication to emotional self-care, exploration and growth.

AT WHAT POINT IN YOUR LIFE DID YOU DECIDE TO CHANGE YOUR DIET? HOW HAS THAT DECISION IMPACTED YOUR LIFE?

I decided to try veganism as a desperate bid to regain thyroid function after a hypothyroid diagnosis. My doctor said I'd be medicated for the rest of my life, and I said, "give me six months." The fear of living with barely-controlled symptoms for the rest of my life eclipsed my fear of alienation from the culinary-arts-focused communities I belonged to. I was very scared of becoming more ill by switching to "high carb" foods, as every doctor I'd seen had stressed that I must eat low-carb and high-protein to control my hypoglycemia. However, their recommendations had made me worse and worse. The first few days were scary, but as my health quickly returned, my confidence grew.

WHAT THINGS HAVE MADE THE MOST DIFFERENCE IN YOUR ABILITY TO LIVE A GOOD LIFE AFTER LIVING WITH OR CURING YOUR DISEASE?

REST. Once I realized humans simply need a certain amount of sleep and rejuvenation every day, and once I started honoring that need, so many of my struggles became exponentially easier to face.

WHAT WAS YOUR DOCTOR'S REACTION AFTER ANNOUNCING YOUR PLANS TO FOLLOW A PLANT-BASED DIET?

My naturopath dismissed me as a patient! Other doctors have been more tolerant, and my current GP is very supportive and encouraging. I've found "alternative" healthcare practitioners are much more resistant to the copious scientific research supporting plant-based diets.

AFTER ADOPTING A PLANT-BASED DIET HOW LONG DID IT TAKE BEFORE FIRST, YOU STARTED TO FEEL BETTER, AND SECOND, YOU KNEW YOU WERE NOT GOING TO LET THIS WIN?

It took a week for my blood sugar levels to normalize. After a month, my energy was higher and stable. Within six months, I felt like a new person. At that point, I thought I had everything figured out (as every 20-year-old does), and though my physical health was much improved, I had a lot more emotional baggage to sort out before I could truly heal.

YOU'VE JUST MET A HEARTBROKEN STRANGER WHO HAS JUST BEEN GIVEN A LIFE-THREATENING DIAGNOSIS. WHAT WOULD BE YOUR TOP FIVE TIPS TO HELP THEM?

Rest like it's your job.

Nourish your cells with lovingly prepared, whole, plant foods.

End toxic/draining relationships now... like, right now, because your life depends on it.

Do something every day JUST because it brings you joy.

Hug it out. Cry it out. Move it out. Scream it out. Just get whatever it is out, so your lifeforce has all the room it needs to heal.

DO YOU TAKE ANY SPECIAL SUPPLEMENTS OR POTIONS? MENTION ANY SPECIFIC BRANDS YOU USE AND WHY YOU THINK THESE HAVE BENEFITED YOU AND YOUR HEALTH.

I take My Kind Methylcobalamin B12 spray and am currently looking for a new brand of Algal EPA/DHA supplement as my previous favorite brand was discontinued. I also eat turmeric and ginger pretty much every day!

WHAT ARE THE TWO OR THREE THINGS YOU HAVE DONE DIFFERENTLY WITH YOUR LIFE AFTER YOUR HEALTH GOT BETTER?

I've learned to be very, very protective of my time. When I was sick, it felt like my life was over before it began. I was devastated. When I "came back to life," I realized we are on this amazing planet for a finite period, and it breaks my heart to imagine the ways we allow ourselves to misuse this precious resource. There is SO MUCH goodness on this earth - people, places, pursuits, pleasure and purpose - and it is our right to fill our days with whatever sets our hearts on fire.

ANY INSPIRING STORIES THAT HAVE HAPPENED TO YOU OR PEOPLE CLOSE TO YOU THAT HAVE NOT BEEN COVERED ABOVE. STORIES THAT CAN HELP OTHERS.

Remember that true transformation doesn't happen during a 28-day plan someone is trying to sell you. It happens during consistently making small choices to prioritize your well-being, long-term health and happiness. Those small choices become habits and habits transform us. Focus on who you want to be one, three, or five years from now and make the small choices necessary to get you there.

66 99

WHEN I TOLD MY DOCTOR I STOPPED
TAKING MY METFORMIN (DIABETES
MEDS), SHE WAS A BIT SURPRISED. I WAS
HER STAR PATIENT. AT ONE POINT SHE
SAID, *"I WISH ALL MY PATIENTS TOOK
THEIR DISEASE AS SERIOUS AS YOU."*

WHEN I ASKED WHY SHE DIDN'T SUGGEST
TO HER DIABETIC, HYPERTENSION,
CARDIOVASCULAR PATIENTS THAT A
WHOLE-FOOD, PLANT-BASED LIFESTYLE
COULD REVERSE THEIR AILMENTS
WITHOUT HARMFUL PHARMACEUTICALS,
SHE REPLIED, *"BECAUSE PEOPLE
DO NOT WANT TO CHANGE THEIR
LIFESTYLES. THEY WANT A QUICK FIX."*

TAMI COCKRELL

TAMI COCKRELL

CONNECT WITH TAMI:
INSTAGRAM: @FORTHEHEALTHOFITTAMI
FACEBOOK: FOR THE HEALTH OF IT TAMI
YOUTUBE: MASTERING DIABETES - TAMI COCKRELL

REVERSED TYPE 2 DIABETES

At 51-years-old, Tami Cockrell was diagnosed with type 2 diabetes, high cholesterol, high triglycerides, fatty liver disease, and vitamin D deficiency. Shocked and disappointed, Tami's competitive spirit kicked into overdrive, and she dove into research to discover how she could bring herself back to life. After trial and error and more trial and error, Tami finally found a program called "Mastering Diabetes," where she learned how food affected her body's every function. Switching to a whole-food, plant-based diet changed Tami's life in ways she didn't fully believe until the weight started melting off and her blood work began to read the best it had in the past 30 years of her life.

AT WHAT POINT IN YOUR LIFE DID YOU DECIDE TO CHANGE YOUR DIET? HOW HAS THAT DECISION IMPACTED YOUR LIFE?

My family decided to eliminate meat after watching several food documentaries, including Forks Over Knives, in January of 2016. Both my husband and I were overweight and on blood pressure medication. He had been recently diagnosed as a prediabetic. We had just come off a year where breast cancer struck my family. We lost my grandmother to her third fight with breast cancer just three days after my mom's lumpectomy. Then, six months later, my husband's mom had a quintuple bypass, and his dad suffered a heart attack just two weeks after she came home. He was unable to undergo surgery because the medication he took for his congestive heart failure caused his kidneys to fail, and he was borderline needing to be on dialysis. At 85, that was not the quality of life he desired.

So, my husband asked his doctor to give him three months without medications to try and reverse his A1C. That's when we cut meat out.

At this point, we went vegetarian, but I only lost four pounds. I weighed 234 pounds when my doctor diagnosed me with hypertension and put me on blood pressure medication. I was so upset with myself for allowing my health to deteriorate. After I left his office, I sat in the car and cried. He had said that if I lost thirty pounds, I could come off of the medication he was prescribing. That year I dropped ten. The next year I dropped ten more. I was still eating dairy, but my blood pressure continued to rise higher the closer I got to my 30 pound goal.

It's funny thinking back now. I recall talking to a friend I hadn't seen for some time and telling her that I was vegetarian. She said, "Gosh Tami. That's great. You must be getting so thin." The truth was that I was not getting thinner at all. Although I had lost 24 pounds over the past three years, I was still wearing a size 20 pants. They just fit a little looser.

My husband and I went to a health fair and had free blood work done. When I went for my consult appointment, my new doctor basically said that I more than likely had insulin resistance and type 2 diabetes. I showed the doctor my numbers: BG 134, blood pressure on medication 149/93 with HR 101, total cholesterol 266, LDL 181, triglycerides 197, weight 210, and BMI 33%. This just confirmed for her that the labs she was ordering would not only confirm insulin resistance and diabetes but more than likely cardiological issues as well. Again there were tears and disappointment in myself.

Later, when we met for my annual check-up with the lab results in hand, she was absolutely correct. I had a vitamin D deficiency, and my A1C was 7.1, I had a fatty liver, I had a high red blood cell count, high hematocrit, high cholesterol, high LDL, low HDL, high triglycerides, not to mention all the other abnormal results I did not understand. My labs were more red than black. She had also run genetic testing on me to see what role they may be playing in my health. It turns out that I carry genes for the highest risk category for cardiovascular disease, diabetes, stroke, high cholesterol, high LDL and if that's not enough, I also carry not one but two genes for Alzheimer's: ApoE3, and ApoE4. ApoE4 is in the highest risk category.

I walked out feeling completely defeated, and arms full of medication, supplements, a glucometer, and meal replacement powder to speed along the weight loss. At first, I had a pity party for myself, then after some research to try and understand what insulin resistance and diabetes were, I decided to take my health into my own hands. I did not want to "stabilize" or "maintain" my diabetes. I knew from the documentaries that I had watched that there was hope in reversing my ailments, despite what my doctor said.

So, in my research to understand my new health issues, I came across a summit put out by this online program called Mastering Diabetes. It's truly all about timing for me. So I got a free two days to access the summit, and I was able to watch about nine hours of it with different doctors. That was the first defining change.

Another moment came after I sent a message to Dr. Esselstyn, and he called me back. I had just finished a pool workout at the gym and drove through Del Taco to get a green bean cheese burrito and nacho fries when my phone rang. It was Dr. Esselstyn on the other end. Divine intervention at its finest. He basically told me that no matter what my genes said on the labs, it was not my destiny. My destiny was what crossed my lips and went into my stomach. I looked down at my food choice and knew I had to figure out what I needed to do. I decided to join the Mastering Diabetes program, and that's when my healing journey began.

You are your only advocate. I truly believe that we need to learn what our lab results mean because our lives depend on it. When I was diagnosed with type 2 diabetes, I asked my doctor, "how is that possible? I'd never been told I was prediabetic before." That night I went home and looked back at my past labs, and for at least three years prior, I was prediabetic. Wow. I had never been told that before. But with that said, I'm not sure it would've made a difference. Timing is everything. After watching the health issue of our families, my bad health came at a time when I was ready for the fight and the challenge.

WHAT THINGS HAVE MADE THE MOST DIFFERENCE IN YOUR ABILITY TO LIVE A GOOD LIFE AFTER LIVING WITH OR CURING YOUR DISEASE?

While living with my diseases, understanding the cause of my diseases was the key to reversal. Learning to eat when hungry and not out of habit, as well as stopping when I was satisfied, were also key behavioral changes to my success.

The Cronometer app helped me to monitor and understand macronutrients, which was very enlightening and a lesson in its own right.

Family support was also huge. It wasn't an easy transition for any of us, but having their support once they understood the importance, was key. It truly helped me to not be overwhelmed when learning how to eat and having trigger foods around me.

Lastly, the accountability and guidance I received from Mastering Diabetes, namely the weekly calls with Cyrus Khambatta and Robby Barbaro, were where the real education came.

After this, curing my disease has been easy. When you see and feel first-hand what a whole-food, plant-based, low-fat lifestyle feels like, there's no question to its role in living my best life. I feel energetic, happy and full of life that I had previously let slip away. I feel 20 years younger.

I want to live life to its fullest. Instead of looking up at the pyramids in

Mexico and taking pictures of my family scaling it. Well, now that's me scaling it. (I may have cried for twenty minutes at the top, but I did it. Just a year before that, I would have never tried it.)

WHAT WAS YOUR DOCTOR'S REACTION AFTER ANNOUNCING YOUR PLANS TO FOLLOW A PLANT-BASED DIET?

In the beginning, she was skeptical. She did not think I'd reverse my diseases via a whole-food, plant-based diet. She asked me to tell her what meals I was eating. Then, she said that beans alone were not a complete protein. She was convinced that I'd be on medications for life and that I could, at best, learn to stabilize and maintain my diabetes for years.

When I reversed my diabetes six months after the diagnosis, she was very excited and pleased that her protocol worked so well. She had no idea I had stopped my Metformin and that I wasn't following the protocol that she and the diabetic counselor set for all patients. When I told her I stopped taking my Metformin, she was a bit surprised. I was her star patient. At one point, she said, "I wish all my patients took their disease as serious as you." When I asked why she didn't suggest to her diabetic, hypertension, cardiovascular patients that a whole-food, plant-based lifestyle could reverse their ailments without harmful pharmaceuticals, and she replied, "because people do not want to change their lifestyles. They want a quick fix."

AFTER ADOPTING A PLANT-BASED DIET, HOW LONG DID IT TAKE BEFORE FIRST, YOU STARTED TO FEEL BETTER, AND SECOND, YOU KNEW YOU WERE NOT GOING TO LET THIS WIN?

I knew right away I was not going to let this win. I have a "competitive spirit" as I like to call it, haha! But I had no idea how to get there.

It's been a long, transitional journey and at first, a series of emotions, failure and anger at myself before finally getting up and facing it head-on. This was when I began my research and started hearing repeated information on the causes of these diseases. They are all linked to the same cause: fat. I wasn't completely certain that all of these testimonials were true. I wondered things like, "did they continue to have good health for many years to come? Could I give up the foods I loved long term?" That's when I found Mastering Diabetes. That was a transition period as well, but once I wrapped my head around it all, the magic began to happen.

My weight melted off and I felt better almost immediately. No more two to three-hour naps in the afternoon. I finally had energy again as I did in my 30s. I no longer had allergy flares and no longer had knee pain. This was most surprising as I just thought the pain was a way of life after my surgeries.

By 19, my right knee was left bone on bone, and I had a complete tear of the ACL. I lived with daily pain and was popping ibuprofen like it was candy. So when my inflammation disappeared, it was unbelievable. It's something I never expected. My acid reflux, plantar fasciitis, and chronic cough also went away. I can't tell you how many performances my kids were in or plays they wrote/directed that I had to walk out of due to a coughing fit. These changes all started within two weeks to three months after eating a low-fat WFPB diet. It was amazing. I also went from a size 20 pant to a size 14.

I missed out on so much over the last 20 years, but this gives me the energy and zest for life, so I don't waste any more time sitting on the sidelines. I'm so very grateful for my disease. It's given me my life back.

YOU'VE JUST MET A HEARTBROKEN STRANGER WHO HAS JUST BEEN GIVEN A LIFE-THREATENING DIAGNOSIS. WHAT WOULD BE YOUR TOP FIVE TIPS TO HELP THEM?

First, understand your diagnosis and to take your health into your own hands. Don't be afraid to question a doctor, or ask a question when you don't understand.

Get comfortable being uncomfortable. What I mean is: you will be swimming upstream and going against what we've all learned about healthy eating. So, get comfortable with being the different one.

Don't be afraid to call ahead to ask the restaurant manager for recommendations to oil-free and sugar-free foods. Or look at the menu. If an ingredient is on the menu, chances are they have it and can steam it. Call resorts you may vacation at and make them aware of your dietary restrictions. Set up an appointment with the chef. Don't be afraid to ask.

Get the cronometer app. It is a game-changer for me and helped me to understand where my fats are coming from. I now make a crockpot chili that has less fat in the whole pot that half an avocado does. Will that half an avocado fill me to satiety? No. But, I can tell you I can get full off that pot of chili for a week. I've really learned how to understand food better.

I'd also explain that your disease does NOT have to be your destiny.

My genetics suck, and yet my diet helped me to change that course. Also, just take the leap of faith. Give it 30 days. Anyone can do 30 days.

" "

THE ONCOLOGIST'S REACTION WAS FIRST, THAT DIET HAS NOTHING TO DO WITH BREAST CANCER, AND SECOND, THAT I COULD NOT POSSIBLY GET ENOUGH PROTEIN AND CALCIUM ON THIS DIET. I'M STILL PROVING HIM WRONG 37 YEARS LATER ON BOTH COUNTS.

DR. RUTH HEIDRICH, PH.D.

DR. RUTH HEIDRICH, PH.D.

STAGE 4 BREAST CANCER SURVIVOR

Already a marathon runner and living what she believed to be a healthy lifestyle, Dr. Ruth Heidrich was in disbelief when she was diagnosed with stage 4 breast cancer. After refusing chemotherapy, radiation, and hormone blockers, Dr. Heidrich chose to revitalize her lifestyle and diet choices, switching to solely plant-based foods. Two years later she crossed the finish line of the Kona Ironman Triathlon, becoming the first vegan and first cancer patient to complete an Ironman. At 84 years young, Dr. Heidrich has now completed a total of six Ironmans, is the winner of over 900 trophies, eight Gold Medals in the U.S. Senior Olympics, and 67 marathons. Named One of the Ten Fittest Women in North America at age 64 (amongst nine other women in their 20s and 30s no less), Ruth has made waves in the plant-based fitness and wellness communities and continues to reach audiences through her books: *A Race for Life, Senior Fitness, The CHEF Cook/ Rawbook, Lifelong Running: How to Overcome the 11 Myths of Running & Live a Healthier Life, and her latest book, Cure, Reverse & Prevent ED: Ten ways to Total Sexual Fitness.*

WHAT ARE YOUR DAILY RITUALS/HABITS WHICH YOU BELIEVE HAVE BEEN KEY TO YOUR HEALTH?

By far, the most important activity in my daily life is a diet of 100% whole plants. This, of course, excludes any animal or animal by-products, all oils, and all refined and processed foods. Second, is daily exercise, which includes a mix of aerobic exercise, running, biking, and swimming, strength training with weights, and stretching.

AT WHAT POINT IN YOUR LIFE DID YOU DECIDE TO CHANGE YOUR DIET? HOW HAS THAT DECISION IMPACTED YOUR LIFE?

The awakening came with a devastating diagnosis of stage four breast cancer. It was especially shocking to me as I'd been a runner for fourteen years at that

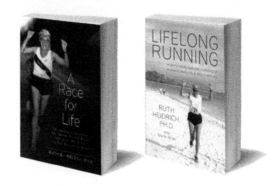

time and had even run marathons. I also thought I knew and followed the "best" diet because of the myths that I was given in my college nutrition course. At that point, I was extremely fortunate to meet Dr. John McDougall, who was starting a research project on the role of the standard American diet (SAD) both initiating and promoting breast cancer. I immediately enrolled in this study, and as a condition of doing this, I had to change to a low-fat vegan diet and decline chemotherapy and radiation. This was necessary to prove that it was the diet alone that was the only experimental variable.

WHAT KIND OF REACTION DO YOU RECEIVE WHEN YOUR PEERS, FRIENDS, AND OTHER "EXPERTS," FIND OUT THAT YOU ARE VEGAN/ PLANT-BASED? ARE THEY INTERESTED AND WANT TO KNOW MORE?

Back in 1982, reactions were mostly very negative. Since I immediately noticed a dramatic change in almost every aspect of my life, I tried to tell them all the good things happening, but they didn't believe me. First off, the signs of the metastases reversed which was, of course, a giant relief. I knew then that the diet was working. Shortly after that, I found out about the Ironman Triathlon and decided to see if I, as a 47-year-old woman, could tackle a 2.4 mile swim, 112 mile bike race, and top it off with a 26.2 mile marathon.
I thought if I could do this, both reverse the cancer and do the Ironman, people would have to notice and hopefully, adopt the same diet.

And people did notice. I started doing athletic events all over the world including China, New Zealand, Japan, Canada, Russia, giving lectures at these same places, as well as Scotland, Greece, and Turkey.

WHAT WAS YOUR DOCTOR'S REACTION AFTER ANNOUNCING YOUR PLANS TO FOLLOW A PLANT-BASED DIET?

The oncologist's reaction was first; that diet has nothing to do with breast cancer, and second, that I could not possibly get enough protein and calcium on this diet. I'm still proving him wrong 37 years later on both counts.

AFTER ADOPTING A PLANT-BASED DIET HOW LONG DID IT TAKE BEFORE FIRST, YOU STARTED TO FEEL BETTER, AND SECOND, YOU KNEW YOU WERE NOT GOING TO LET THIS WIN?

It only took until the very next morning to see some amazing results. I'd been constipated all my life with doctors telling me that moving your bowels three to four times a week is normal for some people. It was that next morning that I found out what "normal" really was!

YOU'VE JUST MET A HEARTBROKEN STRANGER WHO HAS JUST BEEN GIVEN A LIFE-THREATENING DIAGNOSIS. WHAT WOULD BE YOUR TOP FIVE TIPS TO HELP THEM?

1. Change your diet to a whole-food, plant-based diet.
2. Get daily exercise.
3. Make getting good sleep a priority.
4. Handle stress with exercise and mindfulness.
5. Have a new purpose in life and make it to help get this information out to as many people as you can. And that's it!

DO YOU TAKE ANY SPECIAL SUPPLEMENTS OR POTIONS? MENTION ANY SPECIFIC BRANDS YOU USE AND WHY YOU THINK THESE HAVE BENEFITED YOU AND YOUR HEALTH?

Absolutely no supplements other than B12. I also get some daily sunshine. Also, I don't juice anything nor do I "detox," because there is no need to with this clean-living lifestyle.

ANY INSPIRING STORIES THAT CAN HELP OTHERS?

Over the past few years, I discovered that my new diet was having so many more positive effects. My recovery time after training and races was overnight, my adult acne disappeared, my dandruff disappeared, maintaining my ideal weight was effortless, no more heartburn, no more constipation, and maybe best of all, was the effects on my brain! I was motivated, dedicated, and energized to help people realize how powerful this new diet really is! This all started 37 years ago and is still going strong!

Other than my books and a few guest television appearances, the most inspiring opportunity I've had was to have a segment in the wildly popular documentary, Forks Over Knives. I now have many people from all over who come up to me because they recognize me. It's crazy!

I was also named "One of the Ten Fittest Women in North America" when I was 64, and the other nine women were in their 20s and 30s. It's the plants I have to thank for that.

CHANTEL ROBERTSON

CONNECT WITH CHANTEL:
INSTAGRAM: @CHANSHARICE
FACEBOOK: UPFUL BLENDS
YOUTUBE: UPFUL BLENDS
upfulblends.com

MULTIPLE CANCER SURVIVOR

Chantel Robertson is the founder of Upful Blends, a company that creates alkaline herb blends for a healthy mind and body. These herbal blends are inspired by the teachings of Dr. Sebi (a Honduran herbalist and healer) and are 100% non-irradiated, natural herbs from alkaline soils in Iowa and Georgia, and uses indigenous plants from the western cape of Africa, and alkaline herbs from rainforests in Peru, Mexico, and Ecuador.

WHAT ARE YOUR DAILY RITUALS/HABITS WHICH YOU BELIEVE HAVE BEEN KEY TO YOUR HEALTH?

The daily rituals and habits that have been absolute key to my health are these four embodiments: daily rising mediation, moments of awareness and stillness, consuming alkaline herbs, and intermittent fasting.

By daily rising mediation, I'm referring to grounding (also known as Earthing) outside in an open area or wherever I may be at the moment, and being still. Feeling the energy and presence that I AM within this human suit, feeling life that is around me without naming it as a sound or a thing, and just being. From that space, I then get into the mediation of chanting, creativity, manifestation and play. Not only is grounding amazing for spiritual connection, but there is scientific evidence proving the benefits of electrically connecting the human body to Earth because it releases inflammation, supports the immune response, heals organs, eases chronic inflammatory disease and autoimmune diseases.

The moments of awareness and stillness come from my mentor and teacher, Eckhart Tolle. I've read his books for years now and, in this moment, I have the opportunity of receiving support from him in real-time. I spoke with him one day about these beautiful experiences I have when I take breaks throughout the day and come back to stillness. He told me that it is absolutely beautiful AND that he invited me to BE the stillness and the awareness in the doing. So, each day holds for me the opportunity to experience Love/God/Source/Energy while I'm running a business, being in service, waiting in line at the market, or whatever it may be.

Consuming alkaline herbs (which means they have not been manipulated by man/hybridized) serves me in cleansing, purifying, and detoxing my body on an intracellular level. Alkaline herbs help relieve my cells of impurities, metals, and toxins, so inflammation and mucus may be rid from my body.

Intermittent fasting serves me in creating lasting energy, cellular repair, and gives me mental clarity, just to name a few benefits.

AT WHAT POINT IN YOUR LIFE DID YOU DECIDE TO CHANGE YOUR DIET? HOW HAS THAT DECISION IMPACTED YOUR LIFE?

I decided to change my diet when I was 22. It was a quick transition because I never had a liking towards red meat and pork anyways. My family, however, is from the Caribbean, and pork is one of our most famous dishes. At 23, I went cold turkey raw vegan for six months, which means only raw fruits and vegetables as well as nuts and seeds. I then transitioned to a strictly alkaline plant-based diet.

What guided me to this diet goes back to when I was 12 years young and had just moved to South Florida. I began experiencing severe anxiety/panic attacks, along with thoughts and attempts of suicide. I was then put on antidepressants for close to one year. Fast forward to my teen years at age 15. I experienced a few kidney concerns from not consuming water (AT ALL) as well as hormonal imbalances. During that time and up until I was 20-years-old, I was prescribed many medications and birth control. Pumping the body up with medication and not choosing to find the root cause of things is what I was used to experiencing from the medical industry. When I reached 18, I experienced my first breast tumor and had chest surgery. This cancer showed up consistently for the next four years, resulting in a total of four chest surgeries. At 19, I was involved in a car accident that left me bedridden for a year, unable to move. I got hip surgery, had a few muscles snipped, and had my bone shaved down. I had to learn how to walk on my own and was given many medications, such as morphine and oxycodone. This just made things worse in every way. Over the next four years in total, I experienced continued breast tumors, heart disease, severe anemia, hair loss, nerve damage, spine damage, a skin virus, brain damage and mental illness.

All of this made me transition to eating a raw vegan diet. While being on this diet, however, I was becoming weaker, and things were becoming worse. With the doctors not knowing what the cause was and only offering advice in the most uncompassionate way, like, "your heart is just like that. Come back when you're not able to exercise or walk" and "you're a tumor farm, just come back in a few months so we can catch it before it grows rapidly," really pushed me to take matters into my own hands and transition to the alkaline plant-based diet.

WHAT KIND OF REACTION DO YOU RECEIVE WHEN YOUR PEERS, FRIENDS, AND OTHER "EXPERTS," FIND OUT THAT YOU ARE VEGAN/ PLANT-BASED? ARE THEY INTERESTED AND WANT TO KNOW MORE?

The type of reaction that I get from peers and friends is that they can't believe how strict I live my life. They make fun, try to taunt me, and say that I'll become sick if I don't eat meat or starchy foods again. Essentially all the things people say when you begin stepping out of the status quo. They see I can't be swayed and become very intrigued and interested, asking a lot of questions, absorbing this new, profound perspective and way of life. There are also those who, right off the bat, love and respect the discipline, guidance and leadership of truly embodying this lifestyle.

When experts find out that I am plant-based, it's like meeting a long-lost sister/brother. We laugh, we make jokes, and we share tips and experiences. Sometimes, I am still more strict than they are, and they try to ease me out of it because I am consuming a strictly alkaline, plant-based, and only certain water, diet. I even choose to not go into swimming pools, which happened recently at a retreat in Mexico I was a part of.

107

DO YOU TAKE ANY SPECIFIC SUPPLEMENTS? DO YOU RECOMMEND ANY SPECIFIC BRANDS? WHY DO YOU THINK THESE HAVE BENEFITED YOU AND YOUR HEALTH?

The only supplements I consume are herbs and sea vegetables in tea form and capsule form that I get from Upful Blends. The herbs and sea vegetables, such as Irish moss (that holds 92 out of the 102 minerals the body is made of) bladderwrack, kelp, and wakame, are divine in supplying the body all the minerals it needs. This supports me in excellent iron levels, hormonal health, thyroid function, nervous system function, brain health, adrenals and even hair growth.

YOU'VE JUST MET A HEARTBROKEN STRANGER WHO HAS JUST BEEN GIVEN A LIFE-THREATENING DIAGNOSIS. WHAT WOULD BE YOUR TOP FIVE TIPS TO HELP THEM?

My top five tips would be:

Get out into nature and ground yourself daily, multiple times a day.

Incorporate meditation and states of expressing gratitude for the healing that is done at this moment. It's crucial to get the body on the vibrational frequency of love and healing.

Consume Irish moss as a tea and put the gel form on your skin while grounding and absorbing the divine prana. What's happening is that your body is absorbing high amounts of minerals and ridding severe inflammation from the inside out and outside in, while raising your vibration on a cellular level and supporting the ridding of mucus.

Consume only alkaline fruits, vegetables, and get rid of any and all things acidic, including water. Consume 1 gallon of spring water or half your body weight in ounces. Get rid of toxic air fresheners, soaps, cleaning products, all of which are absorbed into the skin and airways going into the body.

If you can juice fast, get a family/friend's support and consume alkaline herbs to support in the healing process of ridding inflammation and mucus.

SHARE A STORY ABOUT THE POWER OF PLANTS THAT YOU USE WITH YOUR CLIENTS TO HELP THEM BELIEVE IN THIS AS AN ALTERNATIVE WAY OF LOOKING AT MEDICINE.

When speaking with a client, I hold the space of letting them know I have been where they are, and I am living proof of the healing power of indigenous plants!

I list all of the diseases that overtook my body as I've mentioned earlier, and then speak on how I chose to go to the forest of Honduras to a healing village to fast for one month with nothing but alkaline water from the mountains, alkaline fruits and vegetables, and alkaline herbs specifically from Mexico, Peru, Honduras, and Africa. I chose to submerge myself in the land to learn about its healing powers for the human body. I was guided by the people there in strengthening this ancient wisdom of internal healing that they have seen and felt.

After that time, all that I've experienced since I was a child has been reversed. The tumors, heart disease, skin disease, nerve damage, mental illness, and severe anemia, are all gone and have not shown themselves since! These high energy alkaline plants hold infinite amounts of energy, power, and wisdom that are experienced as soon as you consume them.

ANY INSPIRING STORIES THAT HAVE HAPPENED TO YOU OR PEOPLE CLOSE TO YOU THAT HAVE NOT BEEN COVERED ABOVE. STORIES THAT CAN HELP OTHERS.

I've mentioned a lot of juicy experiences and transformations above, so what has come to mind at this moment is not a story on plant-based eating per se, but a story focused on how I have cut the cord of mental illness and suicide within an energy state of being and perspective.

A few quick facts on why this is such a critical topic. The AFSP reports that in 2018, there are, on average, 129 suicides per day. The NAMI reports that 46.6 million people experience mental illness. Both of these numbers are increasing daily. There are many factors that play a role in this experience, and what we consume is absolutely one of them along with harbored low vibrational energy and trauma. The body is like a sponge, soaking up so much on a daily basis, like food, thoughts, social conditioning, and the energy of other people.

The last time I felt this emotion of such pain and depression take over me was in the Spring of 2018. After the reversal of my diseases and the immense learning and growth that was done, there was still clearing and acceptance to be done within myself. Now, I will affirm, truly loving yourself through the process of healing is key to allowing healing in finishing its divine work. I cleansed and released many things that overtook my body, yet the love for myself wasn't there, and that fear held itself over me like a black cloud. Complete healing had no space to immerse itself in my life because I didn't clear the hatred I had for myself and the disease, which hindered me from experiencing true God love (or whatever term you prefer).

So, on that day in the Spring of 2018, I was at a park, ready to end it all. In that moment, a presence of indescribable love, warmth and comfort flooded my space with safety and love that I never felt or knew before. In that same instance of me crying, I was laughing uncontrollably. I began having a two-way conversation as I looked to the clearing blue skies above. I began to breathe deeply, to smile and say thank you, I love you too, receiving so much guidance and knowledge.

Everything changed at that moment. I thought that I was in the best health possible when experiencing a reversal of disease, then this experience showed itself. An experience showing me who I am and who we all are. That was just the beginning, too. Every moment, I become stronger physically, emotionally, spiritually and mentally. I have allowed the space for love to be experienced in my life. I allowed myself to purge and come to accept what was. I allowed myself to forgive myself and others. I understood that I held much resentment toward disease and pain, and felt betrayal. With that allowing, I let myself break free from the pain of the body and fully embrace this human life!

Eating an alkaline, plant-based diet has allowed my body to continuously cleanse itself of inflammation and mucus and everything else that clogged the vessel of my body. This has made space for divine connection to source to be experienced in high energy states of being. My body has reconstructed itself. I'm eternally grateful for the healing that's been done on a physical, energetic and intracellular level. Continue persevering and staying grounded within knowing that you are love in its purest form and in the best state of health possible at this moment.

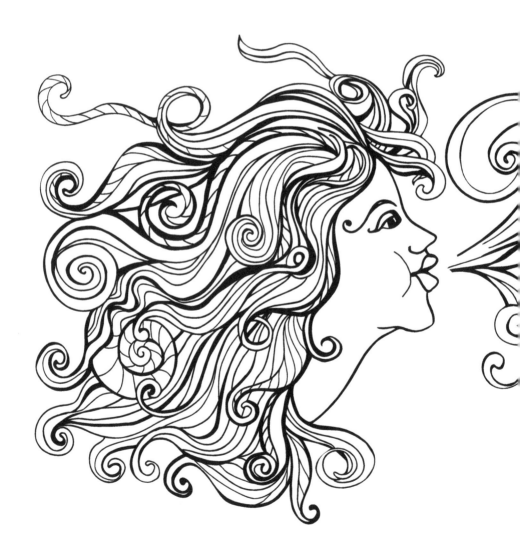

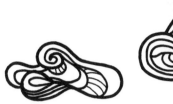

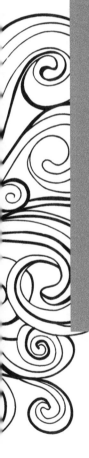

CHAPTER 2

LIFE CHANGING HEALTH:
WEIGHT LOSS

SHANNON LEE

CONNECT WITH SHANNON:
INSTAGRAM: @THEVEGGIENUT
FACEBOOK: THE VEGGIE NUT
YOUTUBE: THE VEGGIE NUT
theveggienut.com

Shannon Lee is the voice behind The Veggie Nut, a social media platform where she offers her plant-based coaching services. Shannon went from suffering every day from various autoimmune diseases, fibromyalgia, IBS, gastritis, high blood pressure, and more, to getting off all medications, losing over 100 pounds, and healing her disorders through the power of plants. Shannon now uses her stories to inspire her clients and social media followers. She is helping others discover just how life-changing a plant-based diet can be.

WHAT ARE YOUR DAILY RITUALS/HABITS WHICH YOU BELIEVE HAVE BEEN KEY TO YOUR HEALTH?

Eating mostly cruciferous and leafy green vegetables make me feel my best. My diet is predominately vegetables, beans, lentils, fruit, nuts, seeds and whole grains. Some other tools I use to make me feel my best is intermittent fasting and drinking lemon water during the day.

AT WHAT POINT IN YOUR LIFE DID YOU DECIDE TO CHANGE YOUR DIET? HOW HAS THAT DECISION IMPACTED YOUR LIFE?

All my life I was pretty much an average size and weight, sometimes fluctuating a couple of sizes. I wasn't thin, but I wasn't overweight either. Weight was never a big issue or concern of mine. As I was approaching thirty, I started experiencing issues with anxiety and had a couple of panic attacks. I went to my doctor, and he prescribed anti-anxiety medication. He also prescribed antidepressants, even though I wasn't experiencing any depression symptoms. He assured me it wasn't a big deal, and the medication helps relieve anxiety too. I ended up having a very negative experience with the antidepressants. They wound up making me depressed and in a constant state of fog. I told my doctor I didn't feel right, but he would just switch me to a different brand. I used three or four different brands, and they all made me feel very off; I wasn't myself. After a while, I just gave in, stuck with the medicine, and listened to my doctor. Some time

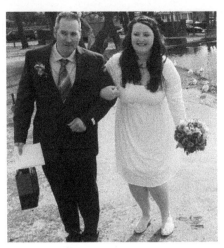
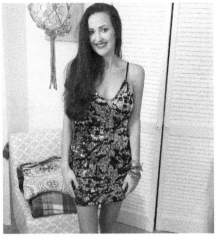

went by and I noticed I was gaining weight but didn't think much of it. I just bought bigger clothes. This continued on for some time. One day, I stepped on the scale, and it read 225 pounds. That was a really big wake up call for me. I had been in such a "fog" with the prescription medications; somehow I didn't realize I gained that much weight. My pant/dress size grew to a size 18. That was a big weight gain for me in a short amount of time. Looking back, it makes perfect sense. Once I was put on antidepressants, I became depressed. I lacked motivation. I just lay in bed, watched television, slept and ate junk food. Once I realized I had let myself gain that much weight, I knew I needed to make a change, right then and there. I told the doctor I wanted to get off the antidepressant and he agreed.

I bought a book and maintained a weight loss journal. I was establishing short term and long term goals. At the time, I was a vegetarian. My diet plan was to cut out fast food and junk food, to lower my carbohydrate intake and up my protein. For protein, I was eating a lot of eggs, cottage cheese and yogurt. I was consuming a lot of animal protein, which I thought was all healthy for me. I started losing weight. I dropped the first twenty pounds pretty fast. Then, one day, my health changed drastically, and my weight was the least of my concerns.

Out of the blue, I started to experience symptoms I've never had before; I felt awful. I started experiencing a long list of very odd, uncomfortable symptoms, all at once. My legs were so achy and weak. I sometimes felt like I couldn't stand on them and feared they might give out under me. I was experiencing the worst kind of backache in my life. The pain was going down my whole spine. I was in excruciating pain all day and night. I swore my spine had to be broken; the pain was that severe. I had bad headaches, brain fog; it was hard to sometimes hold a thought. I experienced skin

"" ""

THE CHANGES WERE SO POWERFUL AND FAST FOR ME

SHANNON LEE

rashes. I had physical problems with my eyes; they stopped producing tears, and my eyelids would swell up. I would have weird red and purplish blotchy discoloration on my face. My body couldn't handle being in the sun anymore. The sun and heat would make me turn red. I felt like I was cooking in an oven; it was unbearable. Parts of my body, like one side of my face, would go numb. My skin would be so sensitive, and even my clothes would feel painful against my body. I had terrible stomach problems, and I was often uncomfortable. I had problems with my blood pressure and heart palpitations. I would have trouble breathing. My breathing would become very shallow, and I would become very lethargic. Due to all of these painful and scary symptoms, I often had trouble sleeping at night. At times I felt so horrible, I seriously thought I was going to die.

During this time, I was going to different doctors, specialists, even taking trips to the hospital. I would sometimes have up to five appointments a week. I would go to one doctor, and they would refer me to see another specialist. I was seeing a rheumatologist, neurologist, cardiologist, gastroenterologist, ophthalmologist, pulmonary specialist, and an ENT. I even tried seeing an acupuncturist and chiropractor. I was constantly getting tests and procedures done. I was prescribed more and more medications but wasn't getting any better. Along the way, I was diagnosed with fibromyalgia, Raynaud's disease, livedo reticularis, IBS, gastritis, chronic dry eye syndrome, and chronic fatigue syndrome. I was told all of these disorders were symptoms of a greater autoimmune disease, but they didn't know which one. They ran tests but said it was sometimes hard to always show up and pinpoint. I had a rheumatologist tell me it sounded like I had lupus. The ENT told me he thought I had Sjogren's disease. At this point, I was sick of going to doctors, getting more tests done, prescribed more medications, but not feeling any better. My husband and I started looking into alternative treatments and answers.

We came across a book called Eat to Live by Dr. Joel Fuhrman, and it was a huge eye-opener. In this book, I learned that there's a big correlation between animal protein and disease. Another book that I read shortly after was The China Study by Dr. T. Colin Campbell, which went into greater detail about the correlation. Everything started to make sense to me. A lightbulb went off. I was eating a lot of animal protein right before I got sick. Like the books explain, we can't change our genes, but we can help determine what happens with them. If we take care of ourselves, the bad genes will remain under control, and we can be healthy. If we eat certain foods like animal protein, it can suddenly bring those bad genes out and make us sick.

As soon as I read those books, I started eating an almost completely plant-based diet. I cut out the eggs, cottage cheese, and yogurt. The only thing I

115

would still have very little of was cheese, here and there. Very shortly after making the switch to a more plant-based diet, I saw a YouTube video that forever changed my life. The video was called "Best Speech You Will Ever Hear" by Gary Yourofsky. I highly recommend everyone seeing this video; it's a real eye-opener. Immediately after watching this video, I knew I was now a vegan for life. There was no going back for me. This video opens your eyes to how cruel, inhumane, and unnatural it is for humans to be consuming animal products. Animal flesh and secretions are inhumane, not necessary, and only make us sick in the long run.

I've always been an animal lover, which is why I was a vegetarian from a very young age. Even I, who thought I was doing right by the animals, didn't know how evil the dairy and egg industry was. The meat and dairy industry go hand-in-hand and are equally as bad. As soon as my eyes were opened, I knew I could never go back to eating or using any animal products again. Being an animal lover, and someone who wanted to be healthier, being vegan was a no-brainer for me. Later that night, I had my husband watch that same video, and he went vegan that day too. I had my mom watch it a couple of days later, and she went vegan also. All three of us have been vegan ever since and couldn't imagine it any other way.

WHAT THINGS HAVE MADE THE MOST DIFFERENCE IN YOUR ABILITY TO LIVE A GOOD LIFE AFTER LIVING WITH OR CURING YOUR DISEASE?

My life is totally different; it's night and day. I used to be in bed most days, and I wasn't hopeful for my future. I thought that's how life was going to be for me; sick and miserable. I was starting to give up hope that I'd ever get better, but I'm so glad I didn't give up. My health has improved so drastically; it sometimes seems surreal, that I was ever once that sick. I hardly have any negative symptoms anymore. The only thing I'm left with is Raynaud's disease and chronic dry eyes, which is nothing compared to the long list of symptoms I once had. I'm proud to say my health is great. I'm off all medications, and I lost over 100 pounds. I went from a size 18 to a size 2.

I used to be afraid to make plans and go anywhere. I'd be afraid that I would wind up being sick and not feel well while I was out, so I hardly left my house, unless it was to go to doctor's appointments. Now I enjoy going out, making plans, traveling, getting out there and enjoying life. It's so liberating being able to go away for days without having to pack any medications or worry about getting sick. Something I wasn't able to do for a while, which I love doing now is going to the beach and enjoying the summer. I used to have a really bad relationship with the sun and heat when I was sick. Now I love it. Summer has become my favorite season, and I'm at the beach whenever I have free time.

Since losing weight, my confidence has greatly improved. I'm more outgoing. I'm more secure in myself. Now when I look in the mirror, I feel like the outside matches the inside. I enjoy shopping for clothes a lot more. I've become more into fashion, makeup, and putting more effort and care into my appearance. I would have never imagined this would be me, but it is and I love it!

WHAT WAS YOUR DOCTOR'S REACTION AFTER ANNOUNCING YOUR PLANS TO FOLLOW A PLANT-BASED DIET? WAS HE/SHE SUPPORTIVE?

Once I discovered that I could heal myself simply by what I put, or don't put in my mouth, I didn't need to go to the doctor much anymore. Now I only go to my doctor once a year for a physical. Which I recently had done, and I'm proud to say everything was perfect. Better than ever, actually. My blood pressure was perfect, and my blood work was perfect. The doctor actually told me that it was some of the best blood work he'd ever seen, especially the cholesterol. He told me that I'm doing great, not to change a thing. My doctor is supportive of my diet and sees first-hand that it keeps me very healthy.

AFTER ADOPTING A PLANT-BASED DIET HOW LONG DID IT TAKE BEFORE FIRST, YOU STARTED TO FEEL BETTER, AND SECOND, YOU KNEW YOU WERE NOT GOING TO LET THIS WIN?

The changes were so powerful and fast for me. I realized around three or four days after switching my diet, my symptoms greatly subsided. It was the first time I was really hopeful that I would get better. I was right. From that point on the symptoms just got less and less. I felt better every day. Knowing eating this way makes me feel my best, and keeps me at a healthy weight, gives me the motivation to keep going with this lifestyle.

117

YOU'VE JUST MET A HEARTBROKEN STRANGER WHO HAS JUST BEEN GIVEN A LIFE-THREATENING DIAGNOSIS. WHAT WOULD BE YOUR TOP FIVE TIPS TO HELP THEM?

Vegetables, vegetables, vegetables, vegetables and more vegetables. Seriously though, whether you're trying to heal a disease, get healthier, or you're trying to lose weight, get into those vegetables! Veggies are great for everything and they are your friends. Especially, cruciferous and leafy green vegetables. Juice them, put them in a smoothie, a salad, or just snack on them. Eat them raw, eat them cooked, just eat them. I also recommend avoiding animal products and highly processed foods, as well as foods that are high in salt, sugar and oil.

DO YOU TAKE ANY SPECIAL SUPPLEMENTS OR POTIONS? MENTION ANY SPECIFIC BRANDS YOU USE AND WHY YOU THINK THESE HAVE BENEFITED YOU AND YOUR HEALTH?

There are a few vitamins I take daily. A women's multivitamin. There are many good vitamins out there, but I personally take the Dr. Fuhrman multivitamin. A probiotic: I take Ultimate Flora Probiotic Women's Complete from Renew Life, I like to take 50-90 billion live cultures. I take a cranberry supplement. I'm not particular and will take any vegan cranberry supplement daily. Once a week I'll take a B12. I personally take the brand Solgar, Vitamin B12 1000 MCG. I also take a vegan DHA+EPA, and I take the one from Dr. Fuhrman.

Everyone should take a good quality multivitamin, and it's just good for overall health. I take a probiotic because it helps avoid stomach problems and yeast infections. A good cranberry supplement helps prevent urinary tract infections. B12 is good for vegans, or anyone middle age and older. DHA+EPA is good for brain health.

I already eat so healthy and most likely don't need to take many of these supplements. Every year when I get my blood work done, my vitamin levels are always high. However, they are water-soluble vitamins, so it won't hurt you. You'll just pee out the extra vitamins. So basically, I have expensive urine. But I always feel it's better to be safe than sorry. Having too much won't hurt you, but having too little will. So I just take them.

WHAT ARE THE TWO OR THREE THINGS YOU HAVE DONE DIFFERENTLY WITH YOUR LIFE AFTER YOUR HEALTH GOT BETTER?

Since getting healthy, I've become very interested in nutrition. I saw first hand the power nutrition can have on the body. I became certified in plant-based nutrition through the T. Colin Campbell eCornell program. I started a YouTube channel, where I share my story, vegan recipes, vegan alternatives, and more. I have the channel to try to help people and to spread the vegan message. For people who want one-on-one help, I offer coaching. It's very rewarding to help others have success with their health, as I've had for myself. The best messages I receive are from people telling me they went vegan because of me. It makes me feel like I am making a small difference in this big world.

ANY INSPIRING STORIES THAT HAVE HAPPENED TO YOU OR PEOPLE CLOSE TO YOU THAT HAVE NOT BEEN COVERED ABOVE. STORIES THAT CAN HELP OTHERS.

To anyone who thinks they are too far gone, whether it be you have a long list of medical problems, or you have a lot of weight to lose, you can do it! Trust me, if I can do it, so can you. Sometimes we reach a point where we think we're too far gone and we lose hope. It can be exhausting just thinking about getting started, so we give up before we even really try.

Don't be that person. Be someone who fights for their life and health. Be someone who knows they are worth it. You only get one life, put in the effort so you can feel good and enjoy your life. You don't have to be unhealthy or overweight. There's a healthier version of yourself just waiting to come out. I've seen and heard stories of people having success in both health and weight loss. Stories from people who have tried everything else and almost gave up hope. You just have to truly want it and believe in yourself. I'm not saying a healthy diet and vegetables will cure everything, but it will definitely improve your health.

How to get started: Just like any change in life, it will take some time to adjust. We are creatures of habit. We don't like change, or to deviate from our daily routine. You have to fight through that and make yourself eat healthy until that is your new routine. You might not be a true veggie-lover, like me, but you will find at least a couple of vegetables and dishes that you enjoy. Have fun with it. Try all types of different vegetables and different ways of incorporating them into your diet. You will find some you like more than others. Some vegetables are an acquired taste. You might not like them at first, but after trying them a few times, your opinion might change. Keep an open mind. Once you know which vegetables, fruits, beans, lentils, nuts, seeds, and whole grains you enjoy, you're all set. You can get into a new, healthy routine. Making meals will be easy, and you will want to continue eating this way because it makes you feel good.

Knowing and caring about what happens to the animals is a big key to going and staying vegan. You might be tempted to cheat on your health once in a while, but it's a lot harder to cheat on your morals and ethics. Sure, you might be able to have a very small amount of animal products and still be healthy, but why bother? You will feel better about yourself, knowing that you're not contributing to the suffering of innocent animals. If you want to treat yourself, reach for a vegan snack. There's a vegan alternative for everything these days. It's never been so easy.

Being vegan is a win-win-win. It's the best for the animals, your health, and the environment.

ANNII KIELEY

CONNECT WITH ANNII:
INSTAGRAM: @ANNIIGETSHEALTHY
FACEBOOK: ANNII GETS HEALTHY
YOUTUBE: ANNII K

Annii Kieley has a dramatic and impressive weight loss story, going from 286 pounds at age 22 to 128 pounds in only eighteen months, then beginning to pack on muscle through heavy strength training. Annii attributes much of her athletic success to adopting a plant-based vegan diet. She now shares her story across a variety of social media platforms, including a radio show on CHMR-FM in Newfoundland and an online podcast called Annii Gets Healthy, available on Spotify, Apple podcasts, Google podcasts, and iHeartRadio

WHAT ARE YOUR DAILY RITUALS/HABITS WHICH YOU BELIEVE HAVE BEEN KEY TO YOUR HEALTH?

I engage in vigorous strength training six days per week on a three day split. I track my food for the following day each night on a tracking app to ensure I am meeting my nutritional goals. I eat very little until I get my lifting done, after which I get most of my food intake. I eat within an eight hour window most days, never going beyond 12 hours. Once per week, currently on Sundays, I rest from strength training and fast anywhere from 24 to 40 hours.

I used to run almost daily but do this much less often now due to my commitment to strength training. When I do run, usually around once or twice per week, I like to do so in a fasted state.

As a recovering addict following a 12-step program, I begin my day with gratitude and a complete surrender of my own self-will. I make sure I am connected with like-minded individuals throughout the day and am vigilant of how I am engaging with the world around me. Attending regular meetings keeps my mind open to new ideas and inspires me to live the best life possible.

AT WHAT POINT IN YOUR LIFE DID YOU DECIDE TO CHANGE YOUR DIET? HOW HAS THAT DECISION IMPACTED YOUR LIFE?

I was overweight from childhood on. I gained even more weight as the years went on until, at age 22, I was 286 pounds and had high cholesterol. Even this was not my call-to-action. My real call-to-action was an attempt to battle my work-related anxiety through a diet where I quit soda and fast food. I was 24 years old and 270 pounds. When I began to lose weight with minimal effort, I added even more changes. I began going to the gym three times per week, became mindful of my carbohydrate intake, and ate lots of vegetables after having an almost carnivorous diet. I eventually transitioned to a vegetarian diet and took up the practice of intermittent fasting. I took up running, and the following year even ran a 10-mile road race.

In around a year and a half, I lost 140 pounds, eventually reaching a comfortable 128-130 pounds. A year prior, in 2017, I lost my father to cancer after a long battle. He was not a drinker or a smoker, so I realized that diet must play a substantial role in cancer progression. It took me almost a year to come to my senses. After I read The China Study by T. Colin Campbell, Ph.D., I realized I needed to act now to reduce my risk.

After going fully plant-based, I gained more energy than I knew possible, and I put this energy into my gym activity. After a long time of resistance training, I started to focus on strength. Building muscle as a vegan woman has been far easier than it is made out to be. All that is required is a proper diet and dedication to improving yourself.

This change was so great that I left my old career and returned to university. I am now studying recreation at Memorial University of Newfoundland School of Human Kinetics and Recreation, minoring in Psychology. I am currently working on two certifications from the International Sports Science Association so that I can pass along what I have learned to others. I also began a new radio show and podcast called "Annii Gets Healthy" on promoting health. Health now makes up a large part of my identity.

I initially transitioned to veganism for health reasons. However, I have since met many activists who have shown me the truth regarding how humans use animals. I now believe that a vegan lifestyle is the best way to care for your body and the world around you.

WHAT THINGS HAVE MADE THE BIGGEST IMPACT ON YOUR WEIGHT LOSS? WHAT THINGS DID YOU CHANGE AND HOW LONG DID IT TAKE BEFORE YOU NOTICED CHANGES IN YOUR BODY?

At first, it was simply eating less and calorie counting, but I have also engaged in intermittent fasting and carb cycling with much success. Eating more vegetables alone was a huge benefit. What had the greatest noticeable effect was physical activity. My food intake, coupled with walking and gym visits, led me to constant weight loss in the first year. Intermittent fasting gave me a second wind of noticeable weight loss, and veganism has helped me gain noticeable muscle mass from my strength training.

WHAT WAS YOUR DOCTOR'S REACTION AFTER ANNOUNCING YOUR PLANS TO FOLLOW A PLANT-BASED DIET? WAS HE/SHE SUPPORTIVE?

I casually mentioned this to my doctor about two months into my transition since I wanted bloodwork done to check for a B12 deficiency. She was rather neutral, but told me to make sure I was getting enough protein and not using too many soy products.

I noted to myself that, as a weightlifter, I am perhaps more aware of my protein intake than many non-vegans. Also, regarding soy, unless one has an allergy to it or is menstruating, there are no adverse effects to consuming normal amounts on a regular basis.

AFTER ADOPTING A PLANT-BASED DIET, HOW LONG DID IT TAKE BEFORE YOU STARTED TO LOSE WEIGHT AND HOW MUCH WEIGHT HAVE YOU LOST?

I lost weight about three to six weeks into my diet change. However I had already "finished" losing weight shortly before transitioning, so I modified my diet to include more carbohydrates before my workouts (carb cycling) and have since gained considerable muscle mass.

HAS THERE BEEN ANY OTHER BENEFITS (APART FROM WEIGHT LOSS) FROM YOUR VEGAN/PLANT-BASED DIET? HAVE YOU FOUND THIS DIET DIFFICULT?

Easily the biggest benefit for me has been an increase in energy levels. I used to find myself lightheaded and sleepy between meals. Even when consuming small portions of meat after training, I would find myself incredibly lethargic. I now am able to push myself harder, with shorter recovery periods. I attribute this to my vegan diet.

I have also suffered from gallstones since my first few months of weight loss. The pain of gallbladder attacks is a pain I could not describe even if I wanted to, and they frequently reduced my quality of life. I am happy to say that on a plant-based diet, it is very difficult for me to get these debilitating attacks. I have only been sick once since my transition, and that was after eating something which unbeknownst to me contained dairy. Before going vegan, I would experience attacks about every two weeks and would experience dull aches perhaps weekly. As of now, I have not had any pain in over six months.

The only thing I truly missed for a good while was eggs. However, I have

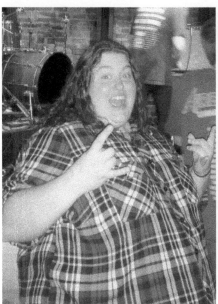 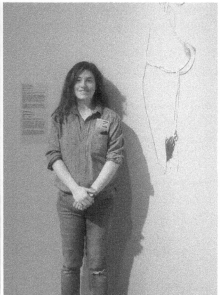

since learned to make a mean tofu scramble (Kala namak salt being the ultimate seasoning). The number of replacements for foods such as cheese and meaty meals is incredible. While I do not think they should be a staple of a healthy diet, they made for excellent treats and can definitely make a transition far easier.

DO YOU TAKE ANY SPECIAL SUPPLEMENTS OR POTIONS? MENTION ANY SPECIFIC BRANDS YOU USE AND WHY YOU THINK THESE HAVE BENEFITED YOU AND YOUR HEALTH.

I use protein powders almost daily as a part of my athletic diet. My favorite powders to date are the vegan line of powders from PEScience, my favorite flavor being the Peanut Butter Delight. I must note that I cannot eat peanuts without a painful stomach reaction, but I do not get that from this product as it contains no actual peanuts.

I take pre-workout on my two most challenging workouts of the week. My favorite brand is Jacked Factory, as their Nitro Surge is a fantastic and vegan-friendly product. I also enjoy two vegan-friendly products from Allmax, one being Aminocore BCAA (which I take daily) and Impact Igniter pre-workout. Last of all, I enjoy Cytogreens Greens Powder, the chocolate flavor being a divine way to feel a bit better on rushed days where I have limited access to fresh green veggies.

WHAT ARE THE TWO OR THREE THINGS YOU HAVE DONE DIFFERENTLY WITH YOUR LIFE AFTER YOU LOST ALL OF YOUR UNWANTED WEIGHT?

Most of the changes in my life revolve around physical activity. When I was obese, I could not walk for more than 15 minutes without becoming tired. This was embarrassing and depressing, as I could not join my friends on hikes without dragging far behind everyone else. Within six months of beginning my weight loss, I found myself keeping up with others, even on more challenging walks. Now, I tend to lead during difficult hikes and am perhaps the most active person in my circle of friends.

Beyond that, I can now eat more mindfully and have gone from living on fast food and microwave meals to taking great pleasure from cooking each day. Feeling stronger each week I lift weights, which is a feeling I cannot possibly describe, and I know for a fact I would not be where I am today if I was still consuming animal products.

ANY INSPIRING STORIES THAT HAVE HAPPENED TO YOU OR PEOPLE CLOSE TO YOU THAT HAVE NOT BEEN COVERED ABOVE. STORIES THAT CAN HELP OTHERS.

I wear many badges on my sleeve. I am a recovering addict who battles with Bipolar Disorder Type 2. My struggles have made me the strong woman I am today, and for these obstacles, I shall be forever grateful. Without the battles I have fought, how could I inspire myself and others around me? Without being obese for so many years, how would I have become so passionate about the joys of movement? If I were not an addict, would I feel the same way about addiction and recovery that I feel today? Absolutely not.

My abdomen now tells the tale of my past obesity-- mostly through my stretch marks and loose skin. People often ask me if I will get the surgery one day to remove my skin. I don't think I ever will. I used to hate my body 90 percent of the time. Now I love my body 90 percent of the time. I'm willing to bear that other 10 percent without expensive surgical intervention with the possibility of complications.

My main wish at this point in my life is to help others. As they say in my program, "the only way to keep what we have is by giving it away."
I am saddened by the growing obesity epidemic where I live, with a baffling one-third of the Newfoundland population being medically classified as obese. We must all work together to create a healthier, happier, and more compassionate society. Otherwise, there will be no society left to change.

HOPE DESROCHES

CONNECT WITH HOPE:
INSTAGRAM: @TRAINWITHHOPE
FACEBOOK: TRAIN WITH HOPE
YOUTUBE: HOPE DESROCHES

"My life has drastically changed for the better. I am now more empowered, confident and happy. I can fit comfortably into any seat, which most people would take for granted. After always being worried I could not fit into a movie seat or airplane seat, it is a big deal! I now love to push myself. I love hiking and always want to see how much further I can go or what mountain I can climb! Also, I enjoy fashion now! It was so hard for me to buy clothes before because nothing fit, but now I have so many options and it is truly exciting!"

At 325 pounds on her 5'5" frame, Hope Desroches was desperate for a change. Trying diet after diet without success, Hope found herself pre-diabetic, with high cholesterol, high blood pressure and a broken spirit. Now, minus 175 pounds, her life has drastically changed. She discovered the benefits of a plant-based diet, started a blog to share her success story and has started a new business to help others do the same.

125

WHAT ARE YOUR DAILY RITUALS/HABITS WHICH YOU BELIEVE HAVE BEEN KEY TO YOUR HEALTH?

Hiking and yoga are a huge part of my life. I hike four to six miles each day and practice yoga for about an hour. Additionally, I follow a fully plant-based diet and stick to a pretty consistent eating schedule for my meals. I avoid snacking.

AT WHAT POINT IN YOUR LIFE DID YOU DECIDE TO CHANGE YOUR DIET? HOW HAS THAT DECISION IMPACTED YOUR LIFE?

I went vegan in June of 2017. It is something that I had wanted to do for a long time, but it was a difficult transition because my family consumed a lot of animal products. I made the choice to go vegan primarily because I was stalling on my weight loss journey, and I wanted to try something different.

Just a few days later, my dog was killed, and it was intensely painful. Relating the pain I felt for my dog to the animals I used to eat made me

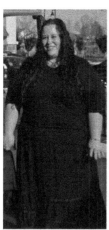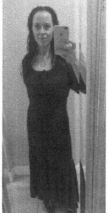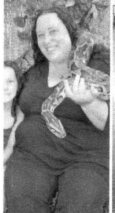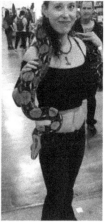

more committed to a vegan diet. Also, as a hiker, I was so in touch with nature and it felt like my diet should reflect that.

WHAT THINGS HAVE MADE THE BIGGEST IMPACT ON YOUR WEIGHT LOSS? WHAT THINGS DID YOU CHANGE AND HOW LONG DID IT TAKE BEFORE YOU NOTICED CHANGES IN YOUR BODY?

I believe that counting calories and staying active are the most essential steps to losing weight. Beyond that, going vegan inspired a love of cooking in me. I felt like I could cook guilt-free since I knew the meals I was preparing caused no harm to myself or the environment. I started being more creative with creating new recipes and meal planning.

WHAT WAS YOUR DOCTOR'S REACTION AFTER ANNOUNCING YOUR PLANS TO FOLLOW A PLANT-BASED DIET? WAS HE/SHE SUPPORTIVE?

My general health doctor was very supportive and simply reminded me to avoid processed food and take certain supplements. However, my OB-GYN was very concerned I would not get enough protein. For that reason, I carefully watch what I eat so I can get as much protein as possible.

AFTER ADOPTING A PLANT-BASED DIET, HOW LONG DID IT TAKE BEFORE YOU STARTED TO LOSE WEIGHT AND HOW MUCH WEIGHT HAVE YOU LOST?

At that point in my weight loss journey, I had already lost about 120 pounds but, I had plateaued for about a month. When I went vegan, I started losing weight again right away and easily got down to my goal weight! Plus, it has been much easier to maintain my weight because of my choice to go vegan.

HAVE THERE BEEN ANY OTHER BENEFITS (APART FROM WEIGHT LOSS) FROM YOUR VEGAN/PLANT-BASED DIET? HAVE YOU FOUND THIS DIET DIFFICULT?

A big part of me still has cravings when I am around ice cream or a cheesy chicken burrito, but I remind myself that if I want that badly enough, I can always make the vegan version of that food to enjoy. Being vegan forces me to be mindful about everything I eat, which is such a great thing.

DO YOU TAKE ANY SPECIAL SUPPLEMENTS OR POTIONS? SPECIFIC BRANDS WOULD BE GREAT AS WELL PLEASE AND WHY YOU THINK THESE HAVE BENEFITED YOU AND YOUR HEALTH?

I actually don't take any certain brands at this time. I take vitamin D and B12 supplements, as well as an all-in-one supplement. I normally buy what's on sale.

WHAT ARE THE TWO OR THREE THINGS YOU HAVE DONE DIFFERENTLY WITH YOUR LIFE AFTER YOU LOST ALL OF YOUR UNWANTED WEIGHT?

My goodness, there is so much! My life has drastically changed for the better. I am now more empowered, confident and happy. I can fit comfortably into any seat, which most people would take for granted. After always being worried I could not fit into a movie seat or airplane seat, it is a big deal! I now love to push myself. I love hiking and always want to see how much further I can go or what mountain I can climb! Also, I enjoy fashion now! It was so hard for me to buy clothes before because nothing fit. Now, I have so many options - it is truly exciting!

ANY INSPIRING STORIES THAT HAVE HAPPENED TO YOU OR PEOPLE CLOSE TO YOU THAT HAVE NOT BEEN COVERED ABOVE. STORIES THAT CAN HELP OTHERS.

In October 2013, I was sitting at a restaurant with my kids. My son, who was five years old at the time, was drawing a picture on the placemat. I was chatting with my husband and seven-year-old daughter while eating an extra cheesy omelet with a large stack of pancakes. I wasn't really paying too much attention to his artwork. When he was done, he handed it to me. It was a family portrait. He drew my husband, his sister, and himself as lean stick figures and me as a big round circle. I looked at the picture and felt very sad, and as if I didn't know, I asked him why he drew me as a circle. He said, "because you're so fat!"

My son was right. I was 325 pounds, on my 5'5" frame. I had tried to lose weight many times, but always gave up on myself and quickly gained it back. My weight was not only a bad influence on my kids, but it kept me from enjoying my life. Getting up from the couch, lifting a gallon of milk from the fridge, and even falling asleep at night, were all difficult because of my large size. I was pre-diabetic with high cholesterol and high blood pressure.

I wish I could say that the story of being drawn as a circle was really my turning point, but it wasn't. It's just an example of the many, many, many times I felt ashamed of my weight. The turning point did not come until 2016, and it wasn't one thing, it was everything. For years I had made excuses, given up on myself, and wished I could find the inspiration to finally lose weight and keep it off forever.

At 35-years-old, I took some time to reflect, and I asked myself what I really wanted for my future. I wanted self-confidence, energy and the ability to do things I have always wanted to do. I wanted to hike, go horseback riding, go tubing in a river, on water slides, or even just sit comfortably in a crowded movie theater. I knew that I could have these things, but it would take a lot of work and dedication.

My website/blog is called *Finally Inspired* because that is how I felt when I started my journey. I was finally inspired to change the way I was living my life so I could have the confidence, energy and the happiness I had always wanted for myself.

When I started my journey, I had a lot of options. I could have chosen gastric bypass, diet pills, or any one of the fad diets that were popular and being pushed down my throat by every other person I met. Instead, I chose to lose weight on my own. At first, I just started by eating a bit less and walking a few times a week. Even then, I wanted to be able to do this without following any program so I could say to people who are struggling, "I did this, so you can too!"

Now, I have lost 175 pounds, and I have a real understanding of what it takes to make real, lasting change and that is why it is my mission to support other people on their weight loss journey.

MARY BETH BRENDEL

15 years of blood pressure medication, Adderall, and on the brink of beginning medication for high cholesterol, Mary Beth Brendel realized that it was time to make a change. Dieting had only led to weight yo-yoing, and nothing was sustainable. After partaking in a 7-day plant-based eating challenge alongside some coworkers and educating herself on the benefits of plant-based eating, Mary's life was drastically changed for the better.

"The weight literally melted off me. Within the first week, I noticed the weight coming off but also that I began to feel better and had more energy. My gums stopped bleeding, my cholesterol fell from 278 to 196 in just a few weeks, and I felt great. Within six months, I lost almost 50 pounds, and I am in the best shape of my life."

WHAT ARE YOUR DAILY RITUALS/HABITS WHICH YOU BELIEVE HAVE BEEN KEY TO YOUR HEALTH?

Staying active by doing something I like that I can sustain and enjoy. Over the past 30 years, my weight cycled up and down. I would exercise on and off. I feel that this time, part of my success has been that I try to work out five days a week for an hour, doing a variety of things that I love. Also, keeping meals simple. I love making wholesome soups and warm, filling chili's. I make extra to freeze that I can grab for lunches or dinners when I don't want to cook. Always having healthy food at hand is a must.

AT WHAT POINT IN YOUR LIFE DID YOU DECIDE TO CHANGE YOUR DIET? HOW HAS THAT DECISION IMPACTED YOUR LIFE?

For the past 15 years, I had been taking Lisinopril for high blood pressure and Adderall for ADD. I had tried Weight Watchers, the TOPS diet, and Nutrisystem, but nothing seemed to be sustainable. I would bounce between 140 and 180 pounds.

In March of 2017, my blood work indicated that my cholesterol was at 278! I told my doctor that I really wanted to take care of this with diet and not add any more medications to my list. All I could think about was the time that my mother had experienced her first heart attack while visiting me in New Jersey when she was about my age.

" "

FAST FORWARD ONE YEAR:
I'M 58 YEARS OLD AND GO IN
FOR A DOCTOR APPOINTMENT.

THE RESULTS?

HYPERTENSION: RESOLVED
ADD: RESOLVED
CHOLESTEROL LEVEL: 167

**NO MORE
MEDICATIONS NEEDED**.

MARY BETH BRENDAL

Thankfully for me, the school I was working in was doing the *Engine 2 Rescue Challenge* (this is a 7-day plant-based challenge that can be found on YouTube), which I took part in. I also educated myself by watching the *Forks Over Knives* documentary, and I made the switch straight away.

The weight literally melted off me. Within the first week, I noticed the weight coming off but also that I began to feel better and had more energy. My gums stopped bleeding, my cholesterol fell from 278 to 196 in just a few weeks, and I felt great. Within six months, I lost almost 50 pounds, and I am in the best shape of my life.

WHAT THINGS HAVE MADE THE BIGGEST IMPACT ON YOUR WEIGHT LOSS? WHAT THINGS DID YOU CHANGE AND HOW LONG DID IT TAKE BEFORE YOU NOTICED CHANGES IN YOUR BODY?

Eating plant-based, no sugar or oil, and being consistently active are all things that have made the biggest impact for me. I felt better within a week, dropped a dress size within a month, and continued from a size 14 to a size 6 in six months.

My cholesterol also started decreasing immediately. After a year, I realized I was much more focused and stopped needing my ADD medication. This was such a great feeling: to feel like I was in control, and I no longer needed medication.

WHAT WAS YOUR DOCTOR'S REACTION AFTER ANNOUNCING YOUR PLANS TO FOLLOW A PLANT-BASED DIET? WAS HE/SHE SUPPORTIVE?

My doctor was very supportive and told me to keep doing what I was doing because it was working. Fast forward one year: I'm 58 years old and go in for a doctor's appointment. The results? Hypertension: resolved! ADD: resolved! Cholesterol level: 167! No more medications needed!

AFTER ADOPTING A PLANT-BASED DIET, HOW LONG DID IT TAKE BEFORE YOU STARTED TO LOSE WEIGHT AND HOW MUCH WEIGHT HAVE YOU LOST?

I started to lose weight during the first week. After six months, I had lost close to 50 pounds. The weight just fell off once I started to eat so clean.

HAVE THERE BEEN ANY OTHER BENEFITS (APART FROM WEIGHT LOSS) FROM YOUR VEGAN/PLANT-BASED DIET? HAVE YOU FOUND THIS DIET DIFFICULT?

I no longer need blood pressure medication, I didn't have to begin medication for my extremely high cholesterol, I have more energy, my skin improved, and my hair is so much softer and healthier. You could say I was glowing.

WHAT ARE THE TWO OR THREE THINGS YOU HAVE DONE DIFFERENTLY WITH YOUR LIFE AFTER YOU LOST ALL OF YOUR UNWANTED WEIGHT?

Cooking has become a new passion of mine. I love to help and encourage others who are ready to learn. I have also taken up running.

These days I always have a week's worth of whole-food ingredients available to grab and throw together quick meals, such as fresh and frozen fruits and veggies, as well as a few baked or microwaved sweet potatoes to add to spinach or kale salad. When I go out to dinner, I bring a small container of homemade, oil-free dressing and a bag of nuts, seeds, and raisins to add to my salad, along with my favorite herbal tea.

ANY INSPIRING STORIES THAT HAVE HAPPENED TO YOU OR PEOPLE CLOSE TO YOU THAT HAVE NOT BEEN COVERED ABOVE. STORIES THAT CAN HELP OTHERS.

It took some patience in the beginning, so I kept it very simple. I was never one to spend time in the kitchen, so my biggest challenge was meal prep. I felt really empowered after watching YouTube videos and cleaning out the kitchen, grocery shopping, and even preparing family meals. It takes time sometimes to get it right, but it is fun finding new recipes that we all love and enjoy. We also have a group at school, and we share recipes and a Facebook page that we all post on.

To stay focused, I watch all the documentaries that are out there, read articles, and buy cookbooks. I also follow the Forks Over Knives Facebook page and love reading all the amazing success stories. I find it easy to stay motivated because I feel so great!

The most difficult part of this journey is watching others suffer unnecessarily. Many people have been open to trying this and others not so much. However, there is no denying the results.

Personally, I needed to lose weight, but my main goal from the beginning was to get off my medications and avoid that heart attack that I knew was just waiting to happen. Win-win!

KATE MANN

CONNECT WITH KATE:
INSTAGRAM: @LOSE_WEIGHT_W_KATE
FB: PLANT-BASED LIFESTYLE & NATURAL WEIGHT LOSS FOR WOMEN
YOUTUBE: KATE MANN
katemannfitness.com

Kate Mann is a holistic lifestyle coach who practices nutritional healing, applying a total body approach to wellness. Kate has shared her weight loss story across her popular social media platforms and has a successful holistic wellness business that focuses on improving women's health through plant-based eating and total lifestyle makeovers.

WHAT ARE YOUR DAILY RITUALS/HABITS WHICH YOU BELIEVE HAVE BEEN KEY TO YOUR HEALTH?

- Some form of mindfulness or breath work each morning
- Stretching
- Daily walks
- Leaving my phone and computer in the office at night

15 years ago, at my heaviest (just shy of 200 pounds), I knew I had hit my threshold. I was so lost and insecure, feeling constant anxiety, and I was using food to cope. One day I woke up and just said to myself in the mirror, "enough! I know you're in there, I'm sorry, and I'm coming to save you!" I put my running shoes on and went for my first jog in years that very day. From that point on, I started exercising more and made an effort to incorporate more healthy foods.

Over the next years, I successfully lost the weight and maintained a regular exercise routine. I was living a pretty "healthy" lifestyle, but I was still yo-yoing through phases of being on and off the wagon with my nutrition and self-care habits. To be clear, I was still eating the standard American diet at this time.

Three years ago, my husband and I watched a series of health documentaries. Forks Over Knives was one I definitely remember. We were pretty inspired by it and were already eating mostly whole-foods, so we said, "why not?," and decided to give the whole-food, plant-based lifestyle a try. We are never going back! It changed our lives.

133

WHAT THINGS HAVE MADE THE BIGGEST IMPACT ON YOUR WEIGHT LOSS? WHAT THINGS DID YOU CHANGE AND HOW LONG DID IT TAKE BEFORE YOU NOTICED CHANGES IN YOUR BODY?

Whole, plant-based foods, daily movement, and maintaining a consistent self-care routine. Those are the three keys to health in my opinion. It all comes down to nutrition and habits. Just by eliminating animal products and processed foods alone, I saw results within the first week. That was honestly the biggest component. It allowed my body AND mind to reset, which allowed me to not only release body fat, but also emotional tension and negative beliefs. I sealed the deal by implementing good, habit-forming techniques, self-monitoring my thoughts and time/energy management.

AFTER ADOPTING A PLANT-BASED DIET, HOW LONG DID IT TAKE BEFORE YOU STARTED TO LOSE WEIGHT AND HOW MUCH WEIGHT HAVE YOU LOST?

From the very beginning of the time when I was at my heaviest (eating a "healthier" standard American diet), I gradually lost 50 or so pounds over a couple of years. However, I stalled at that weight for the next eight years. Then, when I went plant-based, within the first week, I started releasing body fat and noticed my body felt lighter and less bloated. I lost 15 pounds within less than a year WITHOUT trying. It's crazy to think I could have had this success a decade sooner if I had been properly educated about it. That's exactly why I decided to become a coach and help other women have the same success.

HAS THERE BEEN ANY OTHER BENEFITS (APART FROM WEIGHT LOSS) FROM YOUR VEGAN/PLANT-BASED DIET? HAVE YOU FOUND THIS DIET DIFFICULT?

Oh totally! My digestion, skin and energy is AMAZING! I keep feeling like I'm reverse aging! It's great to be 33, and people think I'm still in my 20's.

Also, food is so much for fun now. I have always cooked, but my culinary skills completely switched on when I started cooking with plants. My husband and I joke that we eat like royalty: always so much color, flavor and abundance.

As far as difficulties go, it's mainly just been a lack of understanding or judgment from others about plant-based eating, certain lifestyle choices, etc. Honestly, I just let it roll off my shoulders. I think the best way to teach is not by debate, but rather by example.

DO YOU TAKE ANY SPECIAL SUPPLEMENTS OR POTIONS? MENTION ANY SPECIFIC BRANDS YOU USE AND WHY YOU THINK THESE HAVE BENEFITED YOU AND YOUR HEALTH?

I alternate between several supplements referred to me by Anthony William, the Medical Medium. Instead of listing each of them out, I highly suggest following him and purchasing his books, especially Liver Rescue. I will say I do 16 ounces of fresh celery juice every morning per Medical Medium's protocol, and it is LIFE CHANGING. Again, research his stuff to learn more.

WHAT ARE THE TWO OR THREE THINGS YOU HAVE DONE DIFFERENTLY WITH YOUR LIFE AFTER YOU LOST ALL OF YOUR UNWANTED WEIGHT?

I've slowed down a lot more, and I soak up each day. I am also extremely grateful for everything I have, and a lot more aware of how blessed I am to have good health.

ANY INSPIRING STORIES THAT CAN HELP OTHERS?

Don't pursue health for vanity reasons. Be willing to release negative thinking and inner conflict. If you focus on how you want to FEEL you will look the way you want to look. Every day we have a choice, whether it's in what we eat or how we think. As long as you always choose what's in your highest good you will never make a bad decision.

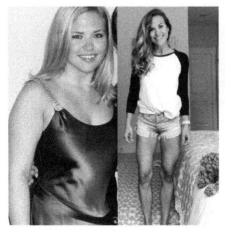
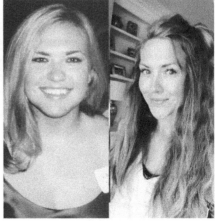

SHEANNE MOSKALUK

CONNECT WITH SHEANNE:
INSTAGRAM: @INDIANROCKVEGANS
FACEBOOK: INDIAN ROCK VEGANS
YOUTUBE: INDIAN ROCK VEGANS

Sheanne Moskaluk and her husband, Dan, were featured in the documentary, Eating You Alive, after both experienced dramatic changes in their health. Switching to a plant-based diet not only led to Sheanne losing 130 pounds, but is the reason the couple cites for Dan winning his battle with stage 4 kidney cancer. Now the couple actively advocates for animal rights, plant-based eating education, and shares their passion for plant-based living through their social media accounts with hopes to inspire others into action.

WHAT ARE YOUR DAILY RITUALS/HABITS WHICH YOU BELIEVE HAVE BEEN KEY TO YOUR HEALTH?

Eating whole plants and drinking lots of water! It's so simple that people tend not to believe the immense and life-changing power of these two rituals. We've become so conditioned by society to believe that we need a technological advance or new scientific discovery to improve or regain our health when actually all we need to do is simplify our food choices to what we evolved to eat – plants. I also walk for an hour a day, at least five times a week.

AT WHAT POINT IN YOUR LIFE DID YOU DECIDE TO CHANGE YOUR DIET? HOW HAS THAT DECISION IMPACTED YOUR LIFE?

Our teenage son joined a gym in the Fall of 2010. He was told that he would never be able to gain muscle without a protein supplement. So, like a good mother, off to the health food store, I went to buy one of those giant tubs of whey protein with the paragraphs of ingredients. While I was browsing the selection, a sales clerk asked whom I was buying it for. She leaned in and quietly whispered, "you need to do some research before you give that to your son." How intriguing.....

I didn't buy the powder, but instead immediately went home to Google, "whey protein." To my good fortune, a YouTube video by Dr. John McDougall popped up titled "The perils of dairy." Dr. McDougall spoke of something completely contrary to anything I'd ever heard or thought I knew about dairy. It absolutely fascinated me, and I began seeking out the work of other physicians and researchers including Doctors Dean Ornish, Caldwell Esselstyn, Michael Greger, Neal Barnard, and so many others. I admit that I became obsessed with the topic. How could I have lived for 46 years having never heard this information before? It was like finding out there was a parallel universe.

The quintessential moment came after reading Dr. T. Colin Campbell's book, The China Study. I realized then that I could no longer continue to feed my family or myself the standard American diet in the manner that I had been. I then adopted a plant-based vegan lifestyle on April 1st, 2011. I cleaned out my fridge, freezer, and cupboards of all animal products and processed foods and began what would be a life-changing journey.

WHAT THINGS HAVE MADE THE BIGGEST IMPACT ON YOUR WEIGHT LOSS? WHAT THINGS DID YOU CHANGE AND HOW LONG DID IT TAKE BEFORE YOU NOTICED CHANGES IN YOUR BODY?

I had struggled with my weight beginning in my early 20s. Like so many women, I gained weight with each pregnancy. I tried every weight loss program out there including, Weight Watchers, Jenny Craig, Nutrisystem, and even Atkins. I would lose some weight while on the program at great financial expense, but as soon as I returned to eating the standard American diet, the weight would return plus some.

By the Fall of 2010, I weighed 300 pounds. I had given up on losing weight and had resigned myself to a lifetime of obesity. I was a spectator in my family's life. I watched from the sidelines while my husband played with our children or took them swimming. I was unable to participate in so many family activities.

So, imagine my surprise when I lost 15 pounds effortlessly the first month of adopting a plant-based vegan diet, all while eating till I was full and satisfied. Granted, the learning curve was huge. There were many epic meal fails, and I often wasn't sure what I would feed my family for the next meal. But, as time passed, it got easier and easier. Now I have as large a repertoire of recipes as I did in the past, perhaps even larger.

The more water I drank daily, the more weight I would lose. The bigger the mountain of veggies I ate, the more weight I would lose. At the beginning, I would easily lose four or five pounds a week. I felt like I was melting! And all without counting calories or points or any other gimmicks – just by eating plants!

WHAT WAS YOUR DOCTOR'S REACTION AFTER ANNOUNCING YOUR PLANS TO FOLLOW A PLANT-BASED DIET? WAS HE/SHE SUPPORTIVE?

After reading many books written by doctors, I have come to learn that nutrition is not taught in medical school. If it is, it's mentioned in passing.

137

I did not include my family physician in my decision to adopt a plant-based vegan diet, as I was not on any medication. Initially, my doctor was fairly neutral stating, "well, it seems to be working for you," but never really giving an opinion. As he witnessed my continued success, improved blood work, and my ability to keep the weight off for many years, he has become much more supportive and has begun to suggest a plant-based diet to any patients struggling with their weight, as well as to his diabetic patients. I believe he has also taken steps in his own personal life to make changes in his diet.

However, over the years, I have dealt with many who have been less supportive. I've been told by several that food doesn't matter or that it's all about carbohydrates. Some have even promoted a paleo or keto diet, further confirming the general lack of knowledge regarding the optimal diet for human health.

AFTER ADOPTING A PLANT-BASED DIET, HOW LONG DID IT TAKE BEFORE YOU STARTED TO LOSE WEIGHT AND HOW MUCH WEIGHT HAVE YOU LOST?

What began as a plant-based vegan diet, soon evolved into a more whole-food plant-based lifestyle as I further educated myself on the topic of nutrition. I eliminated many of the vegan transition foods, reserving them for holidays and special occasions, and focused on "as grown" food, and it worked! Over the next two years, I lost 133 pounds. After struggling for most of my adult life with weight, I finally understood what it was like to be in control.

HAS THERE BEEN ANY OTHER BENEFITS (APART FROM WEIGHT LOSS) FROM YOUR VEGAN/PLANT-BASED DIET? HAVE YOU FOUND THIS DIET DIFFICULT?

The benefits of adopting a plant-based lifestyle have been immense and far-reaching. I made the change purely for health as opposed to specifically weight loss. The weight loss was a lovely "side effect", and I was thrilled to have regained my vitality, confidence and youth.

But that was just the beginning…

My husband Dan was eating plant-based about 95% of the time when he was at home, but he was still eating animal products and processed junk when he was with friends or at work. In his mid-forties, Dan was checking off all the boxes for metabolic syndrome – high blood pressure, cholesterol, triglycerides, etc. He had all the symptoms that lead to an increased risk of heart disease, stroke and diabetes. By eating a plant-based diet, Dan was able to reverse all of those symptoms.

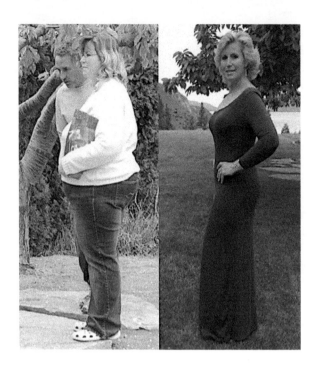
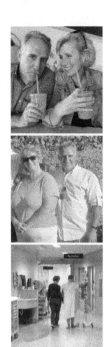

Then, in November of 2013, Dan was diagnosed with Stage 4 renal cell carcinoma. His right kidney was one massive tumor, and the tumor was growing up his vena cava towards his heart and lungs. The cancer had also metastasized to local and distant lymph nodes. We were told that Dan probably had months to two years maximum to live.

Dan had his kidney removed on Christmas Eve of 2013.

The surgeons were able to remove many affected lymph nodes and extract the tumor from the vena cava.

Renal cell carcinoma does not respond to chemotherapy or radiation, so the only hope we were given was the possibility of being accepted to a phase one trial study of an immunotherapy drug. When we asked that it be noted in Dan's file that he was plant-based, we were told that it didn't matter and that nobody cared what we ate. The only question remotely linked to food was, "how's your appetite?"

He was to have the initial treatments every three weeks and then every two weeks for the rest of his life. We were told that these drugs boost the immune system but that it was like "letting the tiger out of the cage." We couldn't be sure what it might attack." And attack it did! After the third treatment, the drugs targeted Dan's liver in a near-fatal attack. He was immediately dismissed from the trial. We were told that we would be naïve to think that the cancer would not grow and spread.

During this time, I continued with what I called "our program of nutritional excellence" focusing on tons of greens and veggies, fruit, unbroken whole grains, legumes, nuts and seeds. I continued to research cancer and nutrition, discovering over one hundred years of data linking animal protein to cancer cell growth.

Dan was diagnosed in November 2013, had surgery on December 24th, 2013, was accepted into a phase 1 study in March of 2014 and was dismissed from the study in May of 2014, after a near-fatal attack. That was the last medical intervention Dan received. By Fall of 2014, his medical team used the word "remission." In the Spring of 2015, Dan's file was closed, as his cancer was radiologically undetectable. At the two-year mark, when his doctors had predicted Dan would most likely die, he went back to work full time. Dan has beaten a 5% survival rate to five years. He is not only surviving but thriving. A whole-food, plant-based lifestyle has changed my life and saved my husband's life.

Due to both of our health recoveries, we were included in the feature-length health documentary called Eating You Alive. We continue to educate people regarding the benefits of a whole-food plant-based lifestyle by speaking at screenings of the documentary, podcasts, VegFests, and other speaking engagements.

When you decide that this lifestyle is non-negotiable, it is never difficult to adhere to. The most difficult part is watching those around you suffer on the standard American diet.

DO YOU TAKE ANY SPECIAL SUPPLEMENTS OR POTIONS? MENTION ANY SPECIFIC BRANDS YOU USE AND WHY YOU THINK THESE HAVE BENEFITED YOU AND YOUR HEALTH.

The only supplements I take are B12 once a week or so as a precaution and D3 during the winter since we live in Canada and are not exposed to a lot of sunshine during the winter months. Supplements are not a substitution for an abundance of fruit, veggies, whole grains, legumes, nuts, and seeds. I believe food is first and foremost the most important element for optimal health

WHAT ARE THE TWO OR THREE THINGS YOU HAVE DONE DIFFERENTLY WITH YOUR LIFE AFTER YOU LOST ALL OF YOUR UNWANTED WEIGHT?

Everything about my life has changed! To pick two or three things would be nearly impossible. Externally, I've taken years off of my appearance, fit back into my wedding dress, and have a wardrobe that reflects my personality rather than clothes that were purchased solely because they were the only ones that fit. I can participate in any activity I want now, perhaps not skillfully, but I'm out there!

Internally, I am so different. I am braver, I am more confident, and I stand up for what I believe in. I speak in front of large crowds with ease, and I am passionate about not letting another person needlessly suffer, emotionally or physically.

ANY INSPIRING STORIES THAT HAVE HAPPENED TO YOU OR PEOPLE CLOSE TO YOU THAT HAVE NOT BEEN COVERED ABOVE. STORIES THAT CAN HELP OTHERS.

I transitioned to a plant-based lifestyle for health. As a result, I lost 133 pounds, and my husband survived stage 4 kidney cancer.

Throughout this transformation, I have continued to educate myself by earning my Plant-Based Nutrition Certificate from the T. Colin Campbell Centre for Nutrition Studies and eCornell University. I've attended the International Plant-Based Nutrition Healthcare Conference and have enrolled in numerous health summits. A deeper understanding has further galvanized my commitment and resolve to not only follow a WFPB lifestyle but to also assist others in adopting this lifestyle.

It was during this time that I fully began to understand how animals actually arrive on our plate and the impact of animal agriculture on the environment. I was shocked that I had lived 46 years consuming animal products, without truly realizing the suffering and misery these sentient beings endured only to, in turn, cause us suffering and misery.

141

Daily, scientists from around the globe are warning of the catastrophic consequences of climate change, much of which can be attributed to animal agriculture. It also contributes to cancer, heart disease and diabetes, all of which have reached epidemic levels, threatening to bankrupt our healthcare systems and topple our economies.

With this awakening, my husband and I have evolved into WFPB health advocates and animal rights activists. Dan has just retired after a 33.5-year career as a police officer with the Royal Canadian Mounted Police, the last ten of which he was a media spokesperson. We work together to help people transition to a plant-based lifestyle, to raise awareness about the plight of farmed animals and their impact on the environment.

Never in my wildest dreams would I have ever imagined that at 55-years-old I would be attending and speaking at animal rights rallies and protests, and participating in marches and street activism. I never thought I would be invited to a Hollywood documentary premiere for a film that I, my husband and Samuel L. Jackson are all castmates in. Or that I'd be speaking on the Holistic Holiday at Sea cruise in the Caribbean or so many other amazing experiences. It's all because I decided to change what was on my fork.

AMBER NICOLE

CONNECT WITH AMBER:
INSTAGRAM: @MCAMMERTIME
FACEBOOK: AMBER NICOLE
YOUTUBE: MCAMMERTIME
ammertime.com

"I started eating WFPB in February 2018, and it was tough, but it's become a part of my life. My starting weight on a WFPBD diet in February was 200 pounds, highest was 285 lbs, and now, in April 2019, I am weighing in at 135 pounds...My weight loss started as soon as I changed from the ketogenic diet to a plant-based one, and I started to feel the effects straight away. My mind became clearer, my skin was soft and clear and I was feeling great. This truly is an amazing way to live, and I will never go back."

Amber Nicole has gained attention across social media platforms as a plant-based advocate who has shared her weight loss journey and how she lost over 150 pounds in a little over one year. Amber is also known as a popular gamer on the Twitch gaming platform and won a qualifying tournament with Twitch Prime Amazon at an event playing PUBG. She was able to play with celebrities such as Ashek, Shroud, Dr. Disrespect, Deadmau5, and Kevin Smith, and was featured in the magazine, RYZE UP.

WHAT ARE YOUR DAILY RITUALS/HABITS WHICH YOU BELIEVE HAVE BEEN KEY TO YOUR HEALTH?

I wake up every morning to an inspirational song. I have quotes on my mirror that remind me to stay humble and change the world and that it starts with one.

Having a good mentality, staying organized and loving myself truly has been key to my health. With a strong foundation, I feel that I can truly find success in all of my goals.

Meal plans and exercise definitely contribute as well, but in order to make that happen, I have to have a good outlook on it and be positive. I'm all about building a healthy foundation to grow from.

AT WHAT POINT IN YOUR LIFE DID YOU DECIDE TO CHANGE YOUR DIET? HOW HAS THAT DECISION IMPACTED YOUR LIFE?

142

I changed my life after a suicide attempt in 2016. I decided to change to a whole-food, plant-based vegan diet in 2018 to truly take on what was best for my body and the environment. I overcame my fears by embracing them and realizing that it takes failure to truly thrive.

WHAT THINGS HAVE MADE THE BIGGEST IMPACT ON YOUR WEIGHT LOSS? WHAT THINGS DID YOU CHANGE AND HOW LONG DID IT TAKE BEFORE YOU NOTICED CHANGES IN YOUR BODY?

The biggest thing that impacted my weight loss was good mental health. It's what separated all the other times I attempted to lose weight and failed. I succeeded in weight loss this time because I changed my outlook to be more healthy and loving. Having true and good reasons for wanting to make the change is what made the difference.

I noticed changes after the first couple of months, but it was after six months that I started to see the muscle come in, and it was the best feeling.

AFTER ADOPTING A PLANT-BASED DIET, HOW LONG DID IT TAKE BEFORE YOU STARTED TO LOSE WEIGHT AND HOW MUCH WEIGHT HAVE YOU LOST?

My journey took one year.

I lost 150 pounds starting from August 2017 to August 2018.

I followed a ketogenic diet from August 2017 to January 2018. I started at 285 pounds. The ketogenic diet is a high protein and no or low carb meat diet. Following this program I lost weight, but eventually I stalled. This is also a diet that makes you more prone to high cholesterol, high blood pressure, cancer, and many other health concerns. Once I cut out meat and dairy, I definitely broke my stall with a vengeance. I also started to build more muscle and feel more healthy overall.

With meat and cheese in my diet, I felt sick and stressed all the time. I didn't even know it until I fully cut it out and started to feel the strong positive effects of a whole-food, plant-based diet.

I started eating WFPB in February 2018 and am still eating this way. My starting weight on a WFPBD diet in February was 200 pounds, and now, in April 2019, I am weighing in at 135 pounds.

My weight loss started as soon as I changed from the ketogenic diet to a plant-based one, and I started to feel the effects straight away. My mind became clearer, my skin was soft and clear, and I was feeling great. This truly is an amazing way to live.

HAS THERE BEEN ANY OTHER BENEFITS (APART FROM WEIGHT LOSS) FROM YOUR VEGAN/PLANT-BASED DIET? HAVE YOU FOUND THIS DIET DIFFICULT?

Yes, many other benefits! I feel cleaner, my skin is nicer, and it helps manage my MTHFR mutation gene. The MTHFR mutation gene (compound heterozygous) basically means it's hard for my body to detoxify processed food, chemicals and folic acid. So switching to a whole-food plant-based diet has worked wonders for my body. It was a bit difficult making the change at first, but it got better with time and research.

DO YOU TAKE ANY SPECIAL SUPPLEMENTS OR POTIONS? MENTION ANY SPECIFIC BRANDS YOU USE AND WHY YOU THINK THESE HAVE BENEFITED YOU AND YOUR HEALTH.

I take a multivitamin and B12 vitamin. The multivitamin is called Seeking Health Chewable Optimal Multivitamin.

WHAT ARE THE TWO OR THREE THINGS YOU HAVE DONE DIFFERENTLY WITH YOUR LIFE AFTER YOU LOST ALL OF YOUR UNWANTED WEIGHT?

1. I've become an actress and am comfortable in front of the camera.
2. I'm running a tough mudder and will eventually run a marathon.
3. I'm so much happier and putting myself out there. I stay very physical and appreciate not being out of breath while walking upstairs.

I love the challenge and want to keep going!

ANY INSPIRING STORIES THAT HAVE HAPPENED TO YOU OR PEOPLE CLOSE TO YOU THAT HAVE NOT BEEN COVERED ABOVE. STORIES THAT CAN HELP OTHERS.

I've done quite a few things in my life that I feel can be inspiring.

I'd love to talk about mental health awareness and how my hate for myself and suicide attempt changed my life.

I also am a huge believer in making your dreams a reality no matter how big and impossible they may seem.

ERIN GREENER

CONNECT WITH ERIN:
INSTAGRAM: @ELGREENER
FACEBOOK: ERIN GREENER

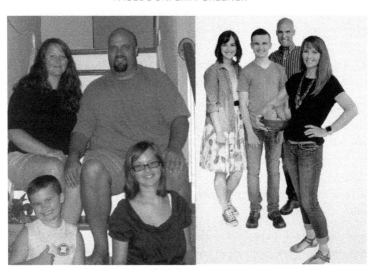

After a cancer diagnosis, Erin's family went plant-based and collectively lost over 335 pounds... from the standard American diet, multiple health concerns including a husband facing thyroid cancer, to a diet comprised of predominantly plants, Erin Greener has discovered the power of eating fruits and vegetables. After switching to a plant-based diet Erin and her husband, Justin, lost over 300 pounds combined, and are now enjoying a more healthful and vibrant life.

"We also noticed changes in the health of our two kids, Hannah and Hayden. Not only did our kids' concentration and grades improve, their moods became more level, Hannah's acne cleared up, Hayden's eczema healed, and Hannah lost around 15 pounds, while Hayden lost 20 pounds. Ever since we switched to plant-based, every year has been more rewarding than the last with more physical activity, family adventures and improved quality of foods in our diet."

WHAT ARE YOUR DAILY RITUALS/HABITS WHICH YOU BELIEVE HAVE BEEN KEY TO YOUR HEALTH?

A daily routine for me seems to be seasonal. I enjoy starting the day with a walk when the weather is nice. When it is colder out, I love doing yoga.

AT WHAT POINT IN YOUR LIFE DID YOU DECIDE TO CHANGE YOUR DIET? HOW HAS THAT DECISION IMPACTED YOUR LIFE?

My inspiration was my husband. He was super obese with many health problems and got diagnosed with thyroid cancer. I was also very obese with many aches and pains and we suffered from sleep apnea, chronic pain, eczema and migraines. We watched the documentary, Forks Over Knives, and it changed our lives forever. The way we view food and eating now is so different from what it used to be and I love it.

WHAT THINGS HAVE MADE THE MOST DIFFERENCE IN YOUR ABILITY TO LIVE A GOOD LIFE AFTER LIVING WITH OR CURING YOUR DISEASE?

Having our whole family (our children made the transition with us) make the transition to a whole-food, plant-based diet was the best thing we did. We were all in it together and held each other accountable. We experimented with our favorite dishes and learned how to turn them plant-based. The changes came quickly. I began to notice my energy increasing almost straight away. I started losing weight quickly, and all of my aches and pains were gradually disappearing.

We also noticed changes in the health of our two kids, Hannah and Hayden. Not only did our kids' concentration and grades improve, their moods became more level, Hannah' s acne cleared up, and Hayden's eczema healed. Hannah lost around 15 pounds, and Hayden lost 20 pounds. They were clearly thriving on this new plant-based lifestyle. We all were!

WHAT WAS YOUR DOCTOR'S REACTION AFTER ANNOUNCING YOUR PLANS TO FOLLOW A PLANT-BASED DIET? WAS HE/SHE SUPPORTIVE?

For me, my doctor was very neutral and on the verge of being not supportive. In fact, I did not even discuss it in great depth with her, as it did not seem that she was much of an advocate of this way of eating.

After some time had passed and after I had lost the weight, I went for a check-up. She actually thought I had lost too much weight and was worried about my health. She sent me to get blood work done, and when the results came back she was very pleased with everything, and I was super healthy! That's when she told me to keep up the good work.

AFTER ADOPTING A PLANT-BASED DIET HOW LONG DID IT TAKE BEFORE FIRST, YOU STARTED TO FEEL BETTER, AND SECOND, YOU KNEW YOU WERE NOT GOING TO LET THIS WIN?

I transitioned into this diet over a few months and became fully plant-based after three months. I lost 100 pounds in about a year and my husband

Justin lost over 200 pounds! This March will be our seven-year anniversary of going plant-strong, and we will never look back. It is so easy once you find new dishes and habits to replace your old ones with.

HAS THERE BEEN ANY OTHER BENEFITS (APART FROM WEIGHT LOSS) FROM YOUR VEGAN/PLANT-BASED DIET? HAVE YOU FOUND THIS DIET DIFFICULT?

Many! No more headaches, (endometriosis) cysts shrunk, more vibrant skin, higher levels of energy and improved quality of life all around.

For me, the most difficult part was finding dishes that were easy to make and still tasted good. But, one by one, we cut out dairy, oil and meat from our diet. We found other dishes that we liked and soon our tastes changed. The last part of the transition was our kids' lunches at school. The total transition took three months. There are also so many more options now and recipes available for free online that make the transition easier than ever before.

DO YOU TAKE ANY SPECIAL SUPPLEMENTS OR POTIONS? MENTION ANY SPECIFIC BRANDS YOU USE AND WHY YOU THINK THESE HAVE BENEFITED YOU AND YOUR HEALTH.

I take a teaspoon of turmeric (with fine ground black pepper) with fresh orange juice every morning. Turmeric is anti-inflammatory and will help fight off disease.

WHAT ARE THE TWO OR THREE THINGS YOU HAVE DONE DIFFERENTLY WITH YOUR LIFE AFTER YOUR HEALTH GOT BETTER?

Having lost the weight, we have really begun to cultivate a love of travel and being outdoors. We are currently living in the UK and are loving exploring areas around us as well as traveling to other countries. We have become plant-based travelers, making our lifestyle work while we explore and travel.

We spend so much more time together as a family. This lifestyle change did bring us all closer. We've become more active and do more activities together. We have even started having family movie nights together to watch documentaries about plant-based lifestyles like Forks Over Knives, Food Inc., and Vegucated. I think this is so important in order to help us stay on track and keep reminding ourselves why we live this lifestyle.

Ever since we switched to plant-based eating, every year has been more rewarding than the last with more physical activity, family adventures and improved quality of foods in our diet. We truly are a happier and healthier family for making the switch.

ENJUNAYA CANTON

CONNECT WITH ENJUNAYA:
INSTAGRAM: @GLOWGIRLWELLNESS
ZuhuriBeauty.com

"My struggles included: irritable bowel syndrome, yeast infections, hemorrhoids, migraine headaches, fibroids, viral infections, depression, severe PMS and heavy flow, extreme sweating without cause, and the constant chafing of my legs. These are just a few of the painful memories I have from being overweight.

I recall lamenting to a woman at a coffee shop about my fibroids and feeling extremely emotionally unstable while on my menstrual cycle. I also shared with her how it seemed that every time my cycle came, I would also get hemorrhoids and a yeast infection. The multitude of problems all at once was horrible to predict and manage. I was willing to do anything to stop years of emotional and physical torment."

She asked me what I ate on a regular basis. In retrospect, it was the S.A.D. (standard American diet), with high consumption of processed and junk food. In the morning I had coffee and either a fast-food breakfast sandwich or a muffin. For lunch, I loved burritos, fried fish, or chicken, along with some french fries. For dinner, I had baked chicken or fish with a heavy cream sauce and some sort of starch. I only drank water when I felt dehydrated.

This woman also asked about my sleeping habits and my social life. I explained to her that I typically slept five to seven hours per night and had a very active social life. I dated a lot. I dined out a lot. I went to a nightclub or a bar at least three times a week. I also had self-destructive habits like smoking cigars, having unprotected sex on occasion, and inhaling second-hand cigarette and marijuana smoke. She calmly explained to me how my diet and lifestyle were creating a toxic environment in my body, leading to so many health problems.

Initially, it was very hard to digest what she was saying because we were of different races and backgrounds. Even though at that time, I was a practicing psychotherapist with a background in human development, I was not open to believing what worked for her and her peers could work for me. I was, however, at my wit's end, and I began to do my own research.

Her quick analysis of each of my symptoms and their connection with food was overwhelming and eye-opening. To know that California's Proposition 65 provided a list of chemicals in foods that cause cancer, birth defects, and neurological problems it was amazing. This proposition makes it mandatory that fast food franchises display a sign that says that certain foods they sell contain acrylamide, and can cause cancer within fetuses, children and adults.

After my initial conversation with this woman, I slowly included her recommendations into my diet. She encouraged me to stop eating animal protein, as well as to follow these guidelines:

· Avoid processed foods or any food that has a label. A label means that more than one ingredient was used to make that food. If you can't pronounce an ingredient on a label, don't put that food in your shopping basket.
· Eliminate refined sugar. Refined sugar provides nothing but calories.
· Eat five or six small meals a day. By eating smaller meals throughout the day you can help speed up your metabolism.
· Cook your own meals.
· Combine protein with carbs. This simple act will fuel your body and mitigate hunger pangs.

For someone who never went grocery shopping, never cooked and never read labels before, this was HARD.

149

I started with eating salads that were mostly comprised of dark, green, leafy vegetables, with other non-starchy vegetables, dressed with juice from a lemon, lime and/or orange. I ate salads all day for about a week and was drinking 64 ounces of water per day. The thought of drinking half of my body weight in ounces of water was very farfetched in the beginning, but I was starting to see I could do it.

To my surprise, I lost five pounds that week. I had tried losing weight through many programs in the past, including Weight Watchers, but I realized that I only ended up losing a certain amount of weight before I quickly regained it. I realized that Weight Watchers was about calorie counting and point counting. It did not teach how one should eat a nutrient-dense diet. It also was not designed to take into account my own unique conditions.

I began adding nuts, apples, berries and tofu to my diet. To avoid hormonal effects from tofu, I began buying organic and sprouted tofu and fermented soy products like tempeh. For some time, I did eat "clean" chicken, cage-free eggs and some fish, but I stopped as I became more conscious about animals. I realized that I could provide myself with all the nutrients society says you can only get from animals, but solely through plant-based products.

" "

IN TWO MONTHS I HAD LOST ABOUT 20 POUNDS AND FELT MYSELF BECOMING A NEW PERSON. PEOPLE COMMENTED ABOUT MY SKIN AND HOW MY FACE WAS SO MUCH SMALLER. I NO LONGER HAD ACNE, NOR DARK CIRCLES UNDER MY EYES. MY DIGESTIVE SYSTEM HAD DRASTICALLY IMPROVED, AND I'D STOPPED SWEATING PROFUSELY.

ENJUNAYA CANTON

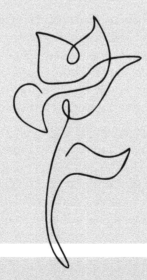

Today a typical day would start with a hemp protein shake (Nurtiv Hemp Protein, organic mixed greens, a small number of frozen pineapples with water or almond milk) or gluten-free waffles with almond butter and an apple. For a snack, I would have a handful or two of cashews, walnuts, almonds or pumpkin seeds. For lunch either a curried pea, mung bean and tempeh dish with hemp protein, or a large salad. Another favorite is a tempeh burger on a gluten-free bun with sweet potato fries or a small salad. An afternoon snack would be a green superfood drink and/or fruit. Dinner would be something like a vegetable curried gluten-free spaghetti. I also drink at least 100 ounces of water, often infused with ginger and lemon as well as liquid chlorophyll. I often drink tea made of lemon, ginger, turmeric, and cayenne powder. I also eat a lot of raw foods and soups.

Before my lifestyle change I exercised off and on during my diets, but it did not seem like it helped. This time, I began walking on the treadmill. As I continued to lose weight and gained more energy, I moved onto the elliptical machine, the stair master and classes. I got so addicted to exercising that I would work out twice a day and take challenging classes back to back. I also picked up yoga, hiking and activities I never imagined I would love.

In two months, I had lost about 20 pounds and felt myself becoming a new person. People commented about my skin and how my face was so much smaller. I no longer had acne, nor dark circles under my eyes. My digestive system had drastically improved, and I'd stopped sweating profusely. As I began to see improvements in my body, I completely stopped drinking alcohol, smoking and became much more selective with who I dated. I had an epiphany about how badly I had been treating myself and how I absolutely had to be the one to take care of me. I realized that if I did not take care of myself, nobody would.

I was transforming in ways that became isolating. I no longer hung out with people who I was friends with for a large part of my life. I had to decide how to handle my problems without alcohol, and I was now the "oddball" of my family and with my peers. I also made the very challenging decision of ending my career as a psychotherapist. I realized that I was not the best person I could be for that job. Though to this day, I am a mentor to many of the young women I was honored to serve as their therapist, but I realized I had developed a passion in the transformation I was going through and that I wanted to teach people how to finally lose the weight (physically, emotionally, and mentally) for good.

In only 3-4 months, I lost a significant amount of weight, and I also eliminated the majority of my health problems, including fibroids. My emotions are stable. My digestive system is healthy. I have not had a

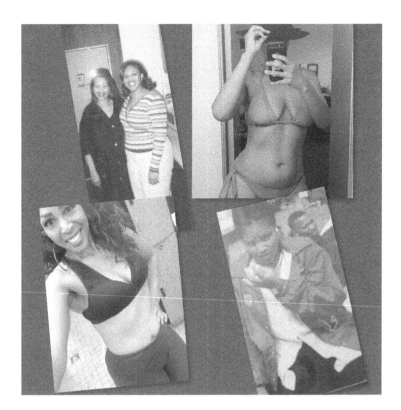

yeast infection or hemorrhoids, and I have not been sick with a cold or a
virus in years. I do not have PMS or challenges with my cycle anymore, and
my legs do not chaff. I have gone from a size 20-22 to a size 8. I have no
stretched skin and a small number of stretch marks. I am still in awe
of the person I have become and who I am becoming.

I have been teaching people how to eat clean as an Eat Right Get Fit
Coach for the past five years. I tell each of my clients every day that the
hardest part is maintenance. There is still the person who I was the majority
of my life inside of me having temper tantrums about why we can't do
what we used to do. I quiet that voice inside of me and remind myself of
the pain I endured as that person, and I REFUSE to ever go back there
again. I tell my clients that being healthy can be very isolating and you
have to decide what is more important. The choice, for me, is very simple.
I choose to live and not die.

BRANDI LEE

CONNECT WITH BRANDI:
INSTAGRAM: @BRANDILEESLIFESTYLE

"I had a very severe binge-eating disorder and bulimia, so it wasn't until I discovered plant-based eating that I really started to make a positive change and heal myself from these disorders. This is when I started to make more of a connection with my food and actually care what was going into my body. I actually started to crave healthy foods versus unhealthy foods."

WHAT ARE YOUR DAILY RITUALS/HABITS WHICH YOU BELIEVE HAVE BEEN KEY TO YOUR HEALTH?

For me, out of all the money I've ever invested into my health, I would say that the most life-changing was my Kangen water ionizer. It's one of the healthiest things that you can have in your daily regime. I'm someone who is into more alkaline, whole, plant-based foods, and it just makes sense to have alkalized water as well. They are expensive machines, but they are well worth it, especially after doing the research into the benefits of alkalinity in the body.

AT WHAT POINT IN YOUR LIFE DID YOU DECIDE TO CHANGE YOUR DIET? HOW HAS THAT DECISION IMPACTED YOUR LIFE? WHAT IS YOUR GO-TO FOOD TO FUEL YOUR BODY?

I started to try diets when I was 11 or 12 years old because I actually was very fat, almost classified as obese by my doctor. They told me that I had to go on a diet, so at that age, I had a very calorie-restrictive diet that was super unhealthy, but I was able to lose weight. After that, I was always aware of dieting, but I wasn't aware of a plant-based/vegan diet until I was in my teens (I am 21-years-old now), and that's when I decided to make a change.

Plant-based eating has really allowed me to follow my true passions in life: to travel the world and spread health, wealth, love, and happiness.

WHO HAS BEEN THE BIGGEST PLANT-BASED INFLUENCER IN YOUR LIFE AND HOW HAVE THEY HELPED YOU?

To be honest, I didn't really have any plant-based influence in my life. My very first boyfriend at age 15 or 16 put the idea of more plant-based and organic eating into my head, but at the time, I thought he was crazy

153

and weird for using "all-natural" products. Eventually, I started to really understand where he was coming from and realize that it made a lot of sense to use more natural products.

However, when I eventually committed myself to eat a plant-based vegan diet, I did so by being my own inspiration. I really took some time to reflect on why I was choosing this lifestyle, and reminded myself of this anytime I was close to slipping up. Really getting clear on the reason why I was doing what I was doing helped me commit to veganism.

HOW DO YOU THINK WE CAN ALL HAVE A BIGGER IMPACT ON INFLUENCING PEOPLE AND HELPING THEM MAKE THE CONNECTION TO HEALTH AND EATING A PLANT-BASED DIET?

This is really easy to answer: lead by example. What I mean by this is not forcing this idea and this lifestyle onto people. This is so important, and it's something that I didn't really realize until recently. You really just have to lead by example. Focus on yourself, and then let the other people follow you. If you keep bringing them to vegan restaurants, eventually they will start to change their minds. You have to take it one step at a time.

IF YOU COULD HAVE A GIGANTIC BILLBOARD ANYWHERE WITH ANYTHING ON IT, WHAT WOULD IT SAY?

A quote by Doctor Sebi (who advocated for the alkaline diet) that says, "A healthy body is worth more than any dollar amount. You don't want to be the wealthiest person on a hospital bed."

HOW HAS A FAILURE, OR APPARENT FAILURE, SET YOU UP FOR LATER SUCCESS? DO YOU HAVE A "FAVORITE FAILURE" OF YOURS?

In regards to my health, the biggest failure I faced was when I initially went vegan. When I first went vegan, I went cold turkey. I didn't prepare. I was vegetarian for about two weeks and thought it was easy, so I decided I'd try going vegan because it would be easy too. After a few days, I noticed that I started to feel sort of starved. It was because I didn't really know what to eat.

At first, the diet felt very restrictive and having struggled with binge eating it made my disorders worse initially. Because of this, I stopped eating vegan for a while, which felt like a huge failure after I had already told so many people that I was going vegan. I didn't want to tell everyone (friends, family, social media, etc) that I was going to take a break from veganism, but I needed to because I was pretending to be vegan while binging non-vegan food when I was alone.

How this set me up for success is by helping me understand patience and the importance of slowly easing into the vegan diet. At the time, this "failure" in adopting a vegan diet felt devastating, but it actually led me to create a better plan of action the next time around. It helped me become stronger and not care what others thought of me as much. This is also something I discuss in my course on the SkillShare platform about how to transition to a vegan diet. The main thing to keep in mind is patience.

When I went back to the vegan diet, I was so much more prepared and had already learned from the multiple mistakes I made the first time around. This time I slowly cut things out of my diet, which made transitioning much easier. After fully transitioning back into a vegan diet, this approach has also helped ease me out of eating things like gluten and sugar, so in the end, I'm very grateful for my initial "failure."

WHAT VEGAN RESOURCE COULD YOU NOT LIVE WITHOUT AND WHY?

This may sound a bit cheesy/selfish, but I would say my own "why," as I mentioned above as well. I do not rely on influencers, books, or documentaries to motivate me to continue what I'm doing. Having my own vision board and having a very powerful "why" (my purpose for being vegan), is really what gives me motivation and reminds me why I initially started eating vegan in the first place. Without this, I wouldn't be here answering these questions.

I think relying on myself and my own "why" in this way has allowed me to become more confident in regards to sharing my own story and leading by example, and showing people that no matter what they've gone through in the past, they can create a new beginning.

WHAT ADVICE WOULD YOU GIVE A SMART AND DRIVEN 18-YEAR-OLD TODAY? WHAT ADVICE SHOULD THEY IGNORE?

My biggest advice for people approaching young adulthood is to be patient. Everything good comes with patience, and I think with each new generation, patience seems to be diminishing because of the instant gratification that comes with social media and technology.

Advice to ignore is anyone putting doubt in your mind about the goals you have for yourself. I think that young people are vulnerable, especially when entering adulthood. It's so easy to be influenced by other people and have others instill doubt in you. Try to not let that influence you and distract you from your own goals and dreams.

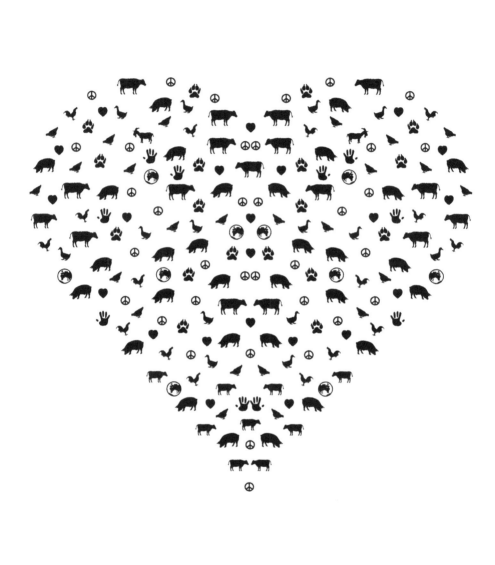

CHAPTER 3

ACTIVISM

INGRID NEWKIRK
CO-FOUNDER & PRESIDENT OF PETA

CONNECT WITH PETA:
INSTAGRAM: @PETA
FACEBOOK: OFFICIAL.PETA
peta.org

"When it comes to having a central nervous system and the ability to feel pain, hunger and thirst, a rat is a pig is a dog is a boy."

Ingrid Newkirk, who turned 70 in June 2019, is the founder and president of *People for the Ethical Treatment of Animals* (PETA), the world's largest animal rights organization. It could be argued that she will one day be remembered as the campaigner who did for animals what William Wilberforce did for slaves, Martin Luther King did for black Americans and Emmeline Pankhurst did for women's suffrage.

Ingrid has dedicated her entire adult life to her passionate mission, and in the 39 years since she launched Peta with four friends in the basement of her Maryland home, she has built her vision into the world's largest – and most controversial – animal rights organization.

PETA has grown to an astonishing 6.5 million members and supporters, with 480 full-time staff, an annual budget of $60m, a dozen offices around the world and a mantra that reads: "Animals are not ours to eat, wear, experiment on or use for entertainment."

AT WHAT AGE DID YOU DECIDE TO BECOME VEGAN AND WHY?

I became an animal cruelty officer and a deputy sheriff in the 1970s. I would investigate horrible abuse, but then return home to have roast chicken for dinner. One day, I investigated a case of an abandoned farm where the animals had been left to starve.

One small piglet was still alive, so I scooped him up and cradled him in my arms. I helped him to sip water, as he couldn't hold his own head up. While driving home that night, I suddenly remembered that I had defrosted some pork chops for dinner. It hit me then. I was no better than the person who had neglected and abused this little piglet. I was paying for this to happen—just behind closed doors, where I couldn't witness the suffering. That little piglet caused me to change my diet, and I went

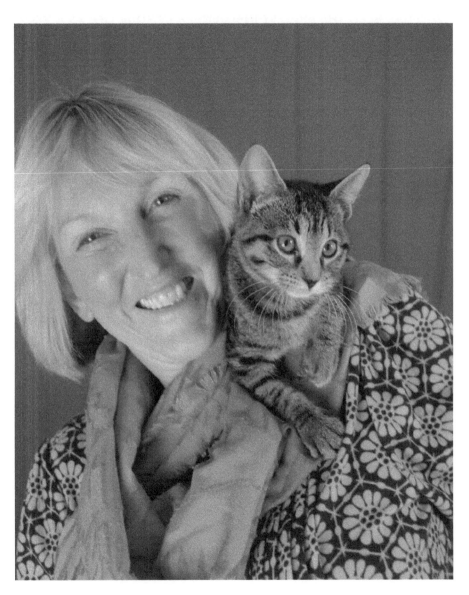

Chapter 3 | ACTIVISM

vegetarian. Later, someone challenged me, asking, "Why do you put milk in your tea?" and explained that calves are taken away from their mothers and killed for veal just so we can steal the milk meant for them. I was horrified and became vegan.

WHO HAS BEEN THE BIGGEST INFLUENCER IN YOUR LIFE AS A VEGAN AND WHY HAVE THEY HAD SUCH AN IMPACT ON YOU?

In my activism, I am inspired by Sojourner Truth, the black woman who, at a time when only white men had power in the U.S., stood up and spoke about civil rights, even when they burned down her boarding house, threw rocks at her and jeered. But what started opening my "animal rights eyes" was reading Animal Liberation by Peter Singer. I realized that in the same way that sexist and racist views allow people to discriminate against women and people of other races—to think of them as less intelligent and less capable—speciesism allows people to confer an inferior status on other animals (humans are not gods, of course—they are animals, too) and to regard them not as individuals with thoughts and feelings but as objects and means to fulfill our own selfish interests and desires. I gave copies of that book to everyone I knew. Coincidentally, at that very time, I was being honored as a Washingtonian of the Year for my work to create the country's first spay/neuter clinic and clean up the appalling city dog pound. During my speech, I spoke from the heart, quoting Animal Liberation, asking the audience to rethink their old habits (like eating the meat on the banquet tables where they sat), to be champions for animals rather than exploiters, and to embrace compassion, respect and understanding for the other species. That year, I cashed out my government retirement fund and used it to start PETA.

IN YOUR OPINION WHICH ACTIVIST IS HAVING THE BIGGEST IMPACT AND WHY DO YOU THINK THAT IS?

The animal rights movement is growing quickly all over the world, and so many wonderful people are doing things, saying things, creating vegan businesses, educating others, influencing companies and otherwise helping animals. It all counts. Ordinary people have become activists in China and are stopping dog-meat trucks; in Spain, people are entering the ring to stop bullfights; in France and Canada, activists are locking themselves inside pig pens in slaughterhouses; in the U.S., animal circuses are going out of business and people are passing laws to stop dogs from being kept chained up. Individuals are raising awareness by complaining to travel companies about the cruelty behind elephant rides and "tiger selfies," and activists in Petra are drawing attention to the plight of overworked donkeys, horses and camels. It takes everyone to do things all the time—and luckily, people are taking responsibility.

Social media has played a large part in giving activists a platform from which to share video footage as well as information on animal cruelty and the benefits of a vegan way of life, from what we eat to what we wear and buy to how we entertain ourselves. These days, investigators make available video evidence of the cruelty they've witnessed and it's reposted on sites to help awaken others' sensibilities and get them involved. Such footage holds the power to bring about positive change in industries and in people's habits.

The number of vegan activists reaching out to the public has dramatically increased, and there is a thriving animal rights community to get involved with. Grabbing the attention of the public is very often the work of many individuals. PETA's exposés are a good example of that. We could not achieve our victories without everyone who chips in.

DO YOU HAVE A FAVORITE ANIMAL AND DO YOU HAVE ANY STORIES ABOUT SHARING A CONNECTION WITH THAT ANIMAL OR ANY OTHER ANIMAL THAT YOU CAN SHARE?

When I was born, there was already a big dog in our family whose name was Shawny. He looked after me from babyhood, and so I grew up thinking of him as my big brother. We went everywhere together, and he slept in my bed or I slept in his basket, and we were both carsick at the same time! He and I knew all about each other and recognized if we were happy or sad, and so I didn't think of him as another species. Through him, I learned to relate to other species just as you might relate to a human. If you had told me you were going to eat him or wear his fur on your coat collar or cut him up to test a chemical, I would have been incredulous and would have fought for him as I fight for other animals today.

161

HOW DO YOU THINK WE CAN HAVE A BIGGER IMPACT ON INFLUENCING PEOPLE?

I value personal activism and believe that every single thing we do makes a difference. The more we do, the more difference we make—and the more quickly animal liberation from exploitation and torment will become a reality.

We can never underestimate the power behind the choices people make in what they choose to purchase. We need everyone to realize how powerful they are and know that if they chose to live as if they cared about animals and actively wished to prevent their suffering, all the corporations would stop producing the cruelly derived things that they now buy. Because everyone eats, washes their hair, puts on clothes, finds amusement in life and buys stuff, it is vital to start setting an example and encouraging others to follow.

So, I encourage everyone to talk to people, even strangers in the grocery store line! Find out their interests and what they care about or are concerned about. Perhaps it is the environment. Perhaps they have a sick relative with heart issues. They could be concerned about the world in which their children are growing up. Find an entry point and an issue they can relate to. Most people don't know how easy it is to change habits that hurt animals. As people become more aware of these issues, they become more serious about putting an end to them.

As advocates for animals, how we present ourselves is very important. Always be pleasant (force yourself if you have to)! If we come across as personable, approachable and helpful, it helps our cause. Being angry is not a clever or persuasive tactic, because the important thing is not how we feel, but what we accomplish.

Being prepared for any debate is vital. So arm yourself with facts along with a few statistics. Spend time each week reading up on animal issues. Never feel intimidated or that you aren't knowledgeable enough for a debate. If you don't know something, be honest and say that you will look into it. Offer to send them information later. After all, no one knows everything!

Lastly, stay motivated! Animals need us!

WHAT ARE SOME PLACES OR EVENTS THAT ARE HAPPENING THAT PEOPLE CAN GET INVOLVED WITH?

PETA has endless ideas for anyone who wants to help—regardless of their age, education, profession or interests. From passing out leaflets to going to demonstrations to giving a school talk or showing a video to a group, writing letters, contacting corporations and advertisers, seeking free services or offering hands-on animal rescue or foster help, the list of volunteer opportunities is endless. Call PETA or explore groups in your area.

Another great way to help is leafleting or tabling. Handing out leaflets to the public is a great way to inform people. Leave a trail of leaflets wherever you go—on the reading rack in your doctor's waiting room, at the laundromat, on the bus, in dressing rooms or anywhere else you're able to leave literature for the public.

IF YOU COULD GET EVERYONE TO SEE ONE FILM OR READ ONE BOOK THAT WOULD HELP MAKE THE CONNECTION, WHAT WOULD IT BE AND WHY?

I would ask everyone to watch Earthlings, starring Joaquin Phoenix. That is a life-changing, wonderful film. For one book, I'd recommend Making Kind Choices, a book that I wrote long ago and that is now available online for a

" "

FIND OUT THEIR
INTERESTS AND WHAT
THEY CARE ABOUT
OR ARE CONCERNED
ABOUT. PERHAPS IT IS
THE **ENVIRONMENT**.
PERHAPS THEY HAVE A
SICK RELATIVE WITH
HEART ISSUES. THEY
COULD BE CONCERNED
ABOUT **THE WORLD** IN
WHICH THEIR CHILDREN
ARE GROWING UP.
FIND AN ENTRY POINT
AND *AN ISSUE THEY
CAN RELATE TO.*

INGRID NEWKIRK

song. Both will help people realize that it is easy to treat animals kindly but that there's more. We have to stop exploiting and killing them—to recognize that they are other individuals like us who deserve respect and who feel pain, joy, love and fear. We must grasp the fact that human domination—speciesism—is a hideous thing that we must shake off, as we have no right to ignore the interests of others just because we fancy a taste of their flesh or want to steal their coats.

CAN YOU SHARE WITH US AN AFFIRMATION THAT YOU LIVE BY?

We are so lucky to have voices and opportunities, to have freedom and to be able to make choices, and we must use those gifts. It's a big task and a heavy burden at times, but we are often the only chance animals have. If something feels uncomfortable or inconvenient or even if it intimidates us, we must still speak up. Opera singer Beverly Sills once said, "You may be disappointed if you fail, but you are doomed if you don't try." Animals need us, and our duty as good people is to help them in every way we can think of.

WHAT IS THE BEST PIECE OF ADVICE YOU HAVE BEEN GIVEN THAT HAS CHANGED YOUR LIFE?

I was born in England, but I spent much of my childhood in India. My father worked as a navigational engineer, and my mother volunteered for Mother Teresa. I remember that as a young child, I rolled bandages for lepers on school breaks and stuffed dolls for the kids in the orphanage. My mother took in all sorts of human and nonhuman waifs and strays—she wouldn't slam the door on anyone who was hungry or ill. "It doesn't matter who suffers, but how," she said. She's the one who taught me that it isn't necessary to rank either humans or animals as more important—any more than it's necessary to kick a stray dog while going to feed a homeless person. All are deserving of our care, love and consideration.

CAN YOU PLEASE LIST SOME SANCTUARIES, CHARITIES, ORGANIZATIONS THAT YOU FEEL WE COULD SUPPORT. THERE ARE SO MANY AND SOMETIMES WE DON'T KNOW WHICH ONES ARE IN IT FOR THE RIGHT REASON'S, WE WOULD LOVE SOME GUIDANCE.

Unfortunately, a lot of zoos, "sanctuaries," and other animal attractions capitalize on tourists' growing demand to see and touch animals, and a lot of the time these facilities are anything but genuine havens. Always research before you travel! Just because a facility claims to be an "elephant orphanage" doesn't mean it actually is one. Ask yourself, "How come all these baby elephants are orphans? And how come there are adult elephants in chains?" Do they allow visitors to touch the animals? No reputable wild-

or exotic-animal sanctuary allows any kind of hands-on interaction, and that includes posing for photos with animals.

The Global Federation of Animal Sanctuaries accredits only genuine sanctuaries, so please always check before deciding to visit one. You can also always e-mail PETA to check.

ANY INSPIRING STORIES THAT HAVE HAPPENED TO YOU OR PEOPLE CLOSE TO YOU THAT HAVE NOT BEEN COVERED ABOVE. STORIES THAT CAN INSPIRE AND HELP OTHERS.

I am at the beach, and a child is excited because he and his friends have caught a fish in a little bucket. They carry the sloshing bucket up the sands to show the boy's family. I go over quickly and admire the fish, and then I say, "Oh, of course, you must put him back quickly, as he will be very scared already, and his own family will be wondering where he has gone. Shall we go and do that carefully now?" I am all smiles, and I wink at the mother as if she will be "in" on this. So off we go and gently release the fish back into the water. I praise the children for helping the fish and for admiring nature's beauty and leaving it in peace. There was no need to be worried about leaping into action to save the fish. People just hadn't thought that way and were accepting.

I don't just dream of a cruelty-free world in which no one will ignore the fact that all animals are flesh and blood like us, that they all have emotions, that they all feel fear and pain and love and joy and want to live, just as we do. I also try to do at least three things every single day that will help bring that about. Perhaps I leave a vegan starter kit (free from PETA) somewhere where people will read it (in a doctor's waiting room, in the seat back pocket on a train, in a magazine rack, or on a bulletin board) or hand it to someone, saying, "You might like this," and talk up some vegan food at a café, in a restaurant or in the grocery store. I may write a letter to the editor, call in to a radio show on an animal topic, give animal newsletters to students, put up a sticker where people can see it, show someone a link to an animal rights video, get friends and family to sign a petition, post things on social media or comment on tourist sites. I want to create a world in which people will pay attention to who animals are and what they need, and we can do it!

165

Thankfully, society is changing as we learn more about animals' awe-inspiring abilities and their feelings, which are just as acute as our own are. More than ever, people—particularly the young—are embracing animal-friendly ways of feeding, clothing and amusing themselves. It is up to everyone to do their part to ensure that the future will be a kinder place for animals. My new book, Animalkind (January 2020), is part of my work to open everyone's heart, eyes and mind.

NATASHA
(THAT VEGAN COUPLE)

CONNECT WITH NATASHA:
INSTAGRAM: @THAT_VEGAN_COUPLE
FACEBOOK: THAT VEGAN COUPLE
YOUTUBE: THAT VEGAN COUPLE
thatvegancouple.com

"Being vegan is the normal thing to do. Whilst eating and exploiting animals may have been normalized, it's not a normal behavior to socially accept the exploitation and needless slaughter of innocent beings... We influence people by making veganism and activism relatable to everyone. We have been to many activist events where families have brought their children, with older people standing right next to teenagers, and professional people in suits are next to hipsters. I believe that once the early majority see that there are people "just like them" who are openly vegan and serious about defending animals, we will see a greater social and cultural shift."

166

Natasha is one half of the influential website and social media accounts of That Vegan Couple. She and her husband, Luca, use their social media influence to inspire people not only to live vegan, but also to take action for animals.

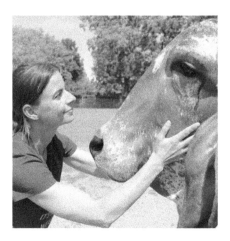
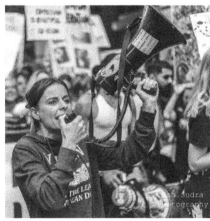

AT WHAT AGE DID YOU DECIDE TO BECOME VEGAN AND WHY?

I went vegan in 2011 at age 31. I decided to go vegan after watching Gary Yourofsky's, "Best Speech You Will Ever Hear" on YouTube. I had been a vegetarian for two and a half years before that, but I didn't fully understand the dairy and egg industries or all the other ways we exploit animals such as for clothing, entertainment, testing and the pet industry. Once Gary's speech connected the final dots for me, the decision to go vegan was easy.

WHO HAS BEEN THE BIGGEST INFLUENCER IN YOUR LIFE AS A VEGAN AND WHY HAVE THEY HAD SUCH AN IMPACT ON YOU? IN YOUR OPINION, WHICH ACTIVIST IS HAVING THE BIGGEST IMPACT ON THE WORLD AND WHY DO YOU THINK THAT IS?

I think the person who inspired me to become vegan has also been the biggest influence in my life as a vegan, so that's Gary Yourofsky. Gary speaks with such conviction and clarity that it's impossible to ignore. Love him or hate him; he will get and hold your attention. He also stays true to the message of animal liberation and doesn't water-down his message to make people feel comfortable - he says it like it is. This resonated strongly with me and has definitely influenced how I go about my activism.

As a new vegan, I remember emailing Gary for help with the typical problems a new vegan often faces. To my surprise, he responded! This blew me away ... someone with so much influence actually took the time to respond to new vegans. This set a great example and because of this, I try to respond to as many new vegan questions as possible.

Having said this, there have been many things and people who have influenced me over the years and who have had an impact on how I advocate for animals. For example, the book, The World Peace Diet - Eating for Spiritual Health and Social Harmony, influenced me greatly in terms of understanding how our culture of using and eating animals shapes our society on a very deep and profound level.

Most recently, I'm influenced by the incredible female activists in Australia who are leading direct actions and showing the animal rights movement what needs to be done in order to achieve maximum mainstream news coverage.

I don't think there is one activist who is having the biggest impact and that's because it takes all of us, advocating in all ways, to reach all people. The question is, how do we measure the "biggest impact"? A social media influencer may upload a video on YouTube or Facebook that gets millions of views, and that's obviously having a big impact. But I've seen activists who aren't social media influencers lead actions that are covered by the mainstream news and have created debate on mainstream platforms, which forces the issue of animal rights into the mainstream agenda - that is having an incredibly big impact too.

DO YOU HAVE A FAVORITE ANIMAL AND DO YOU HAVE ANY STORIES ABOUT SHARING A CONNECTION WITH THAT ANIMAL OR ANY OTHER ANIMAL THAT YOU CAN SHARE?

I've actually always been quite afraid of animals! This is a good lesson that we don't need to be animal lovers to know it's wrong to exploit and kill them. I did have "pets" or companion animals as a child, but I was always very cautious and nervous around them.

I'm also allergic to many animals, so I'm not your typical vegan who wants to have a farm sanctuary, or be a cat lady, or was an animal lover from the very beginning. I don't have a favorite animal, but I do have a least favorite animal... cats! I have always been terrified of cats. As a child, I was petrified that they would jump on me and attack me. As a teenager, my best friend loved cats and her cat knew how afraid I was of him. We would have a stare off in the hallway and I would be too scared to even walk past him. Cats are highly intelligent and intuitive - they definitely know when we don't like them and they have always avoided coming near me.

However, all this changed the day I went vegan. My husband and I were watching Gary's speech on our laptop in a restaurant in Thailand. At the end of the video, we were extremely upset and in tears. At that moment, a cat walked into the restaurant (which isn't uncommon for Thailand) and he or she walked right towards me. It rubbed iself on my leg and stayed with me. This had NEVER happened before in my life! And, for the first time ever, I bent down and petted the cat. I was crying and saying how sorry I was for all the harm I had done to animals over the years as a non-vegan. It was like the cat knew I needed to be comforted by an animal in that moment and be forgiven for all the animals I had eaten and exploited over the years. The cat stayed with me, looking deeply into me until I was ok, and then he/she left. That experience changed my perception and fear of cats. I still don't want to be a cat lady, but I do enjoy being around animals a lot more now.

HOW DO YOU THINK WE CAN ALL HAVE A BIGGER IMPACT ON INFLUENCING PEOPLE AND HELPING THEM MAKE THE CONNECTION TO HEALTH AND EATING A VEGAN DIET? WHAT ARE SOME ORGANIZATIONS OR EVENTS THAT ARE HAPPENING THAT PEOPLE CAN GET INVOLVED WITH?

At the moment I think we have two big jobs on our hands: one is to help non-vegans go vegan, and two is to get vegans to become activists. The resistance for both of these things is actually quite similar. We can have a bigger impact on influencing people to either go vegan, or get active for animals by normalizing both veganism and activism. We have to break the stereotype that vegans look, eat and act a certain way, and the same thing goes for activists.

Being vegan is the normal thing to do. Whilst eating and exploiting animals may have been normalized, it's not a normal behavior to socially accept the exploitation and needless slaughter of innocent beings.

Equally, being a vocal vegan and activist should be the norm. In a social situation, it's unacceptable for someone to be racist, sexist, or homophobic, etc, and people will speak out against such actions and defend the victims. The same thing needs to happen for animals. It's not ok for people to mock the suffering of animals, or the choices of vegans. We need to normalize speaking up against this behavior, defend animals and unequivocally promote a vegan way of life.

The way we normalize defending animals and being an animal rights activist is by getting as many people from all walks of life involved in activism as possible. Taking photos and footage of people from all ages, cultures, genders and occupations getting active for animals will help break down the stereotype that activists are all young people with tattoos and pink hair.

169

We influence people by making veganism and activism relatable to everyone. We have been to many activist events where families have brought their children with older people standing right next to teenagers, and professional people in suits are next to hipsters. I believe that once the early majority see that there are people "just like them" who are openly vegan and serious about defending animals, we will see a greater social and cultural shift.

People can get involved in the animal rights movement by advocating for animals in any way they like. There are three main international groups that are having a great impact, and I encourage people to join. The groups are: Anonymous for the Voiceless, The Save Movement and Direct Action Everywhere.

IF YOU COULD GET EVERYONE TO SEE ONE FILM OR READ ONE BOOK THAT WOULD HELP MAKE THE CONNECTION, WHAT WOULD IT BE AND WHY?

The film Dominion. It documents the brutal truth of how we exploit animals, and I think it should be mandatory viewing for every single human being. Most people are good people who are unknowingly doing bad things. We need to educate people and show them exactly what they're paying for and what they are supporting every time they eat, wear or use animals.

This should also be mandatory viewing for every vegan as well. So many vegans are not active and prefer to keep their food and lifestyle choices to themselves. We need to understand that just living vegan is not what will liberate animals.

Dominion is so horrific and sickening that it has the power to make vegans very angry. That righteous anger is needed - we need to be stirred out of our comfort zones and moved to action. Social change will not happen by people just living vegan and being an example; social change is created by activists. When a quiet vegan watches Dominion and sees activists risking their freedom and lives to plant hidden cameras in slaughterhouses and gas chambers to capture footage for the film, they will hopefully gain some perspective and understand what people are prepared to do for animal liberation. They will hopefully be inspired to speak up and get active themselves.

CAN YOU SHARE WITH US AN AFFIRMATION THAT YOU LIVE BY? WHY DOES THIS AFFIRMATION RESONATE WITH YOU?

"Going vegan is not the most we can do; it's the least we can do."

This has been our tagline on social media for many years now. It means that the very least we can do is not pay people to needlessly slaughter animals (most of whom are babies) for us to eat, whilst destroying the environment on the only planet we call home. Secondly, it means that being vegan is the very baseline of what we can do as human beings, and the next thing that's needed is for vegans to get active for animals and become activists.

Many people think that becoming vegan is a mammoth task that is so hard, which builds needless roadblocks for themselves! What we're saying is that it's not anywhere near as hard, or as big of a deal as many think it is. In fact, it's the very least we can all do. Being vegan is not the end point, it's just the beginning.

WHAT IS THE BEST PIECE OF ADVICE YOU HAVE BEEN GIVEN THAT HAS CHANGED YOUR LIFE?

Around 2005, I was working as a radio journalist. One day I was interviewing someone in the studio about a book. I can't even remember what the book was specifically about, but it had something to do with making changes in one's life. During the interview, the woman said "leap and the net will appear." This absolutely jolted me in that moment! I actually paused the interview and asked her to repeat it, and I wrote it down on a post-it note next to me. At that point in my life, it was exactly what I needed to hear. I did actually leap soon after that, and the net did appear, and I have continued to leap over and over again throughout the years. The net keeps appearing, too.

The point is, just do it. Just make that change, whether it's changing your diet, your health, your job, or your entire life situation... just take that first step and do it. We don't always have it all figured out, and we don't always have all the answers first, but trust that when we're determined enough to leap, the net will somehow appear. If we wait for the net, we may never leap, and we may never discover our true potential and create the life we truly want and deserve.

CAN YOU PLEASE LIST SOME SANCTUARIES, CHARITIES, OR ORGANIZATIONS THAT YOU FEEL WE COULD SUPPORT?

www.dominionmovement.com/donate • *www.edgarsmission.org.au* *www.towerhillstables.com* • *www.sashafarm.org*

ANY INSPIRING STORIES THAT HAVE HAPPENED TO YOU OR PEOPLE CLOSE TO YOU THAT HAVE NOT BEEN COVERED ABOVE. STORIES THAT CAN HELP OTHERS.

We live in a world that is largely based on fear. We fear what other people will think of us, and we fear being judged. This fear is what paralyzes many people from doing what's needed. The truth is that judgment is a normal part of being human, and if we're honest, most people are unconsciously judging others. In fact, isn't criticizing someone for being judgmental a judgment in itself? Considering this, I urge people to stop worrying about what other people will think of them and just do what's needed. Irrespective of what other people in your life will think of you, choosing vegan is the right thing for the animals, the planet and your health. Irrespective of what other people will think, becoming an activist is the right thing for the animals and this movement.

The easiest way to find the courage to do this is to always put yourself in the position of the victim. If you were an animal raised for food or exploited in some other way, would you be concerned about what other people think, or would you want people to just stop participating in the violence and then actively try to intervene in the violence? We always think we can't do something until our life depends on it, or until we put ourselves in the position of someone else whose life depends on it. As Winnie the Pooh says "you're braver than you believe, stronger than you seem and smarter than you think." Each person can be an active vegan in some way, and for the animals, we must.

" "

IT IS MY BELIEF AND MY DEEPEST
HOPE THAT FUTURE GENERATIONS
WILL LOOK UPON OUR TIME
AS ONE WHEN WE MOVED THE
PROGRESS AND EVOLUTION OF
OUR CULTURE FORWARD, WITH
OUR HEARTS, OUR INTELLECT,
OPTIMISM AND DETERMINATION,
AS WE HEALED THE PLANET.

DR. JOANNE KONG

DR. JOANNE KONG

CONNECT WITH JOANNE:
INSTAGRAM: @JOANNEKONGVEGAN
FACEBOOK: JOANNE KONG
vegansmakeadifference.com

"Shifting to a plant-based diet, first as a vegetarian and then vegan, has been the most important decision I have ever made in my life. As I take part in many vegan advocacy activities, giving talks around the world and participating in animal rights activism, I find that veganism is growing around the world because there are so many ways in which it has positive impacts on our lives, whether through improving one's health, caring for the environment, or in my case, desiring to lessen the cruelties committed against innocent beings. Each of us has our own unique vegan journey, and my goal is to plant the seeds of awareness and compassion wherever I go."

Dr. Joanne Kong is a vegan and animal advocate, professor at the University of Richmond (where she received the 2017 Sustainability Leadership Award), and author of the book, If You've Ever Loved An Animal, Go Vegan. Some of her most notable public speaking appearances include the Charlottesville Vegan Roots Festival, Richmond Vegetarian Festival, Asheville VegFest, New York University, Columbia University, VegFest Colorado, Friends Not Food Festival, Ohio State University, Brigham Young University, Green Festival Expo in Washington, D. C., Peace Advocacy Network, National Animal Rights Day in Washington, D. C., Spokane VegFest, MIT, University of Southern California, Yale University, NAVS Vegan Summerfest, and many more. Her highly-praised TEDx talk on veganism is placed on numerous websites internationally and is publicly accessible on YouTube.

AT WHAT AGE DID YOU DECIDE TO BECOME VEGAN AND WHY?

I made an overnight change away from animal products at the age of 28 when I learned about the immense suffering of animals in factory farms. Now an advocate for animals, I point out the roles of society, culture and our upbringing, in reinforcing the overall acceptance of consuming and exploiting animals despite the immense violence and suffering inflicted upon these innocent beings. To me, working towards a plant-based world is about educating others and awakening the innate compassion that we all have within us. It's about the realization that other beings do not need to suffer in order for us to lead sustainable, healthy and compassionate lives.

WHO HAS BEEN THE BIGGEST INFLUENCER IN YOUR LIFE AS A VEGAN AND WHY HAVE THEY HAD SUCH AN IMPACT ON YOU? IN YOUR OPINION, WHICH ACTIVIST IS HAVING THE BIGGEST IMPACT ON THE WORLD AND WHY DO YOU THINK THAT IS?

If I had to name the biggest influencer in my life, I would have to say that it is not one single person, but the beauty, spirit, and life energy in all the animals who have ever been exploited and killed due to the cruelty of humankind's food, entertainment, research and clothing industries.

The total number of humans who have ever existed is about 108 billion, yet every single year, we kill over 150 billion innocent fellow beings. Awareness of such violence inflicted on a massively immense scale gives me tremendous sadness and emotional pain, yet it is also the prime motivator in my continuing to speak out on behalf of non-human animals.

There are so many amazing activists working and making a real difference to create a true paradigm shift to elevate the world to a new level of compassion, kindness and empathy. Veganism is essentially a grassroots movement, and for me it's not about naming individual activists (there are so many!) because it's all about creating community. It's not just the more visible activists, but all the people who make more compassionate choices in their lives that are the collective strength of the vegan movement. All of us together are making a difference and planting seeds of awareness!

DO YOU HAVE A FAVORITE ANIMAL AND DO YOU HAVE ANY STORIES ABOUT SHARING A CONNECTION WITH THAT ANIMAL OR ANY OTHER ANIMAL THAT YOU CAN SHARE?

Some of the strongest and most meaningful relationships we have with non-human animals is with our pets. One of my current pets is an African Grey Parrot (named Jerry), and it is amazing to witness his intelligence, changing emotions, unique ways of communication, his creativity (he loves to sing!) and special personality. He talks and understands what he is saying, has distinct preferences and memories and listens extremely intently to everything that is going on in my house. I personally find it surprising that only in recent years has the general public become more cognizant of the fact that every animal, whether parrot, pig, cow, chicken, dog or cat, is a unique individual. We must celebrate the beauty of life as it manifests in all living beings, and in looking into an animal's eyes never cease to be awed as we see the same life energy that we hold so preciously within ourselves.

HOW DO YOU THINK WE CAN ALL HAVE A BIGGER IMPACT ON INFLUENCING PEOPLE AND HELPING THEM MAKE THE CONNECTION TO HEALTH AND EATING A VEGAN DIET? WHAT ARE SOME ORGANIZATIONS OR EVENTS THAT ARE HAPPENING THAT PEOPLE CAN GET INVOLVED WITH?

I believe that as vegans, perhaps the greatest way we can influence others, is by being healthy and energetic models of the plant-based lifestyle! We can talk about how veganism has enhanced our lives in unique ways, for each of us has our own individual journey and reasons for making a conscious shift in our food choices.

By talking with so many vegans from all walks of life, one important factor I've discovered through my conversations is the knowledge that going plant-based creates an expanded sense of inner calm and peace that comes from living in alignment with one's values. Going vegan IS one of the greatest acts of compassion that we can give as a gift to our world.

The rapidly-growing vegan movement is one that is reaching people all around the world through "veg" fests, documentaries, lectures, conferences and numerous websites. There are so many different ways for individuals to become involved in spreading the vegan message if they are motivated to do so, whether through working with animal rights organizations, volunteering at an animal sanctuary, taking part in supporting the growing numbers of companies that produce plant-based foods and cruelty-free products, or engaging in more public activism such as DXE, Anonymous for the Voiceless and The Save Movement.

IF YOU COULD GET EVERYONE TO SEE ONE FILM OR READ ONE BOOK THAT WOULD HELP MAKE THE CONNECTION, WHAT WOULD IT BE AND WHY?

The one book that I recommend everyone read is Dr. Will Tuttle's *The World Peace Diet*. It eloquently and effectively examines the place of animal exploitation within the history of human culture and how our treatment of animals has disconnected us from our true inner nature of compassion. This in turn, brings harm to ourselves and the planet.

CAN YOU SHARE WITH US AN AFFIRMATION THAT YOU LIVE BY? WHY DOES THIS AFFIRMATION RESONATE WITH YOU?

I have been inspired by this famous statement by Margaret Mead: "Never doubt that a small group of thoughtful, committed citizens can change the world. Indeed, it is the only thing that ever has." It resonates with me because I believe that I am part of a growing group of individuals whose life purpose is to bring people to an elevated awareness of compassion in our lives, to recognize that we and other animals are equal beings, and that we must adopt a greater role as stewards of the beautiful planet on which we live.

WHAT IS THE BEST PIECE OF ADVICE YOU HAVE BEEN GIVEN THAT HAS CHANGED YOUR LIFE?

I am a classical pianist and harpsichordist and when I was in high school I performed in an international competition (I only made it as far as the semi-finals). I was on the phone with my father, telling him about my experience, and he simply told me, "you just have to keep working hard." This advice has really continued to inspire me in any endeavor throughout my life. I really internalized the lesson that, in seeking to fulfill my goals and help others, I must always persevere and not give up.

For me, anything I have ever accomplished has been grounded in maintaining a high work ethic and giving that extra effort that will hopefully help me reach my potential in all areas of my life.

CAN YOU PLEASE LIST SOME SANCTUARIES, CHARITIES, OR ORGANIZATIONS THAT YOU FEEL WE COULD SUPPORT?

I visit a lot of animal sanctuaries throughout the United States, and there are a few I can think of that are worthy of support, especially because they are small organizations that are so deeply committed to the animals (these all have websites):

River's Wish Animal Sanctuary (Spokane, WA)
PreetiRang Sanctuary (Dixon, CA)
The White Pig Animal Sanctuary (Schuyler, VA)
Life With Pigs Farm Animal Sanctuary (Williamsburg, VA; new sanctuary)

ANY INSPIRING STORIES THAT HAVE HAPPENED TO YOU OR PEOPLE CLOSE TO YOU THAT HAVE NOT BEEN COVERED ABOVE. STORIES THAT CAN HELP OTHERS.

I have included two writings below:

1) This is an essay entitled *"Thoughts on Veganism,"* which I wrote in 2017:

The other day, I encountered someone who voiced opposition to animal rights activists, saying that there's no way people are going to quit eating meat—"How are you going to get people to change?" This person implied that advocating for animal rights is a losing battle and that it's not a good or right path.

When alone, I realized that this person had the effect of getting a rise out of me, but even though I felt initial anger towards what the person was saying, I realized that I needed to find a stronger point of focus for my advocacy, which is the essence of what our work is all about. It's not only about motivating people to become vegan, it's not even about right versus wrong or who has the better argument. It's also not only about whether enough people will change to make a difference or whether our society as a whole will ever change. It actually goes way, way beyond this. It is about the fundamental tenets of compassion, and filling every waking moment of our lives with the highest good we possess as living beings: our capacity for kindness, empathy, and seeing ourselves in every other living being who shares our identities as living, sensitive and feeling beings who are aware. This concept seems so simple, yet it has profound implications for the world. As advocates, we give voice to the voiceless, telling the world to bear witness to the tens of billions of innocent creatures who are needlessly killed every year. Who else is going to be kind to these animals, prevent them from enduring a horrendous existence that we would never wish on anyone else? Who else will comfort them and touch them with a loving hand?

The preponderance and inertia of our social conditioning and the power exerted by the animal agriculture industry is such that it would be so easy to do nothing; to simply accept the killing of animals for food as the status quo. But I am not willing to give up and say that it is too difficult or that I can't make a difference. My goal must be to move people to be courageous and open their hearts to the pain they would feel in witnessing what is the most destructive, cruel, exploitative, and oppressive act that happens on our planet today, running like an invisible thread through the fabric of our lives. It is this point of awareness that must be reached, no matter by what path or how difficult it may be.

We as a society, avoid the complicit guilt connected to animal cruelty. How often have we heard the words, "don't tell me, I don't want to think about it!" It is not about having shortcomings or insensitivities, and it is never about judging the actions of others. Rather, these types of responses happen precisely because our capacity to love is so great that we want to look away, to subconsciously and protectively distance ourselves from the cruelty, suffering and death that take place through the industries that exploit animals every second of every day.

People can reach the point of conscious, compassionate awareness through many different paths, and we can encourage them in specific ways, whether it be through their companion animals, visiting an animal sanctuary, watching factory farming videos online, attending a vegan festival or gathering, or viewing a documentary. Bringing about positive change through animal advocacy must be about imploring people to turn inward—to look at themselves, and embrace deeply, fully and consciously their great capacity for love and kindness. Too much of our world is about the material and external aspects of our lives, but we can re-awaken the sensitivity of our true selves to reside within. We all have the power to create a new, transformative and beautiful reality. Only then will we as a society be able to extend that kindness to the fellow beings with whom we walk this earth.

2) Animal Agriculture: *Eating for Compassion, Peace and Sustainability*

As animal advocates we have a critical need to bring to mainstream awareness that animal agriculture is the most destructive industry on our planet and is a leading driver of climate change, species and habitat loss, resource loss and environmental damage. Impending catastrophic climate change is the greatest threat to our existence, and environmental and climate scientists warn that we have very little time to act; ignoring the magnitude of animal agriculture's impacts will be at our own peril.

Planetary healing must include a broad-scale intervention to transform our food production systems, ending the mass killing of animals for food. We must give direct and immediate attention to strategies for animal advocates and environmentalists to work towards common goals, recognize society's disconnect between animal agriculture and the state of our planet, and motivate and empower individuals to shift towards more compassionate, sustainable food choices. It is true that all things are connected - in harming other beings, we harm ourselves.

We must critically and honestly examine our place in the world, for we have reached a point where we can no longer take the natural world and its many gifts for granted. Ending the catastrophic cruelty of industrialized animal agriculture will be a testament to our true compassionate natures as we expand our circle of compassion to sentient beings with whom we share the deepest of connections. It is my belief and my deepest hope that future generations will look upon our time as one when we moved the progress and evolution of our culture forward, with our hearts, our intellect, optimism and determination as we healed the planet.

MARGAUX KHOURY

CONNECT WITH MARGAUX:
INSTAGRAM: @BESTNATURALDEODORANT
FACEBOOK: BESTNATURALDEODORANT
TheBestDeodorant.org

Creator and lover of plant-based and vegan companies, Margaux is the founder and CEO of one of the most popular organic, natural, cruelty-free deodorants, "The Best Deodorant In The World," a company she started out of her kitchen. It's mission is to turn a necessity like deodorant into a force for social impact.

"Our business started a few years ago when we had already changed all our products at home to be 100% natural, from cleaning material all the way through to our mattresses. Deodorant was the last item we couldn't find a natural product for. At the time there really wasn't an option that worked well. In 2017, Joshua, my husband had a health scare. He had to have two surgeries in one week, and he almost didn't make it home. Almost losing my partner and father of our children really made me reconsider what's important in life.

179

I decided then and there to stop treating this company like a hobby and start making it huge. We were global, online and in about 200 retail stores at the time. I made the decision to pull every single product off all store shelves and stop selling it. We re-branded to 100% plastic free and biodegradable (even the shipping material is zero plastic), and we attached a social purpose to the company. We have decided to become an "activist company." Which means we want to fully support those out there in the field doing incredible work for the animals. We want to give all profits (after everyone in the company is paid) to animal rights and human rights activists. We have an amazing mission now, and we wake up every morning so excited to get to work."

AT WHAT AGE DID YOU DECIDE TO BECOME VEGAN AND WHY?

I was 31, this was eight years ago now. It was because I finally woke up to the fact that we don't need animal flesh to be healthy, and also that all products and secretions that come from animals belong only to that animal. Not us. So, it was for ethical and health reasons. I later discovered the environmental reasons to go vegan and I am so happy now that I did.

WHO HAS BEEN THE BIGGEST INFLUENCER IN YOUR LIFE AS A VEGAN? AND IN YOUR OPINION WHICH ACTIVIST IS HAVING THE BIGGEST IMPACT AND WHY DO YOU THINK THAT IS?

When I first discovered Ingrid Newkirk, it inspired me to know there was someone so courageous and bad ass. And of course later, Paul Watson.

I am an activist at heart. I cannot see injustice and simply stand by watching. I have to act. My parents told me I've always been like that, even as a child. Throughout the years, I've taken in really troubled youth and have given them shelter, food, etc.

Before having children of my own, I was a foster parent to over eight boys who needed help desperately. So naturally, once I found out about the hidden abuse humans are inflicting on animals, I became passionate about spreading the truth. I was an organizer for AV, and I do my own outreach at every opportunity.

Our company is now aiming to support animal activists. We will be producing full features on some really well known people doing amazing work. Those truly changing humanity.

DO YOU HAVE A FAVORITE ANIMAL AND DO YOU HAVE ANY STORIES ABOUT SHARING A CONNECTION WITH THAT ANIMAL OR ANY OTHER ANIMAL THAT YOU CAN SHARE?

Mama cow (and baby calves). Actually, it was because of the realization of what we (humans) are doing to cows and calves via the horrific dairy industry that woke me up. Millions of people go vegetarian to avoid animal suffering, but fail to understand that the dairy industry exploits cows on an unimaginable scale.

IF YOU COULD GET EVERYONE TO SEE ONE FILM OR READ ONE BOOK THAT WOULD HELP MAKE THE CONNECTION, WHAT WOULD IT BE AND WHY?

Earthlings and Cowspiracy were powerful for me. Eating Animals by Jonathan Safran Foer is a great book. Also, because I feel children need to be the driving force for good and will lead the way for humanity to change, I love any vegan book for children.

CAN YOU SHARE WITH US AN AFFIRMATION THAT YOU LIVE BY? AND WHY DOES THAT RESONATE WITH YOU?

We are one with the earth and nature. Veganism is love and awareness. Total consciousness and dedication to living as we (humans) are meant to live. My mission is to do as little harm as practically possible.

WHAT'S THE BEST PIECE OF ADVICE YOU HAVE BEEN GIVEN THAT HAS CHANGED YOUR LIFE?

Get your nutrients directly from the source. Where do cows, pigs, buffalos, pandas, horses, goats and apes get their nutrition from? Let's not pretend that eating animals gives us anything that plants cannot.

CAN YOU PLEASE LIST SOME SANCTUARIES, CHARITIES, ORGANIZATIONS THAT YOU FEEL WE COULD SUPPORT. THERE ARE SO MANY AND SOMETIMES WE DON'T KNOW WHICH ONES ARE IN IT FOR THE RIGHT REASON'S, WE WOULD LOVE SOME GUIDANCE.

Great question because I've had some personal experiences with organizations and yes, even sanctuaries that have been less than ethical. First, I would start by encouraging people to buy from ethical brands that support great causes. People are buying soap and clothing anyway. Why not spend the same to get the product and know that the money is doing good in the world. Some people I've worked with doing great things for animals: The Save Movement, Nation Rising, and friends like James Aspey, Paul Watson (Sea Shepherd) and Philip Woolen who supports so many non profits, including the VSPCA in India.

ANY INSPIRING STORIES YOU CAN SHARE?

To me, as a breastfeeding mom of three vegan-since-birth children, it's such a deep, strong connection that's often difficult to put into words.

When I went vegan eight years ago, it was when my first child was in my belly and knowing I'd be nourishing that child with my own milk was powerful. Every baby (human or other) deserves the milk from their own mother. Also, there might be a reason humans chose certain animals for milk because of how much they can produce. Why cow, sheep, goat, etc and not pig, dog or cat? All mammals deserve to retain that which belongs to them and their baby. No one has a right to steal that from them. The crazy thing is, we (humans) don't even need it to survive or thrive.

I'd like to add that we don't feel product choices should fall on the consumer's shoulders. Yes, consumers "vote" with their wallets, so to speak, but I honestly feel it is the responsibility of the small, medium and even larger companies to switch to offer *only* ethical and sustainable products. We need to encourage all companies to think this way, so that consumers have an easier choice. The great thing is, business will only grow as a result. My mission is to show the world you can create and grow huge, sustainable companies without harming people, the Earth or any animals here.

" "

KINDNESS TRUMPS EVERYTHING

HEIDI MUMFORD-YEO

HEIDI MUMFORD-YEO

"My decision was 100% driven by animal rights. However, the more research I did, the more I saw that it is also the single most impactful change anyone can make to protect the planet and environment, and take a stand against global poverty. People sometimes forget that it's very much a human rights issue too."

Heidi Mumford-Yeo is a model, actress and passionate animal rights, advocate. In 2017 she was appointed as an Angel Ambassador for Angels for the Innocent Foundation in London, where she campaigns for animal rights and environmental issues.

AT WHAT AGE DID YOU DECIDE TO BECOME VEGAN AND WHY?

I stopped eating meat as a teenager and slowly started eliminating dairy in my early twenties. I finally decided to give up all animal products in 2015.

Instinctively, I was repulsed by meat from an early age. Then the natural correlation became animal by-products and secretions. Having grown up with animals, it became nonsensical, ludicrous even, to say I loved them while continuing to fund their exploitation and torture. The only logical and moral stance was to become full vegan; it was the single best decision I ever made.

WHO HAS BEEN THE BIGGEST INFLUENCER IN YOUR LIFE AS A VEGAN AND WHY HAVE THEY HAD SUCH AN IMPACT ON YOU? IN YOUR OPINION, WHICH ACTIVIST IS HAVING THE BIGGEST IMPACT ON THE WORLD AND WHY DO YOU THINK THAT IS?

Back in 2015, I started watching Earthling Ed's content and also James Aspey. They were the two most profound influencers on me and my decision.

It was a combination of the brutality and the violence that animals suffer at our hands. This combined with the prevailing logic of veganism, which both Ed and James constructed so powerfully in their respective ways.

Emotional connection and fact-based rationality is a powerful amalgam, and I truly believe it's impossible to construct a sound counterargument against being vegan without appearing either ridiculous or extremely cruel. The logic is infallible.

DO YOU HAVE A FAVORITE ANIMAL AND DO YOU HAVE ANY STORIES ABOUT SHARING A CONNECTION WITH THAT ANIMAL OR ANY OTHER ANIMAL THAT YOU CAN SHARE?

Well, I've grown up surrounded by animals, dogs, cats, horses, rabbits, guinea-pigs and rescue birds. I'd have a menagerie if I didn't live in Central London!

Every animal in my life has been a gift; each one special and unique with their personalities, and each one has left an indelible mark on my life. I had a rescue horse, Duke, who was incredibly special and really defined my childhood. He was dreadfully neglected when we adopted him and to see him flourish and the bond we had, was indescribable. I think you always leave a piece of your soul with the animals that have touched your life. I feel very blessed that I had those relationships.

I now have two dogs. One is a rescued Chihuahua named Freddy, whom I've written a series of children's books about called The Adventures of Freddy! He's the star!

HOW DO YOU THINK WE CAN ALL HAVE A BIGGER IMPACT ON INFLUENCING PEOPLE AND HELPING THEM MAKE THE CONNECTION TO HEALTH AND EATING A PLANT-BASED DIET? WHAT ARE SOME ORGANIZATIONS OR EVENTS THAT ARE HAPPENING THAT PEOPLE CAN GET INVOLVED WITH?

We live in such privileged times of information democratisation, and it's never been easier to spread knowledge. I believe it's incumbent on us to use our platforms wisely. There's so much vacuity and narcissism on social media, but if we embrace it for the positive and use it as a tool for change, then that's incredibly powerful.

Outreach events such as Anonymous for the Voiceless, Surge events, and basically, any animal rights demonstration is a fantastic way to engage people and gain traction. It's also a great way of making friends and supporting each other.

As vegans, we really do need to be there for each other. Living in these dark times with the level of violence that we're subjected to on a daily basis can be utterly overwhelming. This makes having that support system in place critical.

Other than that it's just talking to people, whether it's friends, family or colleagues. We have to remember that no matter how uncomfortable we're made to feel, or however "inconvenient" the facts are, it's our moral duty to keep the dialogue going and to keep speaking up and out for those who cannot.

Lastly, I'd say that what I've learned is that unfortunately, not everyone loves or even likes animals. Perhaps they've never been lucky enough to make the connection or to have experienced the purity of animals. Perhaps, through religious or cultural norms, they were taught to fear animals or view them as objects and commodities. There are many reasons, but what's important to remember is that everyone knows what pain and suffering is. This is why it's important to draw the correlation and to educate people to understand that we are all connected. We share 98% of the same DNA; a central nervous system, eyes, heart and brain. Cognitively and emotionally, we see and experience life through the same prism. In short, getting people to see they are no different to us in their ability to suffer and feel pain.

If that still doesn't resonate, then talking about the impact on their own health and the ecological devastation that animal agriculture wreaks is something most people can relate to or care about.

IF YOU COULD GET EVERYONE TO SEE ONE FILM OR READ ONE BOOK THAT WOULD HELP MAKE THE CONNECTION, WHAT WOULD IT BE AND WHY?

My top three are:

Land of Hope and Glory, which exposes the colossal cruelty on UK farms *What The Health*, which discusses the health implications of eating animals. Finally would be *Cowspiracy* for the environmental atrophy a non-vegan life causes.

CAN YOU SHARE WITH US AN AFFIRMATION THAT YOU LIVE BY? WHY DOES THIS AFFIRMATION RESONATE WITH YOU?

I try to live each moment in the present, to live in a state of gratitude, and to be mindful that every action has a positive and negative. Kindness trumps everything in my book.

WHAT IS THE BEST PIECE OF ADVICE YOU HAVE BEEN GIVEN THAT HAS CHANGED YOUR LIFE?

Never be afraid of not fitting in or needing other people to give you value or purpose. Also, to be the best possible version of yourself and continually refine and improve who and what you are.

CAN YOU PLEASE LIST SOME SANCTUARIES, CHARITIES, OR ORGANIZATIONS THAT YOU FEEL WE COULD SUPPORT?

I support Ed Winters and Surge activism. I believe they do a brilliant job of educating people. Breaking down cognitive dissonance is key, which I believe is a fundamental part of what they do.

There are many sanctuaries that do a wonderful job. Here in the UK, Friend Farm Sanctuary would be one, as well as Hillside.

My friend, Harry Eckman, also does a fantastic job with Change for Animals Foundation. There are so many quality organisations out there.

Personally, I would only support a charity or organisations that is vegan and not single-issue campaigns.

ANY INSPIRING STORIES YOU CAN SHARE?

When I first went vegan it was quite a lonely phase of my life; I didn't know any other vegans, and I had sunk into quite a severe depression having reached saturation point with the horrific reality of what was happening.

The concomitant feelings of despair and hopelessness were overwhelming, and I really had to dig deep to find some inner reserves. However, what this did was teach me that no matter how desolate or hopeless we feel (in any aspect of our lives) the key is to keep going, rest if you have to, but just find that inner strength or inner grace that says there is always hope. Not giving up in the face of adversity and pain is the single most important life lesson I've learnt. When you combine that with empathy and knowledge, then mountains move.

Also, never being afraid of standing alone, of standing up and making your voice heard, even if you are the only one. We're so conditioned as children to conform to societal norms, even when those constructs are morally wrong. I firmly believe that it's our moral obligation to disobey unjust laws and to advocate on behalf of the vulnerable, oppressed and the ones who cannot defend themselves.

MICHELLE CEHN

CONNECT WITH MICHELLE:
INSTAGRAM: @MICHELLECEHN / @VEGAN
FACEBOOK: WORLD OF VEGAN
YOUTUBE: WORLD OF VEGAN
worldofvegan.com

Michelle Cehn is the founder of World of Vegan, a resource, website, and social media influencer, that makes vegan living accessible, delicious and fun. Michelle has reached millions through her social platforms, and is known for her creative, informative, and relatable videos, articles and recipes. She is an outspoken advocate for plant-based eating and has worked with leading nonprofits including Farm Sanctuary, Mercy for Animals, Vegan Outreach, PETA, and PCRM.

AT WHAT AGE DID YOU DECIDE TO BECOME VEGAN AND WHY?

I became a vegetarian at age eight, and vegan at age 20. I picked up a copy of Peter Singer's book, Animal Liberation, at a used bookstore while I was in college. As I read it, my stomach turned, and my eyes were opened to the cruelties inherent in the dairy and egg industries. I had already been a vegetarian for many years, but at that moment, I realized that in order to live in alignment with my values, it was time to go vegan.

WHO HAS BEEN THE BIGGEST INFLUENCER IN YOUR LIFE AS A VEGAN AND WHY HAVE THEY HAD SUCH AN IMPACT ON YOU? IN YOUR OPINION, WHICH ACTIVIST IS HAVING THE BIGGEST IMPACT ON THE WORLD AND WHY DO YOU THINK THAT IS?

This is hard to answer because so many people have influenced my vegan journey, but Peter Singer has had the single biggest impact on me. His book, Animal Liberation, is what inspired me to go vegan in the first place. But more than that, his writings about utilitarianism provided me with the framework of my life's mission—to reduce as much suffering and better as many lives as humanly possible.

All these years later, I still think Peter Singer has an enormous impact on the way animal advocates approach the problems of the world today, and his ethical philosophies help us all make sure the work we do in our lifetime can be the most impactful.

DO YOU HAVE A FAVORITE ANIMAL AND DO YOU HAVE ANY STORIES ABOUT SHARING A CONNECTION WITH THAT ANIMAL OR ANY OTHER ANIMAL THAT YOU CAN SHARE?

My heart has always gone out to the traditionally "unloved" animals. Since I was a small child I've loved pigs, recognizing them as sweet, playful, and highly intelligent beings that are deeply misunderstood. But the first time I ever met a cow face-to-face (at Farm Sanctuary), I fell in love. There is something so healing and peaceful about looking into their deep, connective eyes. I am in awe of how forgiving they can be after all we do to them.

HOW DO YOU THINK WE CAN ALL HAVE A BIGGER IMPACT ON INFLUENCING PEOPLE AND HELPING THEM MAKE THE CONNECTION TO HEALTH AND EATING A VEGAN DIET? WHAT ARE SOME ORGANIZATIONS OR EVENTS THAT ARE HAPPENING THAT PEOPLE CAN GET INVOLVED WITH?

Too often, after we go vegan, we fall into a "vegan bubble." We want all our friends to be vegan, our activities to be vegan, or our outings to be vegan. That's wonderful, and it absolutely feels good to be around like-minded people, but it's such a missed opportunity to connect with people who are not already there.

188

Stay active in all the things you love and embrace, and celebrate the people in your life (and all those you meet along the way) who are not vegan. Simply by being a positive presence in groups, communities, teams, and the lives of others, you can make waves of change.

IF YOU COULD GET EVERYONE TO SEE ONE FILM OR READ ONE BOOK THAT WOULD HELP MAKE THE CONNECTION, WHAT WOULD IT BE AND WHY?

If I could get everyone to do both, I'd choose Earthlings for the film (the fastest way to become awakened to the realities of the world), and Prevent & Reverse Heart Disease, as the book (because heart disease is the number one cause of death in the US, but it's a paper tiger - that single book can save countless lives).

CAN YOU SHARE WITH US AN AFFIRMATION THAT YOU LIVE BY? WHY DOES THIS AFFIRMATION RESONATE WITH YOU?

I've actually never used affirmations (although perhaps I should), but the simplest words I live by are: "Be the change you wish to see in the world."

WHAT IS THE BEST PIECE OF ADVICE YOU HAVE BEEN GIVEN BY A LOVED ONE OR A COMPLETE STRANGER THAT HAS CHANGED YOUR LIFE?

Being a martyr is limiting your ability to impact the world. You can have a far greater impact while enjoying your life to the fullest.

This took me some time to understand, but as I've played with it in practice, I realize it can be so very true.

CAN YOU PLEASE LIST SOME SANCTUARIES, CHARITIES, OR ORGANIZATIONS THAT YOU FEEL WE COULD SUPPORT?

Smaller ones:
Factory Farming Awareness Coalition
Harvest Home Animal Sanctuary
Preetirang Sanctuary
One Step For Animals
The Pollination Project
Food Empowerment Project

(I'm sure you know all the big ones - Mercy for Animals is my favorite of those!)

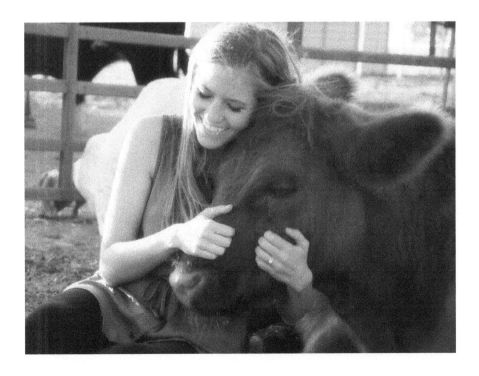

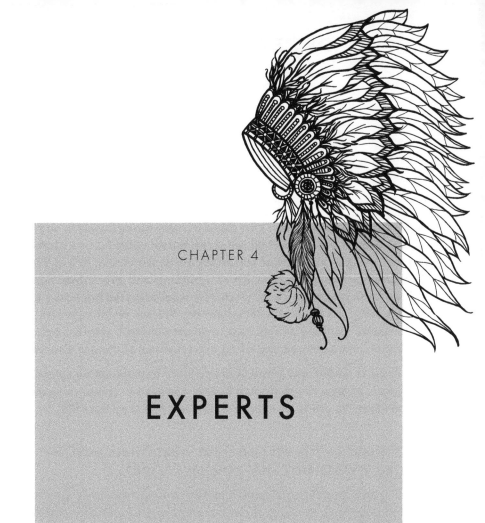

CHAPTER 4

EXPERTS

DR. RENAE THOMAS

CONNECT WITH DR.RENAE:
INSTAGRAM: @DRRENAETHOMAS
FACEBOOK: DR. RENAE THOMAS
drrenaethomas.com

Dr. Renae Thomas has been interested in plant-based nutrition and veganism since she was a child, after her father switched to a plant-based diet, following a diagnosis of metastatic testicular cancer, at just 39. He healed through a combination of traditional and alternative medicine and has been cancer-free ever since. Her inspiration led her down a career path in the medical field, where she focuses on lifestyle and preventative medicine as well as an evidence-based treatment option for prevention, management and often even reversal of chronic diseases.

"My focus is on fad and gimmick-free advice and education to empower individuals to improve their own health. I believe in compassionate care and self-love, to guide people to thrive and live their best life!"

WHAT IS ONE OF THE BEST OR MOST WORTHWHILE HEALTH-RELATED INVESTMENTS THAT YOU HAVE MADE?

Investing time in others. Seriously, It can be so easy in our daily lives to think, "I'm too busy," but it's always those moments where I took a bit of extra time for a patient, stayed back late to chat with a friend in need, replied to that lengthy email or called someone back, that I really felt like I was contributing to this earth with what I was meant to do, which is priceless. Traveling to India to become a yoga teacher was also life-altering for me in far more ways than I could have anticipated!

AT WHAT POINT IN YOUR LIFE DID YOU DECIDE TO CHANGE YOUR DIET? HOW HAS THAT DECISION IMPACTED YOUR LIFE?

My Dad had testicular cancer when I was five years old, and as part of his treatment he became vegan/vegetarian, and I followed suit to "be like my Daddy." When I was 13 I learned the ethical side of animal agriculture and fully understood my choices, which solidified my belief in the way I ate.

I also found out only very recently; actually, he had multiple metastases at diagnosis, he believes it was possibly liver, lung and bone, but cannot

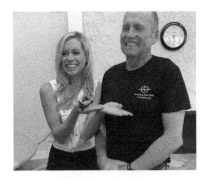

really remember. He's a positive guy and tries not to dwell in the past! He did have traditional chemotherapy (about five treatments he recalls), and a traditional oncologist, however, he also changed to an entirely plant-based nutritional pattern, and incorporated juice fasting and intermittent fasting on his journey to wellness. He has been clear now for nearly 30 years, no recurrence, and metastases have all disappeared.

WHAT KIND OF REACTION DID YOU RECEIVE FROM PEERS, FAMILY & FRIENDS WHEN YOU ANNOUNCED THAT YOU WERE GOING VEGAN?

Everyone I know has known me as a vegetarian/vegan for almost my whole life, and my parents are as well, so I never had to "announce" it. I definitely get a lot of questions such as "where do you get your protein," but I feel like so long as you have solid answers and speak them with confidence, it is relatively easy to reply and move on. A lot of people don't know my food choices as I generally don't attract attention to it. It's just a part of me, the same as my hair colour, or the fact that I like yoga. I don't have to yell it from the rooftops every day. Sure, if asked why I can talk all day, but usually I can tell if someone wants education versus someone who wants an argument. With the latter, I just try to diffuse as fast as possible and direct my energy in more positive pursuits.

DO YOU TAKE ANY SPECIFIC SUPPLEMENTS? DO YOU RECOMMEND ANY SPECIFIC BRANDS? WHY DO YOU THINK THESE HAVE BENEFITED YOU AND YOUR HEALTH?

I do not take any supplements regularly. I focus more on getting the most nutrition that I can from whole plant foods. I treat supplements similarly to any pharmaceuticals: minimal and on an as-needed basis only. I ensure my lab levels of things such as B12, vitamin D, zinc, and magnesium are within the healthy limits and would consider supplementing only if deficient. I feel like my money is best spent on attaining the best quality produce and that that will cover far more than any supplement and work far better in keeping

" "

THE HUMAN DESIGN ISN'T
FLAWED TO NEED SUPPLEMENTS
IN GENERAL, AND WE
GENERALLY ONLY LACK
THROUGH ENVIRONMENTAL
DEGRADATION, ILLNESS,
AND LIVING FAR FROM
WHAT IS NATURAL

DR. RENAE THOMAS

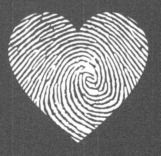

my body healthy. The human design isn't flawed to need supplements in general, and we generally only lack through environmental degradation, illness, and living far from what is natural, in my opinion. The closest thing to a potion I use would be our "sore throat solution," which is warm lemon, apple cider vinegar and ginger. Tastes average, but works like a charm!

WHAT ARE YOUR RECOMMENDATIONS TO YOUR CLIENTS WHEN YOU FIRST SUGGEST THEY SHOULD MOVE TO A PLANT-BASED DIET?

Don't let perfection get in the way of progress! Every extra plant food you eat is doing you good and is a step in the right direction! I usually focus on adding fruits and vegetables, rather than focusing on what one cannot have, as it's more positive. Focusing on making healthy choices, such as adding more fiber, adding a green smoothie, hiding some veggies in the pasta sauce, or trying a new plant-based "milk," because this can be exciting and fun rather than feeling like everything you liked to eat is no longer allowed.

WHAT IS THE MOST INSPIRING OR POWERFUL RESULT THAT YOU HAVE SEEN WITH A PATIENT AND A PLANT-BASED DIET?

SO MANY!!! But, the most near and dear to me, is my Dad. I truly believe that a plant-based diet was an integral part of his recovery from cancer and cancer-free maintenance ever since! He has been clear now for nearly 30 years, no recurrence or metastases, he is so fit and well.

195

SHARE A STORY ABOUT THE POWER OF PLANTS THAT YOU USE WITH YOUR CLIENTS TO HELP THEM BELIEVE IN THIS AS AN ALTERNATIVE WAY OF LOOKING AT MEDICINE?

I usually approach the idea of the power of plants as an adjuvant to traditional medical care and go from there. Sort of a, "did you know that changing your nutrition could also add benefit to your health?" approach. It usually becomes fairly obvious then if the patient is open to this or not, and I try to tailor my approach to what will be most readily accepted by them. A lot of patients dislike being on medications, so offering alternative solutions with the pure motivation to wean off medications can be powerful. It's all about motivational interviewing and figuring out where the patient is at and where you can help them best. I'm all about providing education because many people don't even realize that what they eat affects their health. I have also become super aware that the key power to changing minds is meeting patients where they are at and helping them make changes, no matter how small or far from what I believe is best. This is so that they achieve realistic and sustainable goals, which eventually creates more sizable changes and results.

IF YOU COULD GIVE US JUST THREE ABSOLUTE MUSTS TO INCLUDE IN OUR DIET EACH DAY WHAT WOULD THEY BE?

Fruits, vegetables and low levels of food obsession or stress! Seriously! So many overcomplicate every minor detail and forget the big picture. Most people's health would improve significantly if they just ate more whole plant foods and stopped stressing if they have enough protein or omega threes or too many carbs or the best type of green. Just eat real food and live your life!

SINCE BECOMING VEGAN/PLANT-BASED, WHAT ELSE HAS CHANGED IN YOUR LIFE?

For me, it has been a life-long thing, so it's hard to say. However, I do feel, whether this is good or bad, that I am much more connected to animals and nature, and much more aware of my impact on the world in general. It might sound a little "out there," and I always thought I was just a bit "odd" until I started meeting people who were going vegan and they mentioned similar experiences. I feel like a fog lifts for a lot of people and brings a lot of growth opportunities, which can be challenging since you no longer live in a world of blissful ignorance.

ANY INSPIRING STORIES THAT HAVE HAPPENED TO YOU OR PEOPLE CLOSE TO YOU THAT HAVE NOT BEEN COVERED ABOVE. STORIES THAT CAN HELP OTHERS.

When I was growing up, my parents used to always tell me they didn't care what I grew up to be, as long as I was happy. I think that for a lot of us, this is really the fundamental goal of life, realizing that happiness comes from within and grows when it is shared. I feel like so many of us get caught up in the business, day-to-day work, whining, complaining, comparisons, advertising and the horrors on the news, that we forget to take a step back and appreciate how wonderful and amazing life really is. Learning to love yourself, giving love to others abundantly, and loving the earth and everything in it really is the key to a happy and healthy life.

CANDY MARX

CONNECT WITH CANDY:
INSTAGRAM: @PLANTFEDMAMA
FACEBOOK: CANDY MARX
plantfedmama.com

Candy Marx is a writer, author, registered Master Herbalist, registered plant-based nutritionist, kind living and wellness influencer, intuition mentor, award-winning fashion designer and entrepreneur-turned-social-entrepreneur behind the popular Instagram account, Plantfed Mama. Her work has been featured in national and international press, including The Sunday Telegraph (AUS), The Financial Review (AUS), The Dominion Post (NZ), New Zealand Vegan Magazine (NZ), Digital Journal (USA), Medium (USA), Ethical Style Journal (USA), Raise Vegan (USA), and The Times (USA), to name a few.

"I initially chose to be vegan because of animals, though after learning just how detrimental the livestock industry is, my decision also became about the earth. At the time, I didn't realize that I was also doing my body the BIGGEST favor. I stopped getting sick, I was healthier and fitter, and I felt good all of the time. Things that used to stress me out no longer stressed me out. That's when I realized that physical health, mental health and spiritual health are all very much connected and are impacted by what we eat - plants and lifeforce are literally the keys. When I figured this out it was then crucial for me to study plants from a medicinal side, so I studied Master Herbalism and Human Nutrition. I have just gone through a vegan pregnancy, and I was extremely healthy throughout it, so much that I shocked my doctor. When done correctly, pregnant women can absolutely thrive living a vegan lifestyle. This is why I wrote my book, Plantfed Mama's Holistic Guide to a Vegan Pregnancy, because updated information on plant-based pregnancies is lacking. My book focuses heavily on the nutritional and holistic health aspects, and I wrote the majority of it while I was pregnant. It was important for me to be going through a vegan pregnancy while writing about it. Our food choices directly impact our health and pregnancy-related issues such as morning sickness, gestational diabetes, painful breastfeeding and edema, are less likely to happen on a whole-foods plant-based diet."

197

WHAT IS ONE OF THE BEST OR WORTHWHILE HEALTH-RELATED INVESTMENTS YOU HAVE MADE?

For me, there aren't any gimmicks - the real magic lies in whole-foods. So, the best investment for my health and my family's health has been eating an organic whole-foods, plant-based diet. I say organic because it's crucial to remove as much glyphosate (found in Roundup) from our diets as possible. That stuff is toxic. There are obviously some appliances that make life easier, such as a decent blender, a food processor, and a spiralizer, but you can make do with affordable varieties. It really isn't crucial to have the most expensive blender.

DO YOU TAKE ANY SPECIAL SUPPLEMENTS OR POTIONS? SPECIFIC BRANDS WOULD BE GREAT AS WELL PLEASE AND WHY YOU THINK THESE HAVE BENEFITED YOU AND YOUR HEALTH?

I believe in the power of whole-foods and eating nutrient-dense meals. The majority of supplements are synthetic or are concentrated "part foods," which our bodies have a hard time absorbing and digesting. This means that we don't absorb a lot of the nutrients that are taken via a supplement. With whole-foods, our bodies digest and absorb them much better, making the nutrients more bioavailable. When it comes to supplements, I call this 'wasteful supplementing versus essential supplementing.' When we take unnecessary supplements that our bodies do not absorb, this is wasteful (and super expensive). A large majority of people who take supplements also do not have a deficiency either, they just assume that they do.

Essential supplementing is when there is a deficiency, and different methods are followed to maximize absorption. When looking for a supplement, always choose food-made supplements, since these supplements, preferably from whole-foods, are more bioavailable. Another point to keep in mind is that the majority of calcium is stored in the bones, so a simple blood test from your GP won't show true levels. And if you aren't calcium deficient, taking calcium supplements can cause more harm than good. Minerals and fat-soluble vitamins store in the body and should only be taken via supplement if there is a deficiency. The B-vitamins are another example - the B-vitamins increase the absorption of each other, so taking a B12 supplement by itself also has low bioavailability. You'd be better off taking a food-made B-complex powder, rather than a single B12 supplement.

Vitamin D is another one. It's become super popular to take vitamin D supplements. But, vitamin D is best produced in the body from spending time in the sun. Vitamin D is a hormone, and along with this hormone, our bodies also produce a protein called GCMaF. This protein helps the immune system destroy cancer cells. We absorb LIFEFORCE from the sun as well. If you're relying on supplements, then you miss out on these other vital

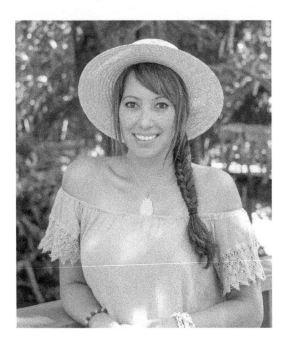

nutrients. Get outside and spend at least 10 minutes per day in the sun, or focus on building up your reserves. If you spend plenty of time in the sun during the warmer months, it will get you through the cooler months. Obviously, be sun smart as overexposure does exist. But if you're out in the sun, wear a hat rather than sunglasses. Blocking our eyes with sunglasses tells our brain that we're indoors, and this message relays to our skin, making it easier to get burnt. If we keep our eyes uncovered, then our brains know we're outside, and this message relays to our skin, meaning that our skin is prepared to be in the sun.

As for potions, there are a few foods that I like to keep handy in case of illness and for overall health and wellbeing: dried elderberries (to make tea and cough syrup), sea moss, a food-made vitamin C powder (this is great to take just before a cold or flu sets in, to help alleviate allergies, and when breastfeeding to help baby if he gets heat rash). I also keep pre/probiotics, chlorella and echinacea handy too. Plantfed Mama is also in the middle of releasing herbal blends that are safe for pregnant and breastfeeding women. A lot of the current herbal supplements can't be taken by pregnant or breastfeeding women, specifically herbal supplements that help raise iron levels (which is super important while pregnant, post-birth and breastfeeding), and to help alleviate colds and flu. Most of the standard iron supplements are sourced from rocks, and contain many harsh additives, which is why they cause constipation in mama and baby; they're super tough on the body! I wanted to change that. Iron supplements, well, all supplements should be made from whole-foods.

HOW DO YOU THINK WE CAN ALL HAVE A BIGGER IMPACT ON INFLUENCING PEOPLE AND HELPING THEM MAKE THE CHANGE TO A PLANT-BASED DIET?

Leading by example. My clients and those I encounter on social media tend to listen to what I have to say because I am walking the talk. They always comment on how healthy I am, or how much my skin glows. From a health perspective, if you don't look healthy, then people won't heed your advice.

As a vegan influencer, it's also important to be able to influence our partners to go vegan too. If we can't influence our own partners to go vegan, then why should strangers listen to us? It's important to have our own house in order, so to speak.

WHAT WERE THE FIRST STEPS YOU TOOK IN MAKING YOUR NUTRITIONAL CHANGES AND WHY DID YOU START DOWN THIS PATH?

I was a vegetarian for 15 years before making the switch to veganism. I grew up around animals, and to me, our pigs were the same as our dogs. I made the connection quite early on. But at first, I didn't know about the hefty cruelty in the dairy and egg industries. We had chickens, and they were always treated with love - they'd run up to us for a cuddle. We also had cows, and they were never artificially inseminated. Their calves lived their lives with their mothers, so finding out what the dairy and egg industries do was a massive wake-up call. That was the day that I became vegan, which was back in 2012.

I've always been a truth-seeker, and I'm always researching topics that most wouldn't think about, so for me, the first steps in making any changes are awareness and knowledge. We have to be willing to ask the hard questions and find out more information to make any change.

IF YOU COULD GIVE US JUST THREE ABSOLUTE MUSTS TO INCLUDE IN OUR DIET EACH DAY WHAT WOULD THEY BE?

Raw fruits and vegetables. These foods aren't only full of macronutrients, micronutrients, enzymes and phytonutrients, but raw fruit and vegetables also contain the highest levels of lifeforce - and lifeforce is the key to mental, physical and spiritual health.

Drinking plenty of filtered and fluoride-free water, and getting plenty of sun while eating your nutrient-dense meal is vital too. Vitamin D increases nutrient absorption. As mentioned, I'm not really into gimmicks, and I do believe the term "superfood" is overused, but the true magic lies in whole-foods.

SINCE BECOMING VEGAN/PLANT-BASED, WHAT ELSE HAS CHANGED IN YOUR LIFE?

My life took on a completely different path once I made the decision to go vegan. I was a high-end fashion footwear designer based in Sydney, and my label was doing really well. I dressed Australia's Next Top Model's Top 20, I showed at Mercedes-Benz Fashion Week, Sydney, in NYC and LA. I dressed a list of celebrities, and my label won a prestigious Qantas award.

When I decided to switch to a vegan diet, I was due to launch my newest and biggest collection (Spring/Summer) in New York. From that trip, I had interest from several US stockists, including two major stockists too - one order from either of them would've been life-changing. But I had two choices: to choose money or to do the right thing. My heart knew what to do, but at the same time, I had worked so hard to get into the US market, and I was throwing all of that away. But I couldn't continue using leather knowing how cruel and toxic it is. I spent 2014 rebranding, which was also tough because I had no new products to sell, so I had to forfeit sales for most of that year. Financially it was tough, but my soul was happy.

What a lot of people don't realize is that leather is listed twice on the World's Top Ten Pollutants, from the livestock industry and leather tanneries. When you truly understand how leather is made, you'll see that ethical and eco (animal) leather simply doesn't exist. Not only are animals and the environment heavily impacted, but the people who work in the tanneries and live near the tanneries are exposed to toxic sludge. The majority of the world's leather comes from India and Bangladesh, and although it helps these countries financially, the tanneries are poisoning the people and the land.

Now, my brand, KSKYE the Label, has rebranded to be eco-vegan and restructured to be a social-label. We launched a BE KIND Series which donates 100% of our profits to animal welfare, conservation and humanitarian charities: International Anti-Poaching Foundation, Rainforest Rescue, Reach Out WorldWide, Sea Shepherd Shelter Ugolyok, and WIRES Wildlife Rescue. We also employ artisans from developing countries.

I've always liked to eat healthy and stay fit and active, and while I rebranded my label, I also began my studies in Human Nutrition and Master Herbalism. Now I'm about to release my book. And I mentor quite a few people as well; I teach people how to strengthen their intuition.

My life completely flipped around for the absolute best after going vegan. You could say I found my soul-calling!

WHAT IS THE MOST INSPIRING OR POWERFUL RESULT THAT YOU HAVE SEEN WITH A CLIENT ON A PLANT-BASED DIET?

A client came to me and she was sickly, experiencing insomnia and found that breastfeeding her baby was painful. She wasn't plant-based, but after following my advice her ailments subsided and she was able to breastfeed without any pain. She also finally got some much-needed sleep.

What most do not realize is that what we eat and what we don't eat, heavily affects our health. So I adjusted her diet and within a couple of days, she was breastfeeding her baby without any issues. This made her see how food was directly connected to the majority of her ailments, and she has kept up the plant-based eating. It only takes one revelation for many people to start digging deeper, and for my client, that was it.

Other clients have healed severe acne, hair loss, IBS, high cholesterol, high blood pressure and eczema, to name a few. Every one of my clients have shown vast improvements simply from changing their diets!

WHAT HAS BEEN THE MOST NOTICEABLE CHANGE AFTER TURNING YOUR FAMILY VEGAN/PLANT-BASED?

Besides being much healthier, I've also noticed spiritual growth as well. Whether you go vegan for the animals, for the earth, or for health, when you take dead, low-vibe-foods off of your plate, it's hard not to spiritually evolve as well.

ANY INSPIRING STORIES THAT HAVE HAPPENED TO YOU OR PEOPLE CLOSE TO YOU THAT HAVE NOT BEEN COVERED ABOVE. STORIES THAT CAN INSPIRE AND HELP OTHERS.

For years I have believed that we can gain every essential nutrient from plants and from the sun. But what I lacked was proof, especially when it came to B12. With every bone in my body, I just knew that we weren't meant to eat animals! And it just didn't feel right knowing that we had to get B12 from animals or supplement it. However, there is growing evidence that bioavailable B12 is produced by small intestinal bacteria, meaning that if you have a healthy gut, your gut will most likely produce B12! This comes after researchers believed that the B12 bacteria was only made in the colon, where it cannot be absorbed. A healthy gut promotes a strong immune system, it's known as our 'second brain' and is linked to our mental health; all illnesses are said to start in the gut. And a healthy gut can produce the very nutrients that we need.

ROBYN CHUTER

CONNECT WITH ROBYN:
INSTAGRAM: @ROBYNCHUTER
FACEBOOK: EMPOWER TOTAL HEALTH
empowertotalhealth.com.au

Robyn Chuter is a health practitioner with a Bachelor of Health Science degree with First Class Honours from Edith Cowan University and a Diploma of Naturopathy from the Australasian College of Natural Therapies, as well as being an Australasian Society of Lifestyle Medicine-certified Lifestyle Medicine Practitioner. If that wasn't impressive enough, she also holds a graduate diploma in counselling from the Australian College of Applied Psychology and holds level three EFT Practitioner and Matrix Reimprinting Practitioner accreditations. In 1995 she began a naturopathic practice with a particular interest in chronic and medically "incurable" health problems like IBS, CFS, migraines, high blood pressure and type 2 diabetes.

WHAT ARE YOUR DAILY RITUALS/HABITS WHICH YOU BELIEVE HAVE BEEN KEY TO YOUR HEALTH?

203

I start each day with a meditation session using the HeartMath emWave device, which gives me real-time feedback on how my thoughts and emotions are affecting me. It also guides me into a state described as "heart coherence," which is an optimal state of synchronization between the mind, emotions and all the systems of the body.

After this, I do some strength training before enjoying a hearty breakfast of fruit, oats and homemade soy yogurt.

After I finish work, I walk my dog for an hour. I'm lucky enough to live near lots of lakes and parks, so there are plenty of places to enjoy nature and to "downshift" after a busy day.

AT WHAT POINT IN YOUR LIFE DID YOU DECIDE TO CHANGE YOUR DIET? HOW HAS THAT DECISION IMPACTED YOUR LIFE?

I became a vegetarian for ethical reasons when I was 15. It just suddenly struck me one day that I was being incredibly hypocritical in calling myself an "animal lover" when there were certain animals that I ate.

Back in the mid-1980s, there were very few information sources available to me for a number of years, so I didn't grasp that dairy and egg production also caused enormous suffering to animals. Eventually, I came to understand the full impact of animal agriculture on human health, the environment and animal suffering, and together with my husband and two children, I made the commitment to be 100% vegan in 2005.

My only regret is that I didn't do it years earlier.

WHAT KIND OF REACTION DO YOU RECEIVE WHEN YOUR PEERS, FRIENDS, AND OTHER "EXPERTS," FIND OUT THAT YOU ARE VEGAN/ PLANT-BASED? ARE THEY INTERESTED AND WANT TO KNOW MORE?

When I first went vegetarian, my family and friends struggled to understand why. I must admit, I was overly militant and judgmental, and probably turned people off who were wanting to learn more. Since then I've learned to approach "pre-vegans" with compassion and curiosity. I find that people are inspired to try a plant-based diet when they observe other people thriving on this way of eating, so I strive to be a healthy role model.

I rarely see doctors, but I find that most are wary of plant-based diets and assume that they will inevitably cause nutrient deficiencies. However, when I start discussing the research literature on plant-based diets and health, it quickly becomes evident to them that they don't know as much about nutrition as they thought they did. Most shut down at this point, but I have encountered a few doctors who want to learn more about this way of eating.

WHAT IS THE MOST INSPIRING OR POWERFUL RESULT THAT YOU HAVE SEEN WITH A PATIENT AND A PLANT-BASED DIET?

I've seen so many people recover their health! The most powerful result I've ever seen was a woman who had such severe ulcerative colitis that she was scheduled for surgery to have her colon removed. After just two days on a plant-based diet (modified for her condition), she stopped bleeding from her bowel. One week later, her bowel movements were completely normal, with no pain, cramping or diarrhea. She cancelled her bowel surgery, and over ten years later she still has her bowel and is free of ulcerative colitis.

YOU'VE JUST MET A HEARTBROKEN STRANGER AND THEY'VE JUST BEEN GIVEN A LIFE-THREATENING DIAGNOSIS. WHAT WOULD BE YOUR TOP FIVE TIPS TO HELP THEM?

1. Adopt a high-nutrient, plant-based diet, high in fruits and vegetables and free of ultra-processed foods such as oils, white flour and sugar.

2. Begin a daily meditation practice and learn to cultivate inner peace, gratitude and equanimity.

" "

OUR STEREOSCOPIC COLOR VISION HELPS
US TO SPOT BRIGHTLY-COLORED RIPE FRUITS,
OUR DEXTEROUS HANDS ENABLE US TO PICK
THEM AND PEEL THEM, AND OUR TASTE BUDS
DETECT SWEETNESS WHICH OUR BRAINS
REGISTER AS PLEASURE.

OUR DIGESTIVE TRACT IS PERFECTLY ADAPTED
TO MOVE FIBROUS PLANT FOODS THROUGH IT.

IT EXTRACTS NUTRIENTS AND SENDS THE
INDIGESTIBLE REMNANTS TO OUR COLON
WHERE OUR GUT MICROBIOTA METABOLIZE
THEM, PRODUCING NUTRIENTS AND
METABOLICALLY ACTIVE BYPRODUCTS
WHICH IMPROVE EVERY ASPECT OF OUR
FUNCTIONING, FROM STABILIZING OUR
BLOOD SUGAR LEVEL, TO REGULATING OUR
IMMUNE SYSTEM, TO STIMULATING THE
GROWTH OF NEW BRAIN CELLS.

PUT WHOLE OR MINIMALLY PROCESSED
PLANTS INTO THE HUMAN BODY
AND IT WORKS AS INTENDED.

ROBYN CHUTER

3. Join a supportive group of people who are taking responsibility for their own health, preferably in person, but online groups can provide effective support too.

4. Seek second, third and fourth opinions about your diagnosis, prognosis, and treatment plan. Ask each healthcare provider that you see, for evidence that supports their treatment plan. Insist on receiving informed consent before agreeing to any diagnostic test, procedure or drug.

5. Read stories of people who have overcome your diagnosis or learned to thrive in spite of it.

CAN YOU SHARE A STORY ABOUT THE POWER OF PLANTS THAT YOU USE WITH YOUR CLIENTS TO HELP THEM BELIEVE IN THIS AS AN ALTERNATIVE WAY OF LOOKING AT MEDICINE?

All you have to do is study human anatomy and physiology; we are beautifully evolved to seek out, gather and enjoy plant foods.
Our stereoscopic color vision helps us to spot brightly-colored ripe fruits, our dexterous hands enable us to pick them and peel them and our taste buds detect sweetness which our brains register as pleasure. Our digestive tract is perfectly adapted to move fibrous plant foods through it. It extracts nutrients and sends the indigestible remnants to our colon where our gut microbiota metabolize them, producing nutrients and metabolically active byproducts which improve every aspect of our functioning, from stabilizing our blood sugar level to regulating our immune system to stimulating the growth of new brain cells. Put whole or minimally processed plants into the human body and it works as intended. Put anything else in and sooner or later, health problems will begin to surface.

ANY INSPIRING STORIES THAT HAVE HAPPENED TO YOU OR PEOPLE CLOSE TO YOU THAT HAVE NOT BEEN COVERED ABOVE. STORIES THAT CAN HELP OTHERS.

One of my most inspiring clients was already vegan when he came to see me, but he was a "junk food vegan." He had type two diabetes, high blood pressure and rheumatoid arthritis. We worked together intensively for six months to replace the hyper-palatable vegan convenience foods with fruits, vegetables, whole grains and legumes. By the end of this process, he was able to stop taking both of his blood pressure medications, all three of his diabetes medications and all three of his rheumatoid arthritis medications. His blood pressure was perfect, his endocrinologist pronounced him non-diabetic, and he was free of all joint pain and swelling. That's the power of plants.

DR. ANGIE SADEGHI, M.D.

CONNECT WITH DR.ANGIE:
INSTAGRAM: @ANGIE.SADEGHI
YOUTUBE: ANGIE SADEGHI MD
DrAngieHealth.com

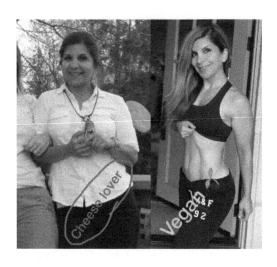

207

Dr. Angie Sadeghi is a gastroenterologist who discovered the power of plant-based eating after clearing her debilitating eczema once she adopted this diet change. She now advises her patients, many suffering from serious bowel diseases, to do the same and has seen drastic life-changing improvements.

"Consider how you want to spend the last ten years of your life. Either you can spend the last ten years as a healthy, active, individual possibly traveling the world, hiking trails, and visiting places, or it can be in-and-out of the hospital taking ten different medicines with a poor quality of life. You can choose!"

WHAT ARE YOUR DAILY RITUALS/HABITS WHICH YOU BELIEVE HAVE BEEN KEY TO YOUR HEALTH?

In May 2014, I decided to start eating a whole-food, plant-based diet (WFPBD), therefore I made lifestyle modifications that have allowed me to continue eating this way for the rest of my life. Simultaneously, I decided to reduce my workouts to a 25-minute duration, but instead, work out every single day. The combination of these two decisions have helped transform my body to be more fit than ever.

AT WHAT POINT IN YOUR LIFE DID YOU DECIDE TO CHANGE YOUR DIET? HOW HAS THAT DECISION IMPACTED YOUR LIFE?

I decided to start eating a WFPBD May 2014 after attending a seminar where health and fitness was discussed. At that point, I was overweight and suffered from several medical problems such as eczema, fatigue and elevated cholesterol. I spoke to my cousin, who is vegan and asked me to watch the documentary, Forks Over Knives, which forever changed my life.

WHAT KIND OF REACTION DO YOU RECEIVE WHEN YOUR PEERS, FRIENDS, AND OTHER "EXPERTS," FIND OUT THAT YOU ARE VEGAN/ PLANT-BASED? ARE THEY INTERESTED AND WANT TO KNOW MORE?

I have seen many different reactions. Some want to learn more and implement changes in their diet, but some are completely resistant to the lifestyle.

DO YOU TAKE ANY SPECIFIC SUPPLEMENTS? DO YOU RECOMMEND ANY SPECIFIC BRANDS? WHY DO YOU THINK THESE HAVE BENEFITED YOU AND YOUR HEALTH?

I am against taking protein supplements, but I do encourage my patients to take vitamin B12 and vitamin D if their levels are low.

WHAT IS THE MOST INSPIRING OR POWERFUL RESULT THAT YOU HAVE SEEN WITH A PATIENT AND A PLANT-BASED DIET?

As a gastroenterologist, I see many patients with inflammatory bowel disease. Since I started helping patients switch to this lifestyle, I have had about 15 patients achieve remission of their disease by switching to a plant-based diet.

YOU'VE JUST MET A HEARTBROKEN STRANGER WHO HAS JUST BEEN GIVEN A LIFE-THREATENING DIAGNOSIS. WHAT WOULD BE YOUR TOP FIVE TIPS TO HELP THEM?

Start eating a whole-food plant-based diet, get more exercise, breathe fresh air, meditate/avoid all stress and laugh a lot.

CAN YOU SHARE A STORY ABOUT THE POWER OF PLANTS THAT YOU USE WITH YOUR CLIENTS TO HELP THEM BELIEVE IN THIS AS AN ALTERNATIVE WAY OF LOOKING AT MEDICINE?

I had chronic debilitating eczema, which had me embarrassed due to pustular lesions on my hands and body. I was so itchy that I couldn't sleep at night. Since I switched to a WFPBD, my eczema completely cleared up, and my skin looks better than ever.

ALIA ALMOAYED

CONNECT WITH ALIA:
INSTAGRAM: @ALIAALMOAYED
YOUTUBE: ALIA ALMOAYED
FACEBOOK: ALIA ALMOAYED
AliaAlmoayed.com

As a nutritional therapist and alternative health activist, Alia Aloayed specializes in health advice geared towards Middle Eastern and Arabic communities. Alia writes health articles for a variety of publications, is the founder and host of an award-winning Arabic TV show, hosts radio programs on health and nutrition, holds health lectures, leads health retreats, and is the author of a variety of books in the health genre including I Want Healthy Kids, I Want a Healthy Pregnancy, and co-author to 101 Ways to Improve Your Health.

WHAT ARE YOUR DAILY RITUALS/HABITS WHICH YOU BELIEVE HAVE BEEN KEY TO YOUR HEALTH?

I start my day with a green juice and a yoga session. The juice energizes me, and it feels like I'm pouring nutrients into my body. The yoga gives me the stability and strength to face what the day brings.

AT WHAT POINT IN YOUR LIFE DID YOU DECIDE TO CHANGE YOUR DIET? HOW HAS THAT DECISION IMPACTED YOUR LIFE?

I switched to a healthier diet almost 20 years ago because of recurrent illnesses. However, I only started to look seriously into the plant-based diet in the past five or ten years. This was mainly because I started having an internal conflict when seeing what the meat industry is doing to the planet and to our health.

WHAT KIND OF REACTION DO YOU RECEIVE WHEN YOUR PEERS, FRIENDS, AND OTHER "EXPERTS," FIND OUT THAT YOU ARE VEGAN/ PLANT-BASED? ARE THEY INTERESTED AND WANT TO KNOW MORE?

To be honest, I prefer not to discuss it. Like politics and religion, veganism has become polarized and usually attracts an uncomfortable kind of conversation. People tend to become defensive and judgmental, but I'm not trying to convert anyone. I respect where people are at in their journeys and their own self-development. What suits me might not suit others.

DO YOU TAKE ANY SPECIFIC SUPPLEMENTS? DO YOU RECOMMEND ANY SPECIFIC BRANDS? WHY DO YOU THINK THESE HAVE BENEFITED YOU AND YOUR HEALTH?

I tend to prefer natural supplements such as wheatgrass and/or spirulina powders; I have those in my green juice daily. I also like Liposomal vitamin C and vegan probiotics. I also use a lot of healing essential oils such as frankincense, tea tree and lavender oils, mainly from DoTERRA.

WHAT IS THE MOST INSPIRING OR POWERFUL RESULT THAT YOU HAVE SEEN WITH A PATIENT AND A PLANT-BASED DIET?

It's amazing to see the effect that a plant-based diet has on balancing hormones and improving heavy periods, period pains, PMS, and polycystic ovaries. As soon as we stop the influx of hormones coming into the body from animal products, a shift happens in the body. Our own hormones start to balance again and find their way to normalcy. The problem is not just that animal products contain naturally-existing hormones from the animal itself, but extra man-made hormones are injected into these animals to make them grow or lactate. These hormones then find their way into our bodies and cause an imbalance in our regular hormonal cycle (in both men and women). In women we see it present itself as early puberty, heavy periods, period pains, PMS, polycystic ovaries, excess hair growth, fertility issues, breast, and ovarian cancers and much more. In men, we see it as abdominal fat, man breasts, mood swings, testicular cancer, low motility and much more. The plant-based diet helps regulate hormones back to what is closer to what is required for optimum health.

YOU'VE JUST MET A HEARTBROKEN STRANGER WHO HAS JUST BEEN GIVEN A LIFE-THREATENING DIAGNOSIS. WHAT WOULD BE YOUR TOP FIVE TIPS TO HELP THEM?

Assuming they ask for advice, I would say:

1) Start with a three-day juice fast (vegetable juices)
2) Lots of good-quality water
3) Look into the Wim Hof breathing method
4) Make sure your diet is alkaline and plant-based (no meat or dairy)
5) Avoid all forms of refined (white) sugar

CAN YOU SHARE A STORY ABOUT THE POWER OF PLANTS THAT YOU USE WITH YOUR CLIENTS TO HELP THEM BELIEVE IN THIS AS AN ALTERNATIVE WAY OF LOOKING AT MEDICINE?

I have a story about a young lady who had severe facial acne and a skin

210

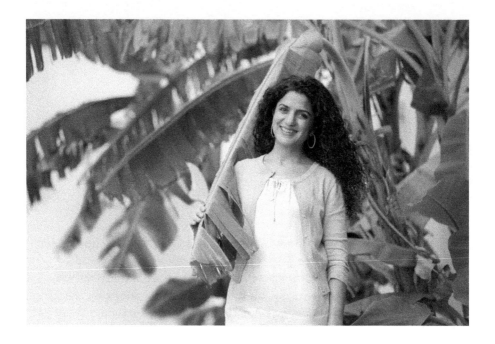

allergy that would not shift no matter what she took for it. She switched to a plant-based diet, which meant no meat and no dairy. She also cut out sugars, started taking probiotics and turmeric, plus daily deep breathing. The results blew her away. Within just a few short weeks the problem that she had suffered from for years had completely vanished.

IF YOU COULD GIVE US JUST THREE ABSOLUTE MUSTS TO INCLUDE IN OUR DIET EACH DAY WHAT WOULD THEY BE?

1) Green juice made with cucumber, parsley, celery, carrot, and green apple (to give the body a boost of nutrients).
2) Turmeric powder mixed with coconut oil (1 tbsp reduces any inflammation in the body).
3) Enough water to produce a big volume of urination.

ANY INSPIRING STORIES THAT HAVE HAPPENED TO YOU OR PEOPLE CLOSE TO YOU THAT HAVE NOT BEEN COVERED ABOVE. STORIES THAT CAN HELP OTHERS.

A quote I love: "we spend our health collecting wealth and then spend our wealth getting back our health." We often go about life forgetting what our priorities are. Health should be our priority at all times, and everything else comes second. This includes physical, emotional and spiritual health.

DR. BANDANA N CHAWLA

CONNECT WITH DR.BANDANA:
INSTAGRAM: @LIFESTYLEDOCS
lifestyledocs.com
peacefulplanetfoundation.org

"I have seen a patient go from 306 pounds to 185 pounds. I have seen diabetes and heart disease reversed. I have seen a morbidly obese sedentary patient transform himself to a plant-based ultramarathon runner. I have seen patients get off depression medications by changing their diet and lifestyle. I can go on and on. I am very fortunate that I get to witness these amazing success stories in my clinic now."

Dr. Bandana Chawla is a board-certified physician in Internal Medicine and Lifestyle Medicine and has practiced as an internist in Houston, Texas for over 20 years. To build upon the success of her lifestyle medicine concept (taking a more holistic approach to wellness), she co-created lifestyledoc.com, a medical practice that focuses on eating well, exercising right, reducing stress and living a balanced life.

AT WHAT POINT IN YOUR LIFE DID YOU DECIDE TO CHANGE YOUR DIET? HOW HAS THAT DECISION IMPACTED YOUR LIFE?

I decided to change at the age of 39. At the end of 2012, the universe kept sending me vegan and plant-based patients. The improvements in their health forced me to do my own research and finally learn nutrition, an important subject that was not emphasized in medical school. Their amazing results got me intrigued, and the fact that I could actually start taking them off some of their medications really made me decide to do more research.

I asked these patients about what made them go vegan, and I just loved the ethical reasons behind it. There was also tons of evidence proving that plant-based diets are optimal for human health. I also came across many ethical and environmental aspects during my research. I decided to go vegan for ethical reasons on February 1st of 2013, and a few years later became completely plant-based, so I could practice what I preach to my patients. Fortunately, my husband became vegan with me, which made it easy to overcome our fears together and take control of our own destiny.

212

DO YOU TAKE ANY SPECIFIC SUPPLEMENTS? DO YOU RECOMMEND ANY SPECIFIC BRANDS? WHY DO YOU THINK THESE HAVE BENEFITED YOU AND YOUR HEALTH?

Vitamin B12 and vegan DHA/EPA - Deva vegan vitamins. I just ordered the new complement capsules from No Meat Athlete.

WHAT ARE YOUR RECOMMENDATIONS TO YOUR CLIENTS WHEN YOU FIRST SUGGEST THEY SHOULD MOVE TO A PLANT-BASED DIET?

Be patient and persistent. Get support from the local community (like vegan potluck) or online community (like specific Facebook groups). Do your own research and find your own "whys." Once you have a deeper connection to it, it becomes a whole lot easier.

SHARE A STORY ABOUT THE POWER OF PLANTS THAT YOU USE WITH YOUR CLIENTS TO HELP THEM BELIEVE IN THIS AS AN ALTERNATIVE WAY OF LOOKING AT MEDICINE?

I often talk about Blue Zones (areas in the world with the longest living populations) and how individuals in these locations live long, healthy, vibrant lives because they eat mainly plant-based foods. We don't have to get old, tired and demented before we die. We can narrow the gap between our health span and our lifespan if we choose to eat a plant-based diet.

213

IF YOU COULD GIVE US JUST THREE ABSOLUTE MUSTS TO INCLUDE IN OUR DIET EACH DAY WHAT WOULD THEY BE?

Greens, beans and fruits. It really is that simple. Eat to live.

SINCE BECOMING VEGAN, HOW HAS YOUR LIFE CHANGED?

I was sedentary before. Now have I done 5Ks, 10Ks, a half marathon, Tour De Houston bike ride and a sprint triathlon. I have so much more energy and vibrancy now, and I love feeling this way.

ANY INSPIRING STORIES YOU CAN SHARE?

After being a physician for 20 years, I am now absolutely loving my job because I actually get to see patients get better on plant-based diets. I am now studying for a Lifestyle Medicine exam to be board certified in Lifestyle Medicine. This new field focuses on nutrition, exercise, stress management, avoidance of tobacco and alcohol, adequate sleep and healthy relationships to help one achieve optimal levels of health and wellness. I am so excited - especially since this is an evidence-based field - that they actually recommend a predominantly whole-food, plant-based diet. This is because it's what the evidence shows.

6 DAILY HABITS FOR HOLISTIC HEALTH

1. Morning routine ≈

I always start with a glass of lemon water, probiotics, Omega supplement,
and vitamin D (during winter). Every morning I leave the house with
a full glass jar of more lemon water and a green smoothie.

2. Daily movement ≈

I love to exercise 4-5 days per week alternating between running,
weight training, biking and yoga. On off days I still move my body but
to a lesser degree. Something like family hikes or walks.

3. Nourishing myself with real food ≈

Ensuring that I always have healthy meals prepped
and ready to eat for me and the family.

4. Self-care ≈

Investing in what my body is telling me it needs. Sometimes self-care
for me is sitting by the water, unplugging and reading a good book.
Other times it's going out to dinner with great friends. I can tell when I
haven't been listening because I will feel out of alignment or "off."
When I feel that way I can easily fix it by getting outside
and enjoying some time in nature.

5. Boundaries ≈

Since I love what I do I have found myself working late and answering
emails anytime they came in, which sometimes led to me prioritizing
work over family and relationships. I knew this had to change, so I created
boundaries in order for my mental and social health to improve.
I now work during specific work day hours and if I need to work more,
I wake up an hour or two before the kids are up so I can get things done.

6. Gratitude practice ≈

Every single morning I write or say three to five things
that I am grateful for that day.

PAMELA ROCCA

MARINA YANAY-TRINER

CONNECT WITH MARINA:
INSTAGRAM: @SOULINTHERAW
YOUTUBE: SOUL IN THE RAW
FACEBOOK: SOUL IN THE RAW
soulintheraw.com

Marina Yanay-Triner is the creator of the popular blog, Soul in the Raw, where she shares her high raw whole-food plant-based journey with the rest of the world. After witnessing the healing from the incredibly painful interstitial cystitis, Marina decided that she wanted to discover the healing magic of whole-food plant-based eating herself to heal from her own health difficulties, including post-traumatic stress disorder. She made the lifestyle switch to a high-raw vegan diet and hasn't looked back since.

"Eating a plant-based diet was my first step in saying "yes" to myself and my needs, and acknowledging that I actually care and want to feel connected again. It helped me regain feeling in my body, and to start listening to its wisdom, bit by bit. It took many years, and it's a process that is still becoming and transforming."

215

WHAT ARE YOUR DAILY RITUALS/HABITS WHICH YOU BELIEVE HAVE BEEN KEY TO YOUR HEALTH?

Eating a whole-foods, plant-based diet is a cornerstone and a basis for everything else: my morning and evening guided meditations, connecting to nature (even if it's in a little way, every single day), Wim Hof breathing, and my alarm clock ringing a few times a day with a mantra I record for myself.

AT WHAT POINT IN YOUR LIFE DID YOU DECIDE TO CHANGE YOUR DIET? HOW HAS THAT DECISION IMPACTED YOUR LIFE?

Seven years ago, my mother healed herself from interstitial cystitis, which is a terrible and extremely painful bladder disease that literally debilitated her and made her not leave the house for eight years. She healed herself through a plant-based diet, and as I watched her do it and literally saw the miracles that it made in her life, I decided to try it too. I wanted to cure myself of terrible and debilitating PMS cramps, as well as PTSD that I was suffering from as a result of being sexually assaulted in high school.

WHAT KIND OF REACTION DO YOU RECEIVE WHEN YOUR PEERS,

FRIENDS, AND OTHER "EXPERTS," FIND OUT THAT YOU ARE VEGAN/ PLANT-BASED? ARE THEY INTERESTED AND WANT TO KNOW MORE?

Absolutely! I think that when my friends see the great impact that this lifestyle has on my life, and how delicious the food I make is, it inspires them to hear more about it and try it, whether it's by going fully plant-based or at least adding more plant-based foods to their diet. I have helped many totally overhaul their diets just by setting an example. This is what I believe in. Rather than being pushy and forcing it on people, leading by example is the best you can do to promote the vegan lifestyle.

WHAT IS THE MOST INSPIRING OR POWERFUL RESULT THAT YOU HAVE SEEN WITH A PATIENT AND A PLANT-BASED DIET?

After just a few days of whole-food, plant-based eating, one of my clients got rid of her arthritic pains! And she went from being obese, eating chicken wings and ordering take-out every single day, to a 100% whole-food, plant-based diet. After a few weeks, her energy levels were so great that she stopped using an alarm clock and she actually started her own business to transform not only her physical health, but her financial health! The most powerful of all her changes was that by the end of our work together (two months), she told me that she finally found true peace as she had never experienced it before in her life.

YOU'VE JUST MET A HEARTBROKEN STRANGER WHO HAS JUST BEEN GIVEN A LIFE-THREATENING DIAGNOSIS. WHAT WOULD BE YOUR TOP FIVE TIPS TO HELP THEM?

1. Eat whole plant foods - plants in their whole form, unprocessed, and as close to nature as they can be.
2. Consult with plant-based doctors who can support you through an evidence-based approach to healing.
3. Take care of your soul and find a daily ritual or practice that will bring you into positive vibes every single day.
4. Spend time outside. There is absolutely nothing better than being in nature, and away from electronics, breathing in the fresh air.
5. Get loads of leafy greens into your diet, as much as three times a day, and switch up the ones you use every day. These are some of the most healing foods.

CAN YOU SHARE A STORY ABOUT THE POWER OF PLANTS THAT YOU USE WITH YOUR CLIENTS TO HELP THEM BELIEVE IN THIS AS AN ALTERNATIVE WAY OF LOOKING AT MEDICINE?

Instead of telling a story, I tell my clients this:

You have contacted me because your intuition and your heart is telling you to try this lifestyle. Maybe you're a little scared, overwhelmed or intimidated. But you know it's the right thing for your body, and you know that it can heal you. What you don't know is how good you can really feel. It's hard to describe because you probably haven't felt it before.

That unknown, even if you think it's probably good, it's a bit intimidating. So, what I encourage you to do is just give this a shot for one or two weeks. I promise you; you'll experience such a profound change that it will be worth all the effort. You'll feel so amazing that this feeling will become your "why" - your reason to keep at it!

IF YOU COULD GIVE US JUST THREE ABSOLUTE MUSTS TO INCLUDE IN OUR DIET EACH DAY WHAT WOULD THEY BE?

Legumes (soaked and then cooked), dark leafy greens and fruits. Make sure to vary up which kind you use in each category every day.

ANY INSPIRING STORIES YOU CAN SHARE?

As someone living with PTSD, I know what it feels like to be entirely disconnected from my body to the point where I lost total feeling in certain areas in my body. While it may sound crazy, having a loss of sensation in the body is an actual scientifically-researched phenomenon that situations of extreme stress bring about. It's an attempt to disconnect from the deep and unyielding pain inside the body.

This disconnection did have some positives: it allowed me to survive something that was almost impossible to comprehend at times. But of course, it also had a major negative: the inability to truly feel. Sometimes this deep feeling that I couldn't feel was pain, and sometimes it was deep joy and pleasure.

Eating a plant-based diet was my first step in saying "yes" to myself and my needs, and acknowledging that I actually care and want to feel connected again. It helped me regain feeling in my body, and to start listening to its wisdom bit by bit. It took many years, and it's a process that is still becoming and transforming.

I believe we all have a place of disconnection in our lives. Sometimes it's physical and obvious like mine. And sometimes it's more hidden.

I encourage you to dive into the world of plants because they will lead you back to building a strong connection with who you are and help you to listen to your real needs and desires. They will lead you back to a place of joy, pain, sorrow and excitement, and to experience a deep, meaningful connection to yourself and your place in the world.

ANJA CASS

CONNECT WITH ANJA:
INSTAGRAM: @COOKINGWITHPLANTS
FACEBOOK: COOKINGWITHPLANTS
YOUTUBE: COOKINGWITHPLANTS
cookingwithplants.com

2015 Vegan of the Year Winner for Outstanding Social Media Outreach, Anja Cass is a popular vegan cook who shares her passion for creating healthy, plant-based recipes via social media and her website, cookingwithplants.com. Her journey towards plant-based eating began after discovering that she had early-onset heart disease. From that point, she set out to discover the best way to reverse the damage to her body. She ended up losing 50 pounds after switching to a plant-based diet and continues to inspire others with her story while helping her followers discover the beauty of healthy, plant-based eating.

218

WHAT ARE YOUR DAILY RITUALS/HABITS WHICH YOU BELIEVE HAVE BEEN KEY TO YOUR HEALTH?

I like to keep things super simple and tasty! My main daily habits include having fresh produce in the fridge as well as pre-cooked grains and potatoes so I can throw a meal together super fast any time I'm hungry! I also make sure that I have my go-to sauces on hand so I can make a quick and tasty meal out of whatever I have in the fridge, freezer and pantry. Easy and delicious!

AT WHAT POINT IN YOUR LIFE DID YOU DECIDE TO CHANGE YOUR DIET? HOW HAS THAT DECISION IMPACTED YOUR LIFE?

In 2012 I had a health scare. After a routine doctor's appointment, I discovered that I had a bulging aorta and the onset of heart disease. With a young son and family history of fatal heart disease on both sides of my family, I researched ways to reverse this. Everything led to a plant-based diet. I also watched the documentary Forks Over Knives and read The China Study. I watched and read everything I could to learn more. I decided to change my eating habits virtually overnight!

At this point, I began cooking plant-based food and saw immediate results. My cholesterol dropped, I had energy again, and I lost over 50 pounds in just five months. I finally felt good again.

My weight loss and healthy glow soon had people questioning what I was eating. In 2013 I started to do quick YouTube videos to explain and show my new meals to family and friends. What happened next I never expected. More and more people started to watch my channel - strangers! People from all around the world were tuning in for my quick, easy and tasty recipes.

WHAT KIND OF REACTION DO YOU RECEIVE WHEN YOUR PEERS, FRIENDS AND OTHER "EXPERTS," FIND OUT THAT YOU ARE VEGAN/ PLANT-BASED? ARE THEY INTERESTED AND WANT TO KNOW MORE?

My parents were initially shocked, but most people were curious. I wasn't pushy or extreme. I always only focused on educating others and sharing my recipes. I think people are often scared of the unknown, so if you can relate this lifestyle to what they already know, it doesn't make it daunting or intimidating for them. I've even had people say, "when I heard you were vegan I really didn't think I would like you, but you're so nice!"

I think the key is to set a good example and let people see that and learn from it. Also, be very informed about the questions you will receive. If there's something you don't know the answer to, then just say "I'm not sure, but that's a fabulous question. Let me find out and get back to you on that."

DO YOU TAKE ANY SPECIFIC SUPPLEMENTS? DO YOU RECOMMEND ANY SPECIFIC BRANDS? WHY DO YOU THINK THESE HAVE BENEFITED YOU AND YOUR HEALTH?

I always make sure I get regular blood tests (every six months) to make sure that everything is on track. I check my iron levels, vitamin D and so forth. However, the one thing that I always supplement (and everyone should, not just plant-based vegans) is B12.

B12 is the one vitamin that is ultra important to our health, and it is something that is not commonly found in our current food and water supplies these days. We used to get it from the bacteria in streams or on food, but almost everything these days is treated and therefore depleted in B12.

YOU'VE JUST MET A HEARTBROKEN STRANGER AND THEY'VE JUST BEEN GIVEN A LIFE-THREATENING DIAGNOSIS. WHAT WOULD BE YOUR TOP FIVE TIPS TO HELP THEM?

First of all, I would give them a BIG HUG! Then I would say:

1. *Breathe.* Take a deep breath. Appreciate that this is actually a good thing. Why? Because you've been made aware that it is actually time to take care of YOU!

2. Do the Opposite. Make a list of all the unhealthy foods, habits and environmental factors you currently have in your life and replace these with healthy substitutes. If you smoke, start dancing instead. If you eat fried meat and dairy, have fresh fruit and vegetables instead. If you have stress in your life, practice meditation! Whatever it is that's been unhealthy in your life, bring in the opposite so you receive the opposite results. You will be amazed at how powerful this can be.

3. Do something for just 15 minutes. This will be a very emotional and draining time for you. It will be hard to focus, but you need to push through and know that small steps will get you to the top of the mountain.
Start by doing things in just fifteen-minute chunks. This way, you will get things done without overwhelming yourself.

4. Practice daily mindfulness. Appreciate all the good things you have in your life. It doesn't matter how simple it is. It could be that you have a warm bed, good friends or clean running water. There is always something to be grateful for.

5. ASK FOR HELP! There is no shame in accepting help from others. Let others be there for you. You don't always have to be the one who is giving to everyone else. And most of all, seek out the help of professionals and people that have been through what you are going through. Copy what they have done! Look on YouTube for people that have overcome or dealt with the diagnosis you have just been given. Especially focus on those that have done it with a plant-based diet because this is what has been scientifically shown time and time again to have the best, immediate, and most importantly, long-term health benefits.

CAN YOU SHARE A STORY ABOUT THE POWER OF PLANTS THAT YOU USE WITH YOUR CLIENTS TO HELP THEM BELIEVE IN THIS AS AN ALTERNATIVE WAY OF LOOKING AT MEDICINE?

In 2012, I went on a three month holiday to Germany. I was actually born there, so most of my relatives are still there. Being the kind-hearted, loving family that they are, they would load me up with mountains of food every day, and I couldn't say no. I just thought I was having fun and enjoying myself, but that couldn't have been any further from the truth. I was actually making myself fat and sick.

Every meal was loaded with meat, dairy and bread, followed by loads of desserts and treats as far as the eye could see. But what was about to happen would change my life FOREVER!

When I came back to Australia, I started getting severe migraines. I couldn't concentrate. I was sluggish, and I felt really flat and low on energy. It was even a struggle to keep on the FAKE smile. I was sick and tired all the time, feeling my energy levels dragging me further and further behind in life. I struggled with diet after diet, only to put on more weight and binge eat myself to sleep at night.

Eventually, I went to the doctor. I told him everything that I was suffering with. He listened carefully and did a full check-up. When he started listening to my heart, his face changed. As he was listening, he looked at me strangely, and then he listened again. Finally, he said, "I think you have a heart murmur. I'm going to send you to get an ultrasound of your heart." I had no idea what all that meant, but I had a pretty good idea that it wasn't anything good.

A few days later, the doctor called me back to his office for an urgent appointment. I nervously walked into his office and sat down. He shuffled his papers around, and then he told me the news that would change my life forever. I still remember his words so clearly. He said, "you have a bulging aorta. If this keeps increasing, it can rupture." I asked him loads of questions and eventually went into shock. This meant that I could die if things didn't change. I needed to find out how I could get healthy again.

After I left the doctor's surgery, I started to do loads of research every day. For weeks and weeks, I searched high and low to find the best ways to reverse heart disease. Everything I found kept pointing to a plant-based diet. I was only 39 at the time, and my son was only nine years old. I was too young to have such an intense health scare. My son needed his mother, my family needed me, and I wasn't ready for an early grave. At this point, there were so many thoughts that were buzzing through my mind. I was confused, and I was flat out scared.

Eventually, I narrowed down a list of whole, plant-based foods and kept that list in my kitchen. I combined it with my cooking skills and kitchen "know how," and started a whole new way of eating: a whole-food, plant-based diet.

It started to change my life; it was actually working! Within five months I lost over 50 pounds, and I've kept it off ever since. Additionally, my cholesterol went back to normal and I started to have so much energy that I actually wanted to start exercising for the first time in my life. I couldn't believe how great I was feeling. Everything just started to fall into place. This way of eating combined with my cooking and kitchen skills finally gave me back time and energy to live my life again.

PAMELA ROCCA

CONNECT WITH PAMELA
INSTAGRAM: @PREPWITHPAM
FACEBOOK: PREP WITH PAM
YOUTUBE: PAM ROCCA
pamrocca.com

Pamela Rocca is a nutritionist, educator, author, and certified yoga teacher who shares her love for plant-based eating through a variety of popular social platforms. Pamela has a passion for crafting delicious and nutrient-packed food on her website, and her passion is to educate others on how to make healthy meals without spending hours in the kitchen.

WHAT ARE YOUR DAILY RITUALS/HABITS WHICH YOU BELIEVE HAVE BEEN KEY TO YOUR HEALTH?

1. Morning routine - I always start with a glass of lemon water, probiotics, omega supplement and vitamin D (during winter). Every morning I leave the house with a full glass jar of more lemon water and a green smoothie.

2. Daily movement - I love to exercise 4-5 days per week alternating between running, weight training, biking, and yoga. On off days I still move my body but to a lesser degree. Something like family hikes or walks.

3. Nourishing myself with real food - Ensuring that I always have healthy meals prepped and ready to eat for me and the family.

4. Self-care - Investing in what my body is telling me it needs. Sometimes self-care for me is sitting by the water, unplugging and reading a good book. Other times it's going out to dinner with great friends. I can tell when I haven't been listening because I will feel out of alignment or "off." When I feel that way, I can easily fix it by getting outside and enjoying some time in nature.

5. Boundaries - Since I love what I do, I have found myself working late and answering emails anytime they came in, which sometimes led to me prioritizing work over family and relationships. I knew this had to change, so I created boundaries in order for my mental and social health to improve. I now work during specific workday hours, and if I need to work more, I wake up an hour or two before the kids are up so I can get things done.

6. Gratitude practice - Every single morning I write or say three to five things that I am grateful for that day.

AT WHAT POINT IN YOUR LIFE DID YOU DECIDE TO CHANGE YOUR DIET? HOW HAS THAT DECISION IMPACTED YOUR LIFE?

I had a really unhealthy relationship with food when I was in high school. I struggled with an eating disorder that consumed me. I wouldn't eat at all, and if I did, I would make myself purge (vomit) after. Sometimes I would exercise for hours until I was certain every single calorie (and then some) was burnt off.

I don't really remember how I "recovered." It was a slow process and took a long time to change my mindset around food. It began when I started to educate myself on the body, health and nutrition. The more I learned about how amazing our bodies were physiologically, the more I knew that I couldn't keep hurting myself.

I went to college for fitness and health promotion, and that was a big turning point. I learned how to eat properly and how to change my mindset. I learned that food was neutral and not inherently "good" or "bad." I continued on to University for Kinesiology and knew it was my life's work to help other people learn to nourish their bodies with real foods in a healthy way.

Since attending college, I became a certified nutritionist, and about three years ago our family moved to a plant-based diet. Our family started out with meatless Monday for the benefit of the environment. My husband and I loved the food, and the way that we felt so much it slowly turned into our lifestyle. The focus is on eating real food that nourishes our body and tastes delicious.

WHAT KIND OF REACTION DO YOU RECEIVE WHEN YOUR PEERS, FRIENDS, AND OTHER "EXPERTS," FIND OUT THAT YOU ARE VEGAN/ PLANT-BASED? ARE THEY INTERESTED AND WANT TO KNOW MORE?

Most people are supportive when they know why we eat this way. If you are trying to help the environment and improve your health, it's hard to not be supportive of that. A few people asked questions like, "where do you get your protein?" or "what do you eat now?" I find that it's easy to educate them with answers. I love inspiring others to try out plant-based meals.

DO YOU TAKE ANY SPECIFIC SUPPLEMENTS? DO YOU RECOMMEND ANY SPECIFIC BRANDS? WHY DO YOU THINK THESE HAVE BENEFITED YOU AND YOUR HEALTH?

Garden of Life probiotics, B12, vitamin D from Ddrops, and NutraSea + D for omega 3s. I take probiotics every morning for gut health and eat foods that are rich in prebiotics. I take omega 3 to reduce inflammation and for heart health. I take vitamin D during the winter months because

I live in Canada and don't get enough sun during the winter months. I take a B12 or B complex supplement because when you are plant-based, it is more challenging to get enough B12. I get my levels tested annually by my naturopath and the first year I was low so I picked up a supplement from her office and have been taking it ever since.

WHAT IS THE MOST INSPIRING OR POWERFUL RESULT THAT YOU HAVE SEEN WITH A CLIENT AND A PLANT-BASED DIET?

I have seen people reduce their bloating, lose weight, improve their complexion, improve their mood and increase their energy. My favorite thing about going plant-based was the increase in energy.

YOU'VE JUST MET A HEARTBROKEN STRANGER WHO HAS JUST BEEN GIVEN A LIFE-THREATENING DIAGNOSIS. WHAT WOULD BE YOUR TOP FIVE TIPS TO HELP THEM?

1. I would talk to them about the power of food and the importance of good nutrition. If they needed help with a nutrition guide or plan, I would help them.

2. Hydration and daily movement.

3. Do all the things you love and surround yourself with people who make you happy. Personally, the things I love would be walks in the forest, stand-up paddleboarding on the water, cooking delicious food and snuggling my husband and children.

4. Put in place a good support system.

5. I'd emphasize the importance of a positive mindset even through the hardest of times. I wholeheartedly believe in the importance of a daily gratitude practice.

CAN YOU SHARE A STORY ABOUT THE POWER OF PLANTS THAT YOU USE WITH YOUR CLIENTS TO HELP THEM BELIEVE IN THIS AS AN ALTERNATIVE WAY OF LOOKING AT MEDICINE?

I had a client who had a heart attack and afterwards adopted a plant-based lifestyle to improve his health. He has been plant-based for four years now and has not had any issues with his heart or cardiovascular system since. He feels fantastic, loves the way he eats, and couldn't imagine going back to the way he ate before.

ERIN LUCAS

CONNECT WITH ERIN:
FACEBOOK: VEGETARIAN HEALTH
veghealth.com

"When my mom was diagnosed with cancer, the doctors said she could change her diet if she wanted, but there isn't any research to support it. As a biomedical engineer, I decided to do some digging into the research to find out for myself. I was amazed when I found study after study showing how a plant-based diet helps prevent cancer. These were big studies following tens of thousands of people over many years. It was amazing, and I couldn't believe the doctors were not aware of this research. I decided right then and there to quit my job and dedicate my life to educating people about the research behind preventing and fighting disease. There is just too much unnecessary suffering out there from a lack of understanding around natural approaches to health. I made the changes myself to help prevent cancer and disease, and I have never felt or looked better in my life."

225

Erin Lucas is the Program Director of VegHealth Institute, an organization dedicated to inspiring and educating people about plant-based nutrition, through nutrition certifications and training programs. With a master's degree in Biomedical Engineering and experience leading large scale programs around medical research, Erin dedicates her work (and life) towards educating people on the research behind lifestyle changes to fight and prevent disease.

WHAT ARE YOUR DAILY RITUALS/HABITS WHICH YOU BELIEVE HAVE BEEN KEY TO YOUR HEALTH?

My daily morning ritual consists of meditation, light yoga and a short run. Each week I also try to plan my meals and do one big grocery shopping trip so that I always have healthy food around. I also never keep unhealthy food around the house to avoid the temptation... apart for the occasional coconut ice cream you'll find in my freezer.

AT WHAT POINT IN YOUR LIFE DID YOU DECIDE TO CHANGE YOUR DIET? HOW HAS THAT DECISION IMPACTED YOUR LIFE?

When I was 22, I learned about factory farming and what happens before our food hits our plates. I was appalled and felt deceived. I turned vegan overnight. For the next ten years, I was an on and off vegan/vegetarian, but things really changed when cancer entered my life.

My Dad was diagnosed with prostate cancer and in the last two weeks of his life, I started learning about the connection between food and cancer.

My Mom was diagnosed with a rare blood cancer around the same time. I was determined to find a natural way to save her and quit my job so I could focus on researching lifestyle changes to fight cancer. I found a clear connection between plant-based eating and cancer prevention/reversal. I decided to switch to a whole-foods, plant-based diet to help inspire my mom and to lower the chance of getting cancer myself. I could never forgive myself if 1) I didn't try as hard as I could to help my Mom fight cancer with natural means and 2) if I didn't make the changes I learned about and wound up with cancer. So for me, the health of myself and my loved ones is my main driving force.

WHAT KIND OF REACTION DO YOU RECEIVE WHEN YOUR PEERS, FRIENDS, AND OTHER "EXPERTS," FIND OUT THAT YOU ARE VEGAN/ PLANT-BASED? ARE THEY INTERESTED AND WANT TO KNOW MORE?

Most people are generally interested to know more. If they have considered a plant-based diet, they will ask me a bunch of nutrition questions. I also get a lot of questions about other diets like the ketogenic diet. If they are not interested, they quickly laugh and defend their choices by saying, "I could never give up [insert meat or dairy product here]."

Generally, if I keep it light, friendly and non-judgmental they are intrigued.

DO YOU TAKE ANY SPECIFIC SUPPLEMENTS? DO YOU RECOMMEND ANY SPECIFIC BRANDS? WHY DO YOU THINK THESE HAVE BENEFITED YOU AND YOUR HEALTH?

Yes, I take B12, vitamin D, omega 3's and a specially formulated multivitamin for vegans (Dr. Fuhrman's Women's Daily). Generally, I don't support multivitamins because there are many risks and it is better to get them from the true source. I take Dr. Fuhrman's supplement because it has been well researched and does not include vitamins and minerals that are harmful in supplement form. It also contains Iodine, which is commonly deficient in our diets.

I have mostly noticed a benefit in terms of my mental state. The supplements have helped my overall mood, including reduced levels of anxiety. It is hard to say whether this is from the B12, D, or omegas, which all impact the mental state or the various components of the multivitamin.

I also take chaste berry and maca root for hormonal health. I was unfortunately on birth control for 20 years, which affected my body's ability to make hormones. These two supplements have made a huge difference in my mood and hormone levels.

WHAT IS THE MOST INSPIRING OR POWERFUL RESULT THAT YOU HAVE SEEN WITH A CLIENT AND A PLANT-BASED DIET?

I really can't point to one, because they are all equally powerful and inspiring to me. With my personal experience with cancer, I tend to be inspired by the stories of people reversing stage four cancers after being told there is nothing that can be done.

YOU'VE JUST MET A HEARTBROKEN STRANGER WHO HAS JUST BEEN GIVEN A LIFE-THREATENING DIAGNOSIS. WHAT WOULD BE YOUR TOP FIVE TIPS TO HELP THEM?

1) Join a mindfulness group and start practicing mindfulness meditation.

2) Cut out ALL toxins from your environment as best as you can. All chemicals from the house, all unnecessary prescriptions, all processed foods, all unfiltered water, all plastics, all toxic kitchen supplies, etc.

3) Get tested. Get a full panel of nutrition, heavy metals and hormones tested to see if it illuminates any underlying imbalances.

4) Eat a whole-foods, plant-based diet. If you don't know how to cook, learn or have friends and family cook for you.

5) Meditate on your will to live. Why do you want to continue living and what will you do? The body has an incredible ability to heal itself, given a will to live.

CAN YOU SHARE A STORY ABOUT THE POWER OF PLANTS THAT YOU USE WITH YOUR CLIENTS TO HELP THEM BELIEVE IN THIS AS AN ALTERNATIVE WAY OF LOOKING AT MEDICINE?

I share two things with people:

1) My personal journey. I was able to overcome both hypoglycemia and gastric reflux disease with a plant-based diet. It is small compared to overcoming something like cancer, but it made a huge difference in my overall wellbeing.

2) The research. Don't believe doctors that say there isn't enough research to support eating one way compared to another. A plant-based diet is the most supportive diet for preventing and reversing disease. We are talking big studies following tens of thousands of people over many years. It has been

227

shown to reverse heart disease, diabetes, some cancers and many many other diseases and health complications. Usually, when I share the health and research side of things, they are interested in learning more.

IF YOU COULD GIVE US JUST THREE ABSOLUTE MUSTS TO INCLUDE IN OUR DIET EACH DAY WHAT WOULD THEY BE?

1) Greens. Add mixed greens to every single meal! They are PACKED with nutrients and do miracles for our health.

2) Cruciferous veggies. They are powerhouses and have been shown to help prevent many diseases.

3) Supplements. It is critical that vegans supplement with B12, vitamin D, omega 3s and iodine (if not eating sea veggies or iodized salt).

ANY INSPIRING STORIES THAT HAVE HAPPENED TO YOU OR PEOPLE CLOSE TO YOU THAT HAVE NOT BEEN COVERED ABOVE. STORIES THAT CAN HELP OTHERS.

I don't really have a story, but more so a lesson that I've learned. It is about trying to change other people. As soon as we learn about the power of a plant-based diet, we want everyone we love to be on this diet.

Unfortunately, change is complicated and we can't force it on other people. People we love don't always want to hear our advice. What I've learned is;

1) Be the change. When people see you living a healthy, plant-based life, it is inspiring to them, and they will start asking questions or quietly follow suit.

2) Give people a book, documentary, or another source of information that they can read so that you aren't teaching them directly. Sometimes people we love are more receptive when information comes from someone else (crazy right?)

3) Be non-judgmental. Everyone has their own journey and their own struggles. People can immediately sense if you are trying to change them from a place of judgment, and they will immediately resist.

4) Unconditional love. When a loved one is sick, we want to do anything and everything we can to help them get their health back. It is important to respect them as individuals and allow them to make their own decisions. Work on helping them from a place of "non-attachment." This means that you remove your personal agenda and help out of pure unconditional love. Unconditional love means we show them love and support even if they do not make the changes we think they should make.

DARCI KINGRY

CONNECT WITH DARCI:
INSTAGRAM: @DARCIKINGRY
FACEBOOK: SIMPLY NUTRITARIAN
thinkintentional.com

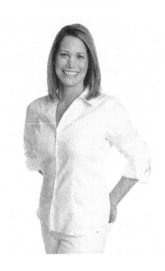

Darci Kingry is a certified life and holistic health coach, bringing passion, experience, and education to clients in a realistic and compassionate way. Darci uses the story of her early life with yo-yo dieting, a heart condition, depression and anxiety to relate to her client's struggles. She supports those who work with her skills in nutrition counseling, meal planning, goal setting and holistic approaches to health, weight and life challenges.

"Nothing has changed my life more than becoming plant-based. It is the best decision I ever made and my only regret is that I did not know about the benefits of it much sooner. My life would certainly have turned out differently."

WHAT IS ONE OF THE BEST OR MOST WORTHWHILE HEALTH-RELATED INVESTMENTS THAT YOU HAVE MADE?

Books: Eat to Live by Dr. Joel Fuhrman, *The Secret to Ultimate Weight Loss* by Chef AJ, and *The China Study* by Dr. T. Colin Campbell and Dr. Thomas Campbell.

Gadgets: InstantPot, Cuisinart 12-Cup Food Processor, Nutribullet RX, cast iron skillets, Santoku knives, strainers with handles, and Pyrex glass snapware.

Supplements: no specific brand but vitamin B12 sublingual is vitally important. Also, Natural Calm magnesium powder. I recommend everyone take this because our stressed out, nutritionally-starved-society is very commonly deficient in this mineral. It helps with sleep, anxiety, digestion, heart and nerve function. I do not take any other vitamin or mineral regularly.

AT WHAT POINT IN YOUR LIFE DID YOU DECIDE TO CHANGE YOUR DIET? HOW HAS THAT DECISION IMPACTED YOUR LIFE?

I changed my diet more times in my life than I can count off the top of my head. I originally attempted to be vegetarian when I was 10 years old because I did not want to eat animals. However, I ultimately was forced to eat fish, and most of my diet was full of dairy and junk food. As an adult, I did not become completely plant-based until about October of 2015 when I found the documentary, Eat to Live, during my heaviest weight. This was my lowest point medically, physically and emotionally. I had lived with chronic knee and hip pain for so many years, even before I was overweight. No other way of eating helped those issues or the lifetime of heart palpitations and daily anxiety that I suffered from.

I chose this because I not only wanted to be healthy and not do harm, but because I didn't want to live in pain anymore. I had no fears because I had tried so many different ways of eating in the past. At the time, I also lived alone and had no one to intentionally or unintentionally sabotage my food choice.

I enjoyed not only weight loss, but also relief from so many long-term medical issues that ended up resolving quickly and permanently. This superseded any negative reactions I got from people at work, friends or family. There were plenty of negative reactions from people asking where I was getting my protein, and about my nutrition (that one is pretty funny), how I was being so extreme, and that I needed to eat dairy for calcium. It went on and on. I lost friends because they were uncomfortable eating around me. Even if I said nothing, just the sheer choices I made compared to their food choices seemed to bother them. They were suffering, overweight, had numerous health conditions, on strong medications, were miserable, and they were mad at me for finding a solution that they felt they "couldn't" do. I was punished for finally finding a true and sustainable way to find better health and increased quality of life.

My success, improved health and lack of sickness and pain, kept me motivated and moving forward. My improved health and wellness were far more important than catering to the misery others wanted me to fall back into to make them more comfortable with their own refusal to make changes.

WHAT WAS THE REACTION YOU RECEIVED FROM PEOPLE WHEN YOU ANNOUNCED THAT YOU WERE GOING VEGAN? WHO WAS YOUR BEST AND WORST SUPPORTER?

Mostly negative reactions. People who felt they "couldn't" make those changes in their own lives and would rather survive on medications and junk food were the meanest to me. I lost most of my friendships with people who were unwilling to change and didn't like my new-found happiness, peace and confidence.

My health improvements started before I lost enough weight for people to really become interested. No one cared about my health improvements, pain, heart condition or the chronic anxiety that was resolved. They didn't care until I lost enough weight to think of me as "healthy." And even then, most did not want to try my "extreme" way of eating or care about how it could change their physical or mental health.

No one cares about your health and nutrition while you are eating McDonald's food or drinking Diet Coke as if it actually is water. No one asks about your protein or vitamins when you are eating pizza, chicken, processed bread, and desserts. The minute I changed my diet and started to succeed in my health goals, people became judgmental, nutrition experts and angry. Many tried to get me to eat the junk they call food. They were still on medications, overweight, tired, depressed and full of anxiety, telling me how extreme I was living and didn't want to hear about my good health and weight loss.

231

YOUR RECOMMENDATIONS TO YOUR CLIENTS WHEN YOU FIRST SUGGEST THEY SHOULD MOVE TO A PLANT-BASED DIET?

I suggest that even if they are not ready to go completely plant-based, that they start shoving leafy greens in their mouth as if their life depends on it. I 100% believe that leafy greens have not only a super-charged nutritional impact on our bodies, but they also affect our mood greatly. When I first started eating purely plant-based, the days and weeks I ate the most greens, I found myself smiling for no reason. I tell clients to literally grab handfuls and shove them in their mouth like medicine if they have to. While all plant foods are important and powerful, greens (and green vegetables) are always at the top of my list. My clients know that at every session I will say, eat more greens several times to reinforce the importance they should place on the nutritional and happiness benefits that greens provide.

I also ask them to drop at least one trigger or comfort food or food group, such as dairy or oil. I explain that abstinence brings about the fastest and most sustainable results and if they are not jumping in full throttle, they have to at least commit to completely eliminating one food or group in order to see the benefits.

WHAT IS THE MOST INSPIRING OR POWERFUL RESULT THAT YOU HAVE SEEN WITH A CLIENT AND A PLANT-BASED DIET?

This is hard because I have seen so many wonderful results with clients. I had one client who was taken off of their diabetes medications within six weeks of working with me and committing to a plant-based lifestyle.

While they had other medical concerns that were improving as well, this was the medication that they most wanted to get off of and to no longer live as a diabetic. It brought me so much joy to know that this client would continue to see their life improve further because of their choice to eat plant-based.

I had another client who was able to avoid thyroid medication for hypothyroid as well as medication for diabetes. She was borderline and headed towards a lifetime of medication, but her commitment to being plant-based thwarted that future and instead has given her the opportunity to have a future of good health.

CAN YOU SHARE A STORY ABOUT THE POWER OF PLANTS THAT YOU USE WITH YOUR CLIENTS TO HELP THEM BELIEVE IN THIS AS AN ALTERNATIVE WAY OF LOOKING AT MEDICINE?

I tell my clients my own story of body image, love of animals and diet history, ultimately ending with how becoming plant-based cured me (at least most of the symptoms) of multiple health concerns and chronic conditions, plus significant weight loss.

I had body image issues from the time I was in my single digits. A family member used to tell me I was fat, even though back then I was quite skinny and lanky. At the age of 10, I decided I would no longer eat animals, and my parents thought it was cute. They had a doctor force me to eat fish, and I consumed mostly dairy and junk food for the next seven years. There were a lot of emotional struggles around my choice in eating brought on by my family's choice to make fun of my choices. However, it was my family that made it possible to live on so much junk food. I did not know anything about being a vegan or eating healthy. I just wanted to save animals.

At 13, I insisted on going to a nutritionist to lose weight because I thought I was fat. I learned so much and began eating in a way that was considered a lot healthier for a while, reducing fat and portions.

At 17, I thought I wanted to try meat again, but I found out that at the time I didn't really like it. I slowly transitioned back to eating mostly chicken and continued to eat dairy. I was never really overweight up to that point, but because I have a more naturally athletic build, I always felt "bigger" than my friends and translated that into being "fat".

At 18, I insisted on going to a nutritionist again to lose weight. Again, I learned a lot about what was considered healthy, though this time I was not a vegan or a vegetarian, but focused on low-fat, low-sugar options.

At 19, I was living with roommates, working two jobs and socializing most nights. My diet consisted mainly of buttered toast and diet coke with shots of tequila as my drink of choice when I hit the bars and clubs.

At 22, I was engaged to get married and again thought I was fat. For my bridal shower, I was on a boiled chicken and vegetable diet with a 1-gallon water requirement for drinking each day. I lost the weight. But my mother and my mother-in-law were less than thrilled that I refused to eat "real" food at my own bridal shower.

Between 22 and 28, I went on and off multiple diets. I was never significantly overweight during that time, but I always thought I was fat. My husband would get tired and say, "if you think you need to lose weight, do something about it."

By the age of 27, I finally found what I thought was the holy grail of health and weight loss. I started with a book called Protein Power, which led me to Robert Atkins' New Diet Revolution. I tried it. It worked! Or so I thought it did. I lost weight fast and people noticed. I felt great, and my blood tests supported my new "healthy" lifestyle. Granted, this was before Atkins, Low-Carb, Paleo and Keto were trendy and, in some cases, didn't even exist as "diets."

I stuck to a mostly high-protein, low-carb, Atkins-style-of-eating for that year. I also started physical therapy for my knees, which, due to being poorly situated, created constant pain and problems with sports as well as sleeping.

At 28, my husband was killed in a head-on collision, and my life fell apart. I stopped physical therapy and at first, was barely eating. I looked great at the funeral, but that was not from a healthy diet. I soon began eating whatever I wanted. I gained and lost and slowly became heavier than I'd ever been. I began to isolate myself.

At 31, I moved across the country, believing that was the answer to my failure; moving forward with my life. I lost the weight, began working nights at a club in addition to a full-time day job and saw my confidence begin to improve a lot. I was wearing short skirts and short tops and was having a great time, but I struggled to support myself. At this time, I wasn't eating healthy. My diet consisted of a lot of 7-Eleven breakfast sandwiches and nightly snacks at the club/bar I worked in.

At 32, I was going to school for yet another certification (I already had my court reporting and skin care/facialist certifications) for massage therapy. I also came into some money and quit my job. I gained a bit of weight during this time and was back to doing low-carb (I loved the steak salads with a side of broccoli at Outback Steakhouse.) While I was having fun in school, working at a spa and hanging out with new friends, I was still not happy with my body, and my continuing health conditions reminded me daily that I was not healthy.

At 33, I quit the spa industry and began work for a software development group in a large financial services company. I ended up staying there for 15 years as a technical writer for this company that was formerly part of the larger organization.

From 33 to 41, I saw my weight slowly increase as I ate poorly and struggled to survive financially. During this time, I tried numerous diets. Some succeeded temporarily, such as the Six Week Body Makeover, consisting of portioned out rice, chicken and vegetables, along with exercise. I lost a lot of weight, but the diet was limited, and my lack of knowledge about how to enjoy vegetables and starch kept me from staying on the diet. I gained the weight back - and a lot more over those eight years.

At 41, I was my heaviest ever. I was sad, depressed, in chronic pain with a heart condition and had daily anxiety that I had since I was a child, but never got treated for. Is it related to my heart murmur that I still live with as an adult? I'm not sure. I know I was tired and had been put on heart medication, which for the first time alleviated my heart palpitations, chest pain and anxiety. Had I not been so overweight with high blood pressure, I am sure my condition would have continued until I found my plant-based life.

In late 2012, again, at my heaviest, I found Dr. Joel Fuhrman on PBS talking about Eat to Live. While it was clearly a way to lose weight, he spent most of the time talking about nutrient density and how eating this way could help with all of my health issues and more. It was the first infomercial-type of program I had seen on eating where the focus was not just on how you can lose weight quickly and easily. I was intrigued and bought the book right away.

My life changed forever. Within three months, I lost 25 pounds and saw many of my chronic health conditions go away. My heart condition and anxiety subsided without meds for the first time in my life. To not feel my heart beating out of my chest in combination with skipping a beat was incredible. To not wake up full of anxiety for no reason was a miracle. My knees and hips no longer kept me up at night, and my chronic eye infection went away forever.

Unfortunately, though I was so happy and successful, over the next year and a half, I slacked off as most "dieters" do, but I never stopped incorporating all the vegetables. I just added more fat and unhealthy options, which prevented me from losing more weight or seeing more health issues dissipate. But I did not regain weight, pain or heart condition.

In January of 2015, I woke up. It was as if God had put it in me to make a permanent commitment not only to my health and happiness but to finding it through a plant-based lifestyle. I immediately got serious and lost 65 pounds within six months. I felt better than ever, and other issues like joint pain and stiffness went away. I had to replace all my clothes - my heaviest being a size 16 (tight) and going down to a comfortable size 6. My blood pressure was low, my heart and anxiety were not bothering me and I had a new life.

Since then, I have become an Integrated Health Coach, certified life coach, and a licensed master practitioner of Neuro-linguistic Programming. I help others find their way to a healthier and happier life. In 2018, I began to volunteer for an amazing organization called Heart2Heart Outreach (www. heart2heartoutreach.org), which matches compassionate volunteers to the lonely elderly residents at care centers. In May of 2019, I accepted an offer to oversee their volunteer program full time and made a career change to fulfill my purpose to serve others. I continue to offer health and life coaching on my own time as well, and to pursue my best health and fitness at the age of 48.

I currently follow a variation of the Eat to Live recommendations because after losing a significant amount of weight and still wanting to reach fitter goals, I discovered that the best plant-based style for me is low-fat, vegetable and starch-based plus fruit. It is restarting my body's fire and pushing me forward to my future healthiest self ever and a true example to my clients and to everyone I meet.

IF YOU COULD GIVE US JUST THREE ABSOLUTE MUSTS TO INCLUDE IN OUR DIET EACH DAY WHAT WOULD THEY BE?

1. An abundance of dark leafy greens and cruciferous veggies.
2. Starchy vegetables - something I limited and was afraid of for so long, but learned to love what they do for me. My weight loss and my relationship improved more when I added back more starchy vegetables than it did during the larger 90-pound weight loss I experienced earlier in my journey.
3. Fruit - people are scared of the sugar, but if you are eating the whole-food, fruit is so important.

SINCE BECOMING VEGAN/PLANT-BASED, WHAT ELSE HAS CHANGED IN YOUR LIFE?

Everything. Everything. Everything. My health, my happiness, my attitude, no medication, no anxiety and no excuses for living my life.

While I will always have body image issues because I grew up believing I was fat and not good enough long before I was actually overweight or before understanding nutrition and the plant-based movement, it does not define me. I am defined by the choices I make today and every day going forward. I am thankful to God for pointing me in the right direction and showing me

" "

OUR HABITS BECOME OUR ADDICTIONS

DARCI KINGRY

my true purpose. If I had not gone through my lifetime of struggles, I would not be able to relate to the people I speak to and coach today. My voice is louder because I know so many others suffer unnecessarily. I will always work hard at eating in a way that promotes a fit and healthy body and mind. I will always be honest with others and let them know that it takes a commitment to change, not just the desire to change. Our habits become our addictions, and it is only through my personal journey that I have learned to look back and see how small moments in childhood can affect your entire life path. I now believe that we can all learn to eat plant-based - but those who suffer from disease, pain, anxiety or depression, benefit even more than those who simply want to lose weight or save our beloved animals around the world.

Through God and the direction I have been led, I have discovered a passion for helping seniors improve their health. The majority of seniors in care facilities today are suffering from numerous illnesses, including Alzheimer's. Most of these conditions can be prevented or reversed with a plant-based diet. I hope to be part of a revolution that will change how we eat so that we can all grow old gracefully and healthfully.

ANY INSPIRING STORIES THAT HAVE HAPPENED TO YOU OR PEOPLE CLOSE TO YOU THAT HAVE NOT BEEN COVERED ABOVE. STORIES THAT CAN HELP OTHERS.

Nothing has changed my life more than becoming plant-based. I lived in chronic pain, anxiety, and with multiple symptoms most of my life that was all unnecessary. It pains me to know that if I had learned as a child or even as a teenager what I know now, my whole life would have been completely different. Because I was told I had to live with my conditions from a young age, I didn't seek treatment or research a way out until I was in my 40s.

A plant-based lifestyle is seen as extreme and controversial, while made-up diets full of fat and processed foods and supplements are revered today. I hope to be part of the solution and show people that you don't have to have cancer or a heart attack to benefit from this "extremely" healthy way of eating. We must be our own advocates and do a lot of research and open our eyes to see that the food that when we fill our bodies with whole-food, plant-based nutrition, we thrive in every part of our lives. Eat more greens. Change your health, change your life.

AILIN DURAN D.S.

CONNECT WITH AILIN:
INSTAGRAM: @SPIRITRAWPICALHEALING
FACEBOOK: SPIRITRAWPICALHEALING
YOUTUBE: AILINDURAN
spiritrawpicalhealing.com

Ailin Duran founded Spiritrawpical Healing with the mission of helping all those in need through healing. She is a certified Detox Specialist and Iridologist that has dedicated her life in guiding thousands of people on their healing journeys in overcoming their health issues over the years

With over a decade of studying the art of detoxification, the human body, raw foods, herbs and fasting, she has become a shining light and a wealth of knowledge to those following the true detoxification path

Ailin has also received amazing praise and is continually mentioned as being one of the best teachers and healers of our time. Through her in-depth articles, videos, and guidance, many have found their way to true healing.

WHAT ARE YOUR DAILY RITUALS/HABITS WHICH YOU BELIEVE HAVE BEEN KEY TO YOUR HEALTH?

Definitely consuming fruits and fruit juices such as grapes, oranges, melons and berries. I see them as the key components of healing. Alkalizing the body with fruits and raw foods, while removing acidity, mucus, and obstructions through detoxification allows the body to completely heal. This leads to all organs, tissues and glands to proper functioning.

AT WHAT POINT IN YOUR LIFE DID YOU DECIDE TO CHANGE YOUR DIET? HOW HAS THAT DECISION IMPACTED YOUR LIFE?

I turned to a vegetarian lifestyle at an early age. This was due to my love of animals as a child. I remember the turning point well. I was in the Dominican Republic with my family and I would cry when I would see them kill the chickens, pigs and goats that I had befriended that summer, for meat. I refused to eat meat after that. In my older years, my health began to decline, and all over body pains and chronic fatigue began to seriously plague my body. I could no longer do the everyday activities I once had. I made several changes and went down many different paths in order to heal myself through the years. I then noticed that the less animal products I ate,

238

the less pain I felt. I turned to a 100 percent raw vegan diet overnight to heal my body of several chronic health issues. Through detoxification, consuming a high fruit diet, eliminating all cooked foods and animal products, my body then had to opportunity it had been waiting for, to deeply hydrate all of its cells and remove that which was causing dis-ease.

WHAT KIND OF REACTION DO YOU RECEIVE WHEN YOUR PEERS, FRIENDS, AND OTHER "EXPERTS," FIND OUT THAT YOU ARE VEGAN/ PLANT-BASED? ARE THEY INTERESTED AND WANT TO KNOW MORE?

Veganism is becoming more mainstream these days. I'm glad that it is becoming more understood and accepted. This was not the case a few years back. As a detoxification specialist, I consider becoming vegan as the minimum step one can take towards healing. It is my belief that everyone should at the very least be vegan for good health, and the closer you eat towards a simple and natural diet, consuming foods grown from the earth in their natural form, the healthier you will be.

It is great that more people are becoming more interested in alternative healing modalities. I have seen time and time again in my own clients that so many have been let down by the medical system in healing their health issues. More and more people are taking healing into their own hands and realizing that health and healing all starts with the foods they consume! 239

DO YOU TAKE ANY SPECIFIC SUPPLEMENTS? DO YOU RECOMMEND ANY SPECIFIC BRANDS? WHY DO YOU THINK THESE HAVE BENEFITED YOU AND YOUR HEALTH?

Before one aims to fix a deficiency due to a lack of a certain vitamin or mineral in their diet, they must ask themselves the following:

1. Are they digesting and breaking down their foods properly and completely?
2. Are they absorbing the nutrients from those foods completely in the bowels?
3. Is their utilization strong within their glands?
4. Are they eliminating wastes out of the body properly?

Nutrition can be found in all plant foods. Deficiencies arise when any of the following processes begin to fail in the body; they are digestion, absorption, utilization and elimination. I have found most people have a weakness in one or more of these areas.

I tried many supplements and isolates during my healing journey. For many years I had worked at Whole-foods in their supplement department, which provided the ability to try everything in order to help heal myself. Many of the supplements I tried only provided temporary relief, but no long term healing. All supplements failed me and I didn't find true healing until I began digging deep into my detoxification with a raw vegan diet. Through incorporating high fruits and strong herbal formulas, I was able to provide support to those glands and organs that needed assistance during healing.

Over the years, I have found isolated compounds in supplements to be detrimental and acidic to the body in many people. I have seen these isolates stay stuck in the body, irritating tissue, either creating hyper or hypo conditions in the tissues and glands. My main goal is to fix every root cause of dis-ease in the body, so as to not need isolated supplementation.

WHAT IS THE MOST INSPIRING OR POWERFUL RESULT THAT YOU HAVE SEEN WITH A CLIENT AND A PLANT-BASED DIET?

I have seen countless healing stories in my clients of more than hundreds of different dis-ease conditions. There are too many to count. Some examples being the body pushing cancer out through every opening: the skin, the colon, urine, etc., to clients healing from severe skin issues like eczema, psoriasis, fungal issues, to the healing of heart palpitations, brain fog, tumors, headaches, several chronic issues like Lupus, Lyme's, Arthritis, and degenerative diseases like M.S., and Parkinson's.

Many have gone down the medical path and even several naturopaths for several years without finding an answer that heals. Once they find detoxification, we are finally able to provide an answer! We see all types of different illnesses walk through our door. I have seen stage 4 cancer gone in six weeks, eczema healed in two months, and even those with neurological weakness regain feeling and mobility of their body in just a few months.

As the body regains life in all of its cells and the cause of death and decay is pushed out, the disease-reversal process begins. I have helped children as young as a few years old, teenagers, adults and the elderly all heal from various health issues. As detoxification is a natural process of the body, there are no limits to what the body can heal itself from!

YOU'VE JUST MET A HEARTBROKEN STRANGER WHO HAS JUST BEEN GIVEN A LIFE-THREATENING DIAGNOSIS. WHAT WOULD BE YOUR TOP FIVE TIPS TO HELP THEM?

1. Incorporate more fruits into your diet.

2. Get your entire case, health history and irises analyzed to acquire a personalized diet and herbal protocol specific to your body's weaknesses. This is where most people fail in their healing journey because they do not know their exact organ and gland weaknesses to address in order to heal.

3. Follow your diet & herbal protocols and continue simplifying your diet to heal.

4. Incorporate necessary detox tools into your daily life to open up the channels of elimination and move the lymph system.

5. Help others find true healing after you have gained your health back!

CAN YOU SHARE A STORY ABOUT THE POWER OF PLANTS THAT YOU USE WITH YOUR CLIENTS TO HELP THEM BELIEVE IN THIS AS AN ALTERNATIVE WAY OF LOOKING AT MEDICINE?

I have my own journey of when I was diagnosed with Fibromyalgia, a debilitating disease. I had stabbing chest pains, leg pains, uterus pains, back pains, kidney pains, head pains, colon pains, stomach pains, neck pains, nerve pains, muscle pains, joint pains and more! I felt trapped in my body, in constant pain that I could never get away from. I also had many other diseases like chronic fatigue syndrome, endometriosis, chronic back pain, depression, anxiety attacks, extreme allergies and sensitivities to certain foods and chemicals, chronic headaches, chronic constipation and more.

If it were not for finding detoxification and changing my entire way of life to heal, I would most likely be in a wheelchair or perhaps even dead. My own healing journey continually inspires me to help those that are suffering. It is because I have gone through so much suffering in my own life that I am able to relate to my client's suffering and pull them out of this pain and fear onto the other side of vitality and healing.

IF YOU COULD GIVE US JUST THREE ABSOLUTE MUSTS TO INCLUDE IN OUR DIET EACH DAY WHAT WOULD THEY BE?

1. Dry Fasting
2. Fruits - grapes, watermelons and oranges are the most powerful
3. Herbal Support

ANY INSPIRING STORIES YOU CAN SHARE?

I believe detoxification to be the true path to healing the body. I have seen every single person who goes on a detoxification program have their illnesses completely healed and their lives transformed! Many people dream of finding the answer to their health every day, and they spend years searching for that answer and never find it. If you are reading this, I want to let you know how lucky you are.

It is because you are reading this that the universe knows you are ready to move on to the next step in your healing. Whatever illness you have, for however long you have had it, there is always hope. Never give up. I have seen miracles with detoxification. With dedication, focus and an open heart, everything is possible.

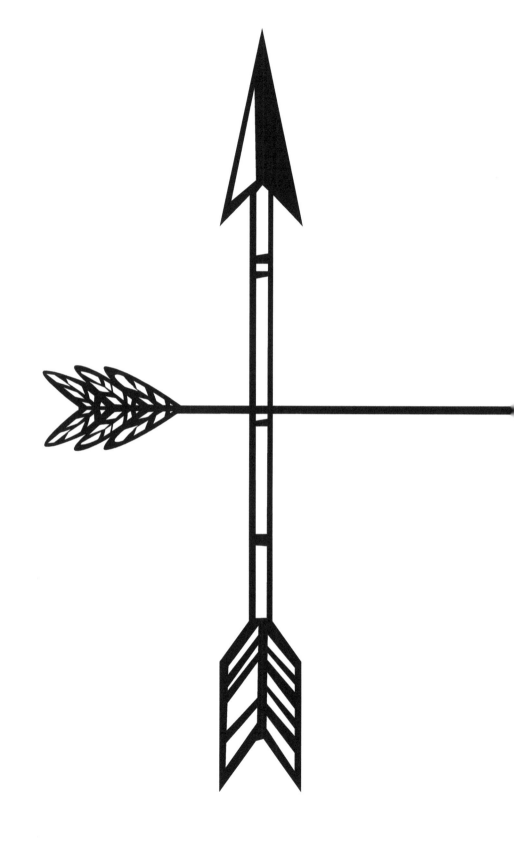

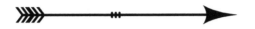

CHAPTER 5

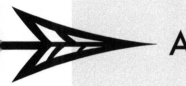

ATHLETES

HEATHER MILLS

CONNECT WITH HEATHER:
INSTAGRAM: @HEATHERMILLSOFFICIAL
FACEBOOK: @HEATHERMILLSOFFICIAL
vbites.com

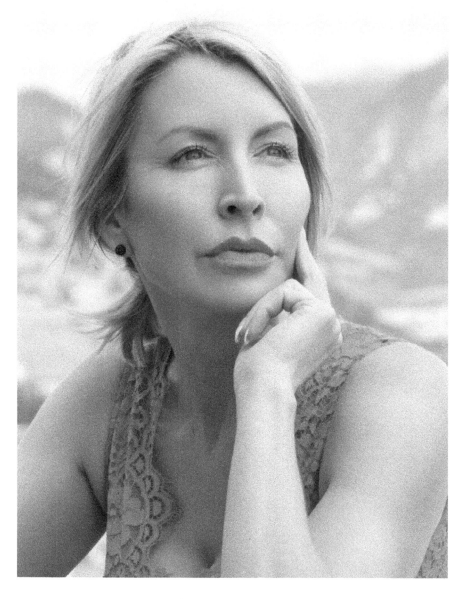

A woman that has an innate ability to defy and conquer anything that falls in her path... Heather Mills is a widely-recognized former model, entrepreneur, and world-leading athlete who had her leg amputated after colliding with a police motorbike in 1993. After the amputation, a spreading infection in her leg had doctors continuing to amputate, moving up her leg, until they were at the point of amputating her knee. Before letting this happen, Mills made the switch to a plant-based diet, which she credits to the infection in her leg disappearing within weeks, much to the surprise of her medical team. Now Mills runs a successful meat-alternative business called V-Bites, with 74 products in 24 countries, making it one of the biggest vegan faux meat companies in the world.

WHAT IS ONE OF THE BEST OR MOST WORTHWHILE HEALTH-RELATED INVESTMENTS THAT YOU HAVE MADE?

The best investment I ever made was to put my money into pioneering the development of meat, fish and dairy-free alternate products by creating the vegan company, V Bites, 25 years ago. It has helped hundreds of thousands of people with their health, animal cruelty, and environmental issues. As well as making the transition to a plant-based diet easier.

245

HOW IMPORTANT IS NUTRITION FOR A TOP-LEVEL ATHLETE? AT WHAT POINT DID YOU DECIDE THAT A PLANT-BASED DIET WAS THE BEST DIET FOR YOU?

I decided to become plant-based after losing my leg, crushing my pelvis, and puncturing my lungs in a road traffic accident. They kept amputating my leg more and more because of an infection and I wanted to save my knee. My girlfriend, who had claimed she cured herself of breast cancer, was the one who pushed me to go on a vegan diet. My leg healed in two weeks. After three months in the hospital, the pharmaceutical drugs could not heal the infection. After turning vegan, I have never looked back.

DO YOU TAKE ANY SPECIAL SUPPLEMENTS? SPECIFIC BRANDS WOULD BE GREAT AS WELL. WHY DO YOU THINK THESE HAVE BENEFITED YOU AND YOUR HEALTH/PERFORMANCE?

I take hydrochloric acid and a digestive enzyme that I have developed, which will come on the market in 2019 as well as an Algal Oil available on vbites.com. These supplements, a B12 supplement, in addition to a good plant-based diet, are the only other supplements generally needed.

" "

I HAVE CONVERTED MANY
ATHLETES, AND YES, THEY ARE
NOW WORLD CHAMPIONS AND
AGREE THEIR PERFORMANCE
HAS GONE UP. I HAVE BEEN
VEGAN FOR 25 YEARS, AND
IT IS DEFINITELY THE REASON
I AM AN OLD AGE WORLD
RECORD HOLDER.

HEATHER MILLS

WHAT IS YOUR GREATEST STRENGTH? WHAT DRIVES YOU AND KEEPS YOU AT THE TOP OF YOUR GAME?

Caring that I do everything for the right reasons with the greatest effort. I am convinced that creating a world speed ski record at the age of 47 happened because I lived for many years on a plant-based diet and remained at optimal fitness levels.

HOW DO YOU HANDLE THE UPS AND DOWNS OF GOOD AND BAD DAYS? WHAT STRATEGIES DO YOU USE?

A great sense of humor and a lot of life experience in war zones where real problems happen. I have a good comparison to get my head out of the goldfish bowl. Anyone interested in learning should go and do more charity work. They will feel less stressed and less sorry for themselves.

WHAT KIND OF TIME COMMITMENT DOES YOUR TRAINING AND TRAVELING SCHEDULE DEMAND? HOW DO YOU BALANCE THAT WITH FAMILY, FRIENDS AND EATING HEALTHILY?

Luckily, I only sleep four or five hours per night.

I get all my emails done from 4 am to 7 am, then I get the family ready for school and turn my phone off. Then it's back on when school starts and back off when school finishes for three hours and then back on till midnight. I generally travel by flying in the morning and flying back at night or in the holiday period and take the family so they can have fun, but I am full on and full off. There is no in-between when you're running your own business. I love to be in the moment rather than rushing ahead so I can enjoy the experience and it took me years to perfect. It is one of my proudest achievements in the equilibrium balance that is needed in life.

I have a training schedule that I stick to and fit that around everything else four times per week in the gym. When I was a Ski Racer, I trained and raced in the morning and did business in the afternoon.

WHAT KIND OF REACTION DID YOU RECEIVE WHEN YOU ANNOUNCED THAT YOU WERE GOING VEGAN? FROM YOUR COACH, FAMILY AND FRIENDS?

My sister had been a vegetarian since the age of 15. After seeing my infection heal so quickly, many of them have followed the plant-based path, and none of us have ever looked back.

SINCE TRANSITIONING, HAS YOUR PERFORMANCE LEVEL GONE UP? WHAT'S YOUR ADVICE TO OTHER ATHLETES OR WOMEN WHO MAY

BE INTERESTED IN TRYING A PLANT-BASED DIET?

I have converted many athletes, and yes, they are now World Champions and agree their performance has gone up. I have been vegan for 25 years, and it is definitely the reason I am an old age world record holder.

WHEN YOU SET A GOAL, HOW DO YOU STICK TO IT?

You just get on with it and remain focused, and you must love it, or you will not achieve it. My body gives up before my mind does, which helps.

WHAT IS YOUR FONDEST MEMORY OF YOUR SPORTS CAREER?

I was told I was too old to become a Ski Racer and the coach said I will never make it. The coach then left and worked for another country. I then went to race in that country and won my first silver medal in a slalom ski race, and the coach was at the bottom of the mountain in total shock. That moment was priceless for anyone who has ever been told something is not possible.

DO YOU HAVE OR HAVE YOU HAD A MENTOR IN YOUR LIFE? IF SO, WHO WAS IT AND WHAT IMPACT HAVE THEY HAD ON YOU AND DO YOU STILL HAVE THEM?

I have never had a positive mentor, but I did have many negative influences in my life that drove me to be successful and get away from them. Even a negative can be turned into a positive. Anger can be a powerful thing if you use it positively.

ANY INSPIRING STORIES THAT HAVE HAPPENED TO YOU OR PEOPLE CLOSE TO YOU THAT HAVE NOT BEEN COVERED ABOVE. STORIES THAT CAN HELP OTHERS.

The most important thing in life is to be healthy as without health, we ultimately are not happy. A lesson I have learned is to never judge others. You were once not fully plant-based yourself, so take them with a kind hand and feed them great food.

Conversion happens slowly for many people who are not forced into a healthy lifestyle when they have had no illness. It's important to gently spread the word by example and problem-solving, not criticizing.

Monuments were never built for the critics, only the criticised.

ANAIS ZANOTTI

CONNECT WITH ANAIS:
INSTAGRAM: @ANAISZANOTTI
FACEBOOK: @ANAIS ZANOTTI
YOUTUBE: @ANAIS ZANOTTI
anaisfit.com

Anais Zanotti is a NASM certified personal trainer, skydive coach and fitness model who started bodybuilding at age 15. Anais attributes much of her fitness success and overall health to her plant-based diet, which has improved her battle with hypothyroidism as well.

"A few months after I started eating vegan, one of the trainers at my gym came to me saying that I was looking younger and asked what I did to my face. I am 36 years old, and the only thing I have done was change my diet by going vegan. I guess I have the vegan glow."

AT WHAT POINT IN YOUR LIFE DID YOU DECIDE TO CHANGE YOUR DIET? HOW HAS THAT DECISION IMPACTED YOUR LIFE? WHAT IS YOUR GO-TO FOOD TO FUEL YOUR BODY?

I love animals! I became a vegetarian when I was ten years old, but back then, we did not have information as we do now through social media and online. When I was little, I did not know what to eat as a vegetarian, which is why I went back to fish. This lasted until last year when I decided to go vegan because I was already making a lot of vegan meal plans for clients. I wanted to try it out.

My go-to food is usually tempeh, sweet potatoes and broccoli. Or a quinoa bowl with roasted cauliflower, black eye peas and pumpkin seeds.

WHAT IS YOUR GREATEST STRENGTH? WHAT DRIVES YOU AND KEEPS YOU AT THE TOP OF YOUR GAME?

I am very driven. Once I have a goal, there is nothing that can stop me from achieving it.

HOW DO YOU HANDLE THE UPS AND DOWNS OF GOOD AND BAD DAYS? WHAT STRATEGIES DO YOU USE?

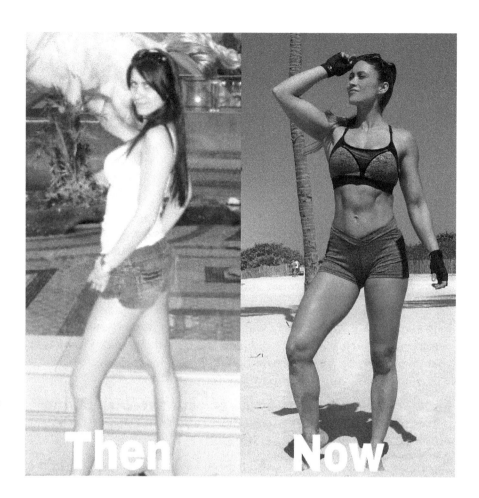

Then   Now

I am always trying to stay positive. What helps me is listening to some good music and going to the gym. I have had days when I had a terrible start and exercising helped me to really clear my mind. If I don't have the option to stop by the gym, going for a 20-minute walk with my headphones has helped me to feel better on bad days.

WHAT KIND OF REACTION DID YOU RECEIVE WHEN YOU ANNOUNCED THAT YOU WERE GOING VEGAN? WHAT DID YOUR COACH, FAMILY AND FRIENDS SAY? WHAT IMPACT HAS THIS HAD ON YOUR PERFORMANCE? RECOVERY?

A lot of my followers on social media were very excited to see my results and my new vegan lifestyle. I had a lot of positive people around me

Chapter 5 | ATHLETES

who were happy that I chose to go vegan. A few months later, I got my husband to go vegan as well.

My mom was a bit worried at first because a lot of people think that vegans don't get enough protein. But after I showed her my meals and how much protein I was getting, she was pretty impressed.

It's amazing how much better I feel. My recovery is much faster than before, I have more energy, I can train longer than I used too and I have more endurance.

Another big thing for me is no more upset stomachs. When I used to eat fish and eggs, I would feel tired after my meals. Now I have a ton of energy and even my skin is better than ever. There are so many benefits. I will stop here because I could write pages about all the good things.

SINCE TRANSITIONING TO A VEGAN/PLANT-BASED DIET HAS YOUR PERFORMANCE LEVEL GONE UP? WHAT IS YOUR ADVICE TO OTHER ATHLETES OR WOMEN WHO MAY BE INTERESTED IN TRYING A PLANT-BASED DIET?

I am able to do 25 pull-ups now. Before I was stuck at 16-20. I'm definitely getting stronger.

My best advice for someone that would like to try out a plant-based diet is to slowly remove animal products. That way, you have time to learn and try out plant protein to replace them. Let's say you eat chicken, fish, and eggs. In the first week, stop the chicken and add some alternative, like seitan, tempeh, tofu and legumes. In the second week, now that you are more familiar with the food you have available on a plant-based diet, you can remove the fish. In the third week, remove the eggs and dairy. I know eggs can be hard for a lot of people and I thought it would have been for me, but just wait until you try out a tofu scramble that is absolutely amazing!

One thing that I require is to keep track of macros at the beginning with the Myfitnesspal app. That way, you can check if you are getting your daily macros requirements.

For protein, I use EHPLabs Blessed Protein by Clear Vegan. It's made with pea protein. It's easier on the stomach than whey protein, so no more bloating! :) Plus, the taste is amazing! My favorite is Vanilla Chia.

WHAT IS YOUR FONDEST MEMORY OF YOUR CAREER IN THIS SPORT?

When I was a trainer on the floor. Now I only coach online. I had so many fun days at work. Not that I don't love what I do now, but it was so fun interacting with my clients.

DO YOU NOW OR HAVE YOU HAD A MENTOR IN YOUR LIFE? IF SO, WHO WAS IT AND WHAT IMPACT HAVE THEY HAD ON YOU? ARE THEY STILL YOUR MENTOR TODAY?

My mentor was my manager, Claude. He has helped me a lot in my career and pushed me to do big things. He gave me a lot of guidance. Because of him, I was able to take my modeling career to the next level and get published worldwide in the biggest mainstream magazines. Now I am no longer modeling, but I am still in contact with him. He is always there when I need advice.

ANY INSPIRING STORIES THAT HAVE HAPPENED TO YOU OR PEOPLE CLOSE TO YOU THAT HAVE NOT BEEN COVERED ABOVE. STORIES THAT CAN HELP OTHERS.

Since the age of 13, I have had thyroid issues. I have been taking 175mg of Levothyroxine for over 15 years. After a month of going vegan, my dosage has dropped to 125mg!! That has never happened!

My B12 was above normal as well, even though all I take is a multivitamin and BCAA during training.

CRISSI CARVALHO

CONNECT WITH CRISSI:
INSTAGRAM: @VEGANFITNESSMODEL & @GOODNESS.GRACIAS
FACEBOOK: VEGANFITNESSMODEL
veganfitnessmodel.com

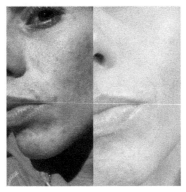
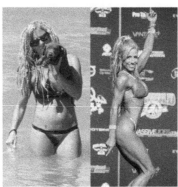

Crissi Carvalho is a holistic vegan fitness coach, model, chef, author, owner of Vegan Fitness Studio, and an Australian Ninja Warrior. She won the Arnold Classic in 2016 and is known for promoting a healthy, high-carb diet whenever she can.

"I made the switch at 38 years old to veganism for a number of reasons. First, there was a cancer health scare when I was 36 years old, on top of the fact that I had constant acne, bloating and migraines. Then I lost my best friend, Zinni, to cancer at the young age of 38. I became even more committed to veganism when I became aware of the animal cruelty involved in the meat and dairy industry. Shocked that I could be part of this system, I decided to stop eating meat forever."

WHAT IS ONE OF THE BEST OR MOST WORTHWHILE HEALTH-RELATED INVESTMENTS THAT YOU HAVE MADE?

The best money I have spent is on a juicer and blender that I purchased in 2011. These two items enabled me to clean out my inner terrain and reset my entire body back to a healthy homeostasis.

AT WHAT POINT IN YOUR LIFE DID YOU DECIDE TO CHANGE YOUR DIET? HOW HAS THAT DECISION IMPACTED YOUR LIFE? WHAT IS

253

YOUR GO-TO FOOD TO FUEL YOUR BODY?

Nutrition is key for any athlete, but even more so for older athletes, as the body will no longer allow for any short cuts. After I switched to plant-based eating, I have been able to compete at the top level in both Australia and around the globe in Europe, Hong Kong and the USA. If I was following the traditional BRO bodybuilding diets, I would need time off to reset and detox my body. I have now competed without an offseason for five years back to back, getting better in each and every competition.

DO YOU TAKE ANY SPECIAL SUPPLEMENTS?

I competed the first two years supplement-free. I wanted to prove that first, I could successfully compete as a vegan. I didn't want to add supplements to skew my results, and I found it was very possible. Then I started having Prana On protein, mixed in my oats or smoothie bowls. This made me hit macros easier, and it tasted so good! This has now become a staple in my diet. I play around and sometimes take herbs like guarana, dandelion, reishi, chaga, maca and camu camu.

WHAT IS YOUR GREATEST STRENGTH? WHAT DRIVES YOU AND KEEPS YOU AT THE TOP OF YOUR GAME?

My greatest strength and the thing that makes me tick is to inspire people to make a change in their health and wellness and to help them transition to veganism while thinking more environmentally.

HOW DO YOU HANDLE THE UPS AND DOWNS OF GOOD AND BAD DAYS? WHAT STRATEGIES DO YOU USE?

When competing, it is all about MINDSET. As a coach and athlete, one needs to be in control of their emotions, their thoughts, their self-talk, their responses and their reactions. When self-doubt and negativity enter your mind, your body responds. I practice positive thoughts and gratitude daily, and when competing I trust the process. Most of all, I practice patience.

WHAT KIND OF TIME COMMITMENT DOES YOUR TRAINING AND TRAVELING SCHEDULE DEMAND? HOW DO YOU BALANCE THAT WITH FAMILY, FRIENDS AND EATING HEALTHILY?

My training takes around one and a half hours per day in offseason and around two to three hours a day when I am in complete prep mode. I train around six days a week and do cardio around three to six times a week. I also do calisthenics, pilates, bouldering and ninja warrior obstacle training when I can fit it in. My training and dieting fit in with my lifestyle, as it is my career, and my family loves to eat as I do - just a whole lot more! Travelling can be hectic and therefore I travel to only two competitions per year and I usually build in an annual vacation, so it balances out.

WHAT KIND OF REACTION DID YOU RECEIVE WHEN YOU ANNOUNCED THAT YOU WERE GOING VEGAN? WHAT DID YOUR COACH, FAMILY AND FRIENDS SAY? WHAT IMPACT HAS THIS HAD ON YOUR PERFORMANCE? RECOVERY?

Most of my family doesn't know what to think, and my husband knew I needed to for health. He loves eating the food I make and loves eating plant-based. Most people accepted my new lifestyle, and many have gone vegan now too!

SINCE TRANSITIONING TO A VEGAN/PLANT-BASED DIET HAS YOUR PERFORMANCE LEVEL GONE UP? WHAT IS YOUR ADVICE TO OTHER ATHLETES OR WOMEN WHO MAY BE INTERESTED IN TRYING A PLANT-BASED DIET?

I became an athlete due to my new thriving lifestyle! I truly don't think I would have competed and still be competing at 45 if I hadn't gone vegan and eaten a whole-food, plant-based diet. Many women that I have competed against for the past five years are now transitioning. I feel if you lead by example, you don't need to offer advice.

255

WHEN YOU SET A GOAL, HOW DO YOU STICK TO IT?

Head down, glutes up! I am stubborn, therefore if I set a goal, it's like a freight train on auto-pilot! I truly am very driven and careful when it comes to goal setting because I keep going until it's accomplished or I feel I let myself down.

YOUR FONDEST MEMORY OF YOUR CAREER IN THIS SPORT?

Too many to list, but here are two;

1. Transitioning many women to veganism through my online programs and ebooks. Many have had their husbands and families also transition. To change people's lives for the better is VERY memorable, and I am so honored to be part of their journey.

2. When my clients win or place in their competitions! Plus now having four-time PRO card Bikini Bodybuilding winning clients. Vegans can do it!

DO YOU NOW OR HAVE YOU HAD A MENTOR IN YOUR LIFE? IF SO, WHO WAS IT AND WHAT IMPACT HAVE THEY HAD ON YOU? ARE THEY STILL YOUR MENTOR TODAY?

No mentors in my life except for the people I have come across that are happy and at peace. These people are the ones that make me feel ultimately how we should be. Though I am a go-getter, I also have a very grounded aspect to my life. Nature, love and animals are my inner peace.

ANY INSPIRING STORIES THAT HAVE HAPPENED TO YOU OR PEOPLE CLOSE TO YOU THAT HAVE NOT BEEN COVERED ABOVE. STORIES THAT CAN HELP OTHERS.

A vegan whole-food, plant-based diet has been life-changing for not only myself but for many others that I have coached and many others that I have crossed paths with.

The motto "you are what you eat" is so very true. What we eat directly affects how we think and how we think affects how we feel. I believe that in the past, many of my "cranky, sad and depressed" moods and my illnesses were directly a result of what I would put into my body. Eating oxygen-rich and nutrient-dense foods and drinking good clean water is ultimately what gives us a thriving life. Why be average when you can thrive?

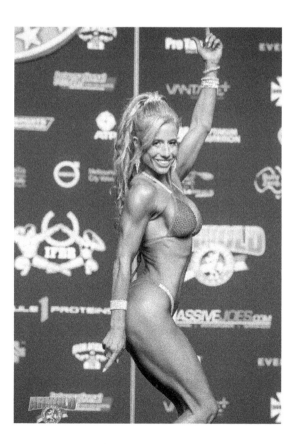

" "

MANY WOMEN THAT
I HAVE COMPETED
AGAINST FOR THE PAST
FIVE YEARS ARE NOW
TRANSITIONING.

I FEEL IF YOU LEAD BY
EXAMPLE, YOU DON'T
NEED TO OFFER ADVICE.

CRISSI CARVALHO

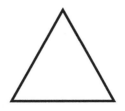

KOYA WEBB

CONNECT WITH KOYA:
INSTAGRAM: @KOYAWEBB & @GETLOVEDUP
YOUTUBE: KOYA WEBB
koyawebb.com

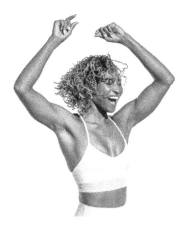

An internationally recognized yoga teacher, personal trainer, holistic health and wellness coach, author, motivational speaker and professional fitness model, Koya Webb has taken the holistic living world by storm. As a "transformational specialist," Koya has helped countless individuals to reach their personal goals through encouraging positive and sustainable lifestyle changes, whether it is through cultivating a self-love practice, fitness practice, or diet change, weight loss, or reversal of life-threatening conditions to experience optimal health.

WHAT IS ONE OF THE BEST OR MOST WORTHWHILE HEALTH-RELATED INVESTMENTS THAT YOU HAVE MADE?

The best health investment I've made is studying the power of herbs, taking the Institute for Integrative Nutrition course and following the electric diet.

AT WHAT POINT IN YOUR LIFE DID YOU DECIDE TO CHANGE YOUR DIET? HOW HAS THAT DECISION IMPACTED YOUR LIFE? WHAT IS YOUR GO-TO FOOD TO FUEL YOUR BODY?

I decided to change my diet when I realized what I was eating was harmful to my body and the planet. I decided to be vegan because I wanted to experience optimal health, I didn't want to contribute to the suffering of animals and I wanted to reduce my carbon footprint.

WHAT IS YOUR GREATEST STRENGTH? WHAT DRIVES YOU AND KEEPS YOU AT THE TOP OF YOUR GAME?

My greatest strength is unconditional love. My commitment to constant evolution keeps me at the top of my game.

HOW DO YOU HANDLE THE UPS AND DOWNS OF GOOD AND BAD DAYS? WHAT STRATEGIES DO YOU USE?

I meditate every day to stay at the top of my game. I practice yoga to strengthen my mind, body and spirit and to heal mentally, spiritually and physically.

WHAT KIND OF REACTION DID YOU RECEIVE WHEN YOU ANNOUNCED THAT YOU WERE GOING VEGAN? WHAT DID YOUR COACH, FAMILY AND FRIENDS SAY? WHAT IMPACT HAS THIS HAD ON YOUR PERFORMANCE? RECOVERY?

My family thought my veganism was just a phase. My friends missed me cooking all the things and eating the same things they ate.

My health is the best it's ever been.

SINCE TRANSITIONING TO A VEGAN/PLANT-BASED DIET HAS YOUR PERFORMANCE LEVEL GONE UP? WHAT IS YOUR ADVICE TO OTHER ATHLETES OR WOMEN WHO MAY BE INTERESTED IN TRYING A PLANT-BASED DIET?

I think the most important thing in transitioning to a plant-based diet is to make sure you're getting all the vitamins, minerals and nutrients you need to survive.

WHAT IS YOUR FONDEST MEMORY OF YOUR CAREER SO FAR?

My fondest memory in yoga is when I first started and felt super intimidated, but decided to breathe through my fears and continue. Now every time I get scared, I just breathe my way through the fear.

DO YOU NOW OR HAVE YOU HAD A MENTOR IN YOUR LIFE? IF SO, WHO WAS IT AND WHAT IMPACT HAVE THEY HAD ON YOU? ARE THEY STILL YOUR MENTOR TODAY?

My mentor is Spirit. Spirit guides me through meditation or when I tune into my intuition and allow myself to be guided.

ANY INSPIRING STORIES YOU CAN SHARE?

My first yoga class was incredibly frustrating. I looked around the room and was completely intimidated by how flexible everyone was. I was very strong and fast, but so tight I couldn't even touch my toes. Then, the instructor had us do a headstand. This was my first class! Plus I had a stress fracture. I wasn't sure I should even try it, but I didn't have the energy to resist. I just went along with it and hoped for the best. I managed to get my legs up and didn't feel discomfort in my back, but I did feel as if my brain was going to ooze out of the top of my head. So many thoughts swirled in my mind: this is not for me . . . I can't do this.

I'm not made for this . . . I'm not bendy. . . there's no way . . .

The instructor must have noticed how much I was struggling because she came over to me, looked me in the eyes, and said, "breathe with me." She took a deep inhale. I inhaled with her, and then we both exhaled together. It felt so good. I don't think I'd taken a deep inhale or exhale since I'd felt that sharp pain. At that moment, I felt at peace. A tingling sensation spread across my body. And I remembered that that was the feeling that I'd had when I was baptized as a child. That was the Holy Spirit! I was amazed. I felt a connection with Spirit for the first time since my injury.

From that moment, yoga became my best friend.

I started going to class regularly, and slowly, my muscles relaxed and my yoga improved. Breathing deeply during my practice, I continued to feel connected to Spirit. My stress and anxiety levels dropped. I felt better enough to start swimming and biking to help my body strengthen and recover. After six months, I felt lighter, more optimistic, and more confident. My body was fit and powerful. Healthier mentally, spiritually, and physically, I was able to return to the track a year after my injury. I went on to win three championship titles in the high jump, heptathlon, the mile relay and to lead Wichita State to their first Women's Track and Field Championship title. All because of yoga.

When I got injured, I was so afraid; afraid of being a failure, afraid of being judged and afraid of who I'd be without track. By opening myself up to change, I discovered yoga and my capacity to heal and adapt. I was able to come back stronger and thrive in a completely unexpected way. I let my fears make me fierce, and years later wrote a book about how I process fears. It's called *Let Your Fears Make You Fierce: How to Turn Common Obstacles Into Seeds For Growth*.

DOTSIE BAUSCH

CONNECT WITH DOTSIE:
INSTAGRAM: @VEGANOLYMPIAN
FACEBOOK: DOTSIE BAUSCH
dotsiebauschusa.com / *switch4good.org*

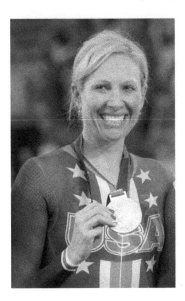

With a prolific professional cycling career that produced a medal at the 2012 London Olympic Games, eight U.S. National Championships, two Pan American gold medals, and a world record. Not only was she vegan, but she was almost 40 years old when she triumphed at the Olympics – the oldest ever in her discipline. Dotsie Bausch has become a powerful plant-based eating role model for athletes and non-athletes alike.

Dotsie's accomplishments are extraordinary, but more remarkable is the hard-fought road this exceptional athlete trudged to achieve such heights. Ultimately, Dotsie's greatest achievement isn't athletic. Her biggest victory is the battle won to resurrect her life from the depths of an eating disorder so severe it very nearly claimed her life.

Long before embodying radiant health and becoming an influential game-changer, Bausch struggled for years with a severe eating disorder and a recreational drug habit that ultimately led to a suicide attempt. It was during her recovery that she discovered her gift and love for cycling.

HOW IMPORTANT IS NUTRITION FOR A TOP-LEVEL ATHLETE? AT WHAT POINT DID YOU DECIDE THAT A PLANT-BASED DIET WAS THE BEST DIET FOR YOU?

I suffered from anorexia and bulimia in my early 20s. When I found cycling as one of my pathways towards healing, I started to understand the effect nutrition could have on my performance. It has been an evolution, but I can honestly say that my whole-foods, nutrient-dense, plant-based, organic food choices have me recovering at almost double the rate of my teammates who are ten years younger than I am.

The golden egg of any sport is finding a natural way to produce the maximum workload to encourage the most growth potential and adaptation to reach a new level. If you recover quickly, you can wake up and train hard again day in and day out. If you are not recovering well, you have to take too many rest days, losing valuable advantages over your competitors.

Because of my history, I created a promise to myself that no food in the whole wide world is off-limits. With that comes freedom of choice. Nowadays, I choose foods that are nutrient-dense and filled with the biggest bang for their buck per gram of food, and that is always food in the plant world. I don't want empty food, and by that, I mean anything that's a filler but not a "doer" inside my body. As an athlete I want all of my food to be healing something, replenishing everything and growing new features within my muscle structure to increase my aerobic and muscular capacity.

DO YOU TAKE ANY SPECIAL SUPPLEMENTS OR POTIONS? MENTION ANY SPECIFIC BRANDS YOU USE AND WHY YOU THINK THESE HAVE BENEFITED YOU AND YOUR HEALTH.

For pre-workout, I load with electrolytes and glycogen and always rice and some plant protein (lentils, almond butter or a veggie sausage). I need a little protein to ward off hunger yet simple to digest, and a full bottle of electrolyte mix.

Post-workout is refueling my muscles with glycogen immediately for accelerated repair, then I go into my protein for recovery about 45 minutes later, which is a shake I make of Vega performance protein, Vega antioxidant omega oil blend, blueberries, half a banana, maca powder, cacao nibs, cinnamon, unsweetened almond milk and ice.

WHAT IS YOUR GREATEST STRENGTH? WHAT DRIVES YOU AND KEEPS YOU AT THE TOP OF YOUR GAME?

I think my greatest strength might be resilience. My whole life has been a series of ups and downs, like everyone else's life, but my ability to rapidly bounce back from disappointing and heartbreaking situations has kept me flexible and in the game. Being able to successfully cope with disappointment, despair and pain is definitely a strength I lean on almost daily.

HOW DO YOU HANDLE THE UPS AND DOWNS OF GOOD AND BAD DAYS? WHAT STRATEGIES DO YOU USE?

Cycling has been a true gift to me from day one. I used it as a healing vehicle in the beginning. When I was ready to re-integrate activity and exercise back into my life, my therapist wanted me to try something that I had never done before and had no negative connotations with, because one symptom of an eating disorder is over-exercise. I chose cycling. I chose it out of the blue, really. It just seemed like it would feel good with the wind in my hair and the feeling of freedom would be welcomed. I never stopped.

In part, cycling saved my life.

Training as a professional athlete constantly makes me feel like I am working on the edge of my abilities, which is an exhilarating and terrifying place to be. My coach is consistently pushing me up against the wall, and it's not just physical. He also asks so much of my mental capabilities. I feel stretched to the max most of the time, trying to balance life, work and my athletic career. But competitive cycling has truly seen me through so many situations and if it weren't for it, I would have never lived in this place where I feel bold and competent, inadequate but capable, valuable and invaluable and so in control yet out of control.

Competitive cycling and all of its ups and downs is the biggest mirror to life that I can find. Every lesson I have learned in cycling transfers over to my relationships and my work, and infuses me with the confidence I need to live life fully each day. It's an honor to be doing this. I recognize there are others who would like to be in my shoes. That is single-handedly what motivates me on days when I don't feel like training.

SINCE TRANSITIONING TO A VEGAN/PLANT-BASED DIET HAS YOUR PERFORMANCE LEVEL GONE UP? WHAT IS YOUR ADVICE TO OTHER ATHLETES OR WOMEN WHO MAY BE INTERESTED IN TRYING A PLANT-BASED DIET?

Everything in my life improved when I went plant-based.

Yes, my performance improved as my blood flow increased, my power output increased my ability to recover in between strenuous workouts increased, but, my hormones also came into balance, which was great for training, but also for my daily experiences. My PMS almost completely disappeared and my skin cleared up.

263

There is something really powerfully wonderful that happens when we eliminate all animal foods from our diet. When all of the hormones we were ingesting before that wreak havoc on our internal emotional compass and then suddenly leave, a new sense of self emerges.

WHEN YOU SET A GOAL, HOW DO YOU STICK TO IT?

I have never thought much about this question. My personality is fairly gritty by nature and as I mentioned, I tend to be fairly resilient. I set a goal, and then I just start working towards it. Each day is a new day and I work towards that goal, and some days I get closer to it than others. The days where I don't feel I made much progress, I just let them go and I know that in order to eventually reach my goal, I have to just keep going. Some days are baby steps and others are giant leaps, but they all count.

WHAT IS YOUR FONDEST MEMORY OF YOUR CYCLING CAREER?

The Olympic podium. I will simply never forget the feeling of seeing the American flag raised. I can still "bring it up" if I close my eyes and imagine. I don't want to ever lose what that felt like.

The thing that is a slight bummer is that it's just you up there, and the truth of the matter is you did not get there alone. You get there with the support of your family, friends, coaches and sponsors. I remember wishing that they were all up there with me getting to experience the high.

ANY INSPIRING STORIES THAT HAVE HAPPENED TO YOU OR PEOPLE CLOSE TO YOU THAT HAVE NOT BEEN COVERED ABOVE. STORIES THAT CAN HELP OTHERS.

Today I no longer view food as something to battle; those eating disorder days are behind me. Now I'm excited about eating, and I feel a deep sense of empowerment and pride each time I sit down for a meal.

Beauty unfolds in my heart every time I eat when I think about my choice to not include violence in my meal. That beauty blooms into other parts of my life: in how I treat other people, my friends, my colleagues, my animals at home. I feel connected to my food in a more soulful way because I know that with every bite, I'm choosing peace and making a statement for something I believe in. That connection between my food and values, that feeling of being emboldened by what I'm putting on my plate is true freedom, true strength, true happiness.

" "

I DON'T WANT EMPTY FOOD,
AND BY THAT, I MEAN ANYTHING
THAT'S A FILLER BUT NOT A
"DOER" INSIDE MY BODY. AS AN
ATHLETE I WANT ALL OF MY FOOD
TO BE HEALING SOMETHING,
REPLENISHING EVERYTHING,
AND GROWING NEW FEATURES
WITHIN MY MUSCLE STRUCTURE
TO INCREASE MY AEROBIC AND
MUSCULAR CAPACITY.

DOTSIE BAUSCH

SAMANTHA SHORKEY

CONNECT WITH SAM:
INSTAGRAM: @SAMSHORKEY
FACEBOOK: JACKED ON THE BEANSTALK
YOUTUBE: SAMANTHA SHORKEY
jackedonthebeanstalk.com

Samantha Shorkey is a certified personal trainer and certified weight management specialist who is the first-ever vegan to win the INBL South-Western Natural Championship for the bikini pro category. She now helps others succeed in their fitness goals through her successful coaching platform, Jacked on the Beanstalk.

WHAT IS ONE OF THE BEST OR MOST WORTHWHILE HEALTH-RELATED INVESTMENTS THAT YOU HAVE MADE?

The most obvious health-related investment would absolutely be my gym membership. I definitely get my money's worth out of that monthly charge, seeing as I'm in the gym six days a week. I'm also a huge fan of my yoga wheel for daily stretching and bending while listening to a guided meditation or an inspiring podcast. I am forever grateful for investing in a Vitamix (game changer for all your blending needs) and my stackable dehydrator trays (for making tofu jerky.) I also can't forget my air fryer (which is awesome for making crispy, oil-free cauliflower or tofu/tempeh bites) as well as my Instant Pot (for making dried beans and lentils from scratch).

WHAT WERE THE FIRST STEPS YOU TOOK IN MAKING YOUR HEALTH / NUTRITIONAL CHANGES AND WHY DID YOU START DOWN THIS PATH?

One of the first steps I took in making my health and nutrition a priority was getting my head in the right frame of mind, which is a BIG part of my coaching too. I often say that a "joy and inner peace plan" is far more crucial than an exercise or nutrition plan, in order to actually feel sexy and confident in your own skin for the long term. Anyone can follow a diet plan or a training plan for a couple of weeks or months.

Like many others, what initially sparked my urge to compete in bikini competitions was getting out of a toxic relationship and feeling like I needed to make a change in order to feel happy again. Like most people, I saw myself as this constant self-improvement project. I was always setting high standards and expectations for myself and thinking that WHEN I lose ten pounds or WHEN I sculpt the perfect butt, THEN I'll show my ex how amazing I am and THEN I'll FINALLY be happy. This is what initially sparked my interest in fitness competing.

I worked my ass off (literally) going from zero to hero with two-a-day workouts and six tiny, bland, boring vegan meals per day. But honestly, that was not the path that led me to my best state of health and nutrition. I had many struggles and "all or nothing" cycles along the way.

To truly achieve long-term, SUSTAINABLE, healthy habits and daily routines, I literally had to achieve a so-called "perfect" body to learn that this is NOT where true satisfaction and fulfillment come from. I had to accept and love myself exactly where I was at, through thick or thin and wake up every morning and acknowledge something I was grateful for and something I loved about myself. I realized that this is because you have to approach any health and nutrition change from a place of love and not hate. I had to focus on what I wanted to learn rather than what I wanted to change, and suddenly, this whole eating healthy and being active thing got a lot easier.

WHAT HAS BEEN YOUR BIGGEST RESOURCE FOR COOKING RECIPES? WHO HAS BEEN YOUR BIGGEST INFLUENCER FOR YOUR VEGAN/ PLANT-BASED DIET CHANGE?

The first vegan diet book I ever read was Brendan Brazier's, Thrive Diet. It's about whole-foods and eating for athletic performance. I wouldn't say that I ever followed a similar diet to what he recommends in the book, but it was where I first learned about protein balls, protein smoothies and superfoods galore! I've been a vegan hippie meathead ever since. The main difference in my diet is that I just eat a lot more protein than Brendan. FUN FACT: I met him a couple of years later and was super shy and awkward only to discover that he was also shy and awkward. That was kinda cool. :)

WHAT IS YOUR GREATEST STRENGTH? WHAT DRIVES YOU AND KEEPS YOU AT THE TOP OF YOUR GAME?

Honestly, my greatest strength is the fact that I've always remained true to myself and my ethics, and I'm not just talking about being vegan. It means always being real and authentic with my clients, blog readers and podcast subscribers about my own personal struggles and experiences. I'm by no means perfect with diet and exercise despite being a vegan coach and pro bikini competitor, and I'm more than okay with that. I firmly believe that with anything we pursue in life, we'll have much better results when we focus on what we want to LEARN rather than what we want to CHANGE about ourselves.

Rather than getting caught up with "perfecting" my physical appearance, I've always put more focus on self-discovery and less focus on self-improvement. It's amazing how much easier eating healthy and staying fit becomes when you get out of that pressure-filled, all-or-nothing, obsessive drive to be "perfect."

I'd also like to credit my willpower as one of my greatest strengths. Like any muscle, the more you use it the stronger it will get.

YOUR FONDEST MEMORY OF YOUR CAREER IN THIS SPORT?

Being able to repeatedly break the stereotypes that exist about all vegans being weak, scrawny and protein-deficient. I always say that I don't preach; I inspire. Being a fit vegan (not to mention the first-ever Vegan World Naturals bikini pro) in the protein-obsessed, meat-heavy world of competitive bodybuilding allows me to do just that.

What's even more awesome is having one of my clients win the 2015 12-Week Transformation Challenge put on by bodybuilding.com and winning $200,000 for it (beating out 345,000 contestants worldwide). And most recently in 2018, one of my clients won Lee Labrada's 12-Week Lean Body Challenge. After her big win, I had my own personal hero (world famous fitness model relic Jamie Eason) send me a message congratulating me on my coaching. That felt pretty damn awesome too.

DO YOU NOW OR HAVE YOU HAD A MENTOR IN YOUR LIFE? IF SO, WHO WAS IT AND WHAT IMPACT HAVE THEY HAD ON YOU? ARE THEY STILL YOUR MENTOR TODAY?

The woman who inspired me to become the animal-loving fitness freak I am today is my very own mother: Nora Shorkey. You know that scene from the movie, Ace Ventura: Pet Detective, when he enters his apartment and says, "come to me, my animal friends"? Then a billion birds and beasts suddenly appear and flock to him? Well, that's my mom. Ever since I can remember, our houses have been home to countless strays and rescued animals. I was only eight years old when I told my mom that I didn't want to eat animals anymore. She knew nothing about a vegetarian diet, but being the huge animal lover that she was, she respected my decision and said she'd try her best to accommodate. Surprisingly enough, my mom never tried to dissuade me from being vegetarian. I think because deep down, she knew it was her own compassion and love for animals that influenced this dietary choice. Although she continually referred to me as a "pain in the ass vegetarian," she was proud of me for standing up for what I believed in. If it weren't for her teaching me to love and respect all animals from such an early age, I'm quite certain that I wouldn't be where I am today.

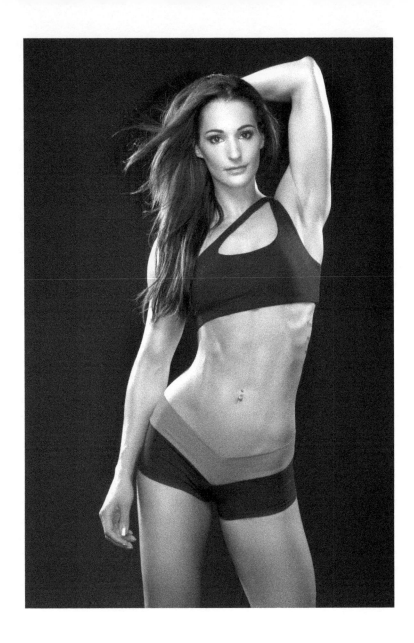

269

WHAT HAS BEEN THE MOST NOTICEABLE CHANGE AFTER TURNING YOUR FAMILY VEGAN/PLANT-BASED?

I like to think that being vegan enhances my life in every way except at family dinners and BBQs where no matter what, you're always that "pain in the ass vegan."

It's so true that when you eat healthy, you feel healthy and when you eat like crap, you feel like crap. I know this sounds gross, but I always had phlegm in my throat when I'd drink milk as a vegetarian before going vegan. Every morning I'd start my workday with a whey and skim milk protein shake and one of my co-workers used to always complain that I'd be clearing my throat non-stop for the first couple of hours. Literally, as soon as I stopped drinking milk it went away. I also think my skin looks better and younger than many other women my age. It's also easy for me to maintain a healthy weight, eating a balanced vegan diet complete with carbs and fats.

I definitely have more energy as a vegan, and I just can't help but feel good knowing that everything going into my body is clean, unprocessed and grown from the earth. I tell people all the time "I can be perfectly healthy without contributing to the death and suffering of others, so why would I?"

ANY INSPIRING STORIES THAT HAVE HAPPENED TO YOU OR PEOPLE CLOSE TO YOU THAT HAVE NOT BEEN COVERED ABOVE. STORIES THAT CAN HELP OTHERS.

My own inspiring story is that I am a two-time winning vegan bikini athlete and the first-ever VEGAN World Naturals Bikini pro.

I'm also proud to say that I've seen many successful and inspiring client transformations. My favorite client transformation at this point was coaching a meat-eater who turned vegan for a hugely popular worldwide challenge. As I mentioned above and as luck would have it, she also became the grand prize winner of Bodybuilding.com's $200,000 12-Week Transformation Challenge in 2015 (beating out 345,000 contestants worldwide.) If that's not inspiring and awesome, I don't know what is!

FIEN LAMMERTYN

CONNECT WITH FIEN:
INSTAGRAM: @PEDALINGPINKPANTHER

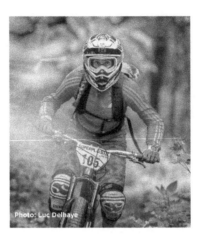

Photo: Luc Delhaye

"My family and friends had a hard time accepting my changes. They didn't really get it, and they never expected me, a former meat-lover to go vegan. I have a feeling that I unlocked a door they wanted me to keep shut and ignore. I am an animal lover and an athlete, so it makes complete sense for me to live this lifestyle. I am living in line with my beliefs as an animal lover and as an athlete, I am stronger and fitter than ever, and I believe this is due to eating a plant-based diet."

WHAT IS ONE OF THE BEST OR MOST WORTHWHILE HEALTH-RELATED INVESTMENTS THAT YOU HAVE MADE?

Taking a vegan bodybuilder as a coach. His name is Puru Schout, and he's an inspiring human. He helped me make sure I did the vegan lifestyle right.

AT WHAT POINT IN YOUR LIFE DID YOU DECIDE TO CHANGE YOUR DIET? HOW HAS THAT DECISION IMPACTED YOUR LIFE? WHAT IS YOUR GO-TO FOOD TO FUEL YOUR BODY?

I got into the bodybuilding world and had to eat chicken all day every day. After one year of doing that, I just felt that it wasn't really good for my body. I shortly realized after this decision that I wanted to get my proteins from a solely plant-based diet.

I got into this lifestyle because of health reasons, but I stayed in it because

I discovered the horrible truth about the meat and dairy industries. Now I am living the plant-based lifestyle because of my health, as well as for the animals and the environment.

I've always been a big animal lover, yet I didn't blink an eye when I had to eat them. Now, it makes more sense when I say I'm an animal lover. I don't feel like a hypocrite anymore.

I wasn't born vegan, and I wasn't raised vegan, so I do know what it's like to eat meat. I used to eat it every day and I used to love it. At this point, the thought of eating meat again disgusts me.

HOW DO YOU HANDLE THE UPS AND DOWNS OF GOOD AND BAD DAYS? WHAT STRATEGIES DO YOU USE?

I'm quite a spiritual person. I truly believe that the universe has got our backs and that all good and bad things happen for a reason. Knowing it's some higher power who wants it as that gives me peace of mind.

WHAT KIND OF REACTION DID YOU RECEIVE WHEN YOU ANNOUNCED THAT YOU WERE GOING VEGAN?

First, I changed my coach so I got the support I needed.

My family and friends were pretty difficult to tell. They don't really get it and they never expected me, a former meat-lover, to go vegan. I have a feeling that I unlocked a door they wanted me to keep shut and ignore.

One of my main strengths is that when everyone believes I am going to fail, I step up my game even more. The more obstacles people throw in my way, the more likely I will overcome them and feel more motivated than ever.

SINCE TRANSITIONING TO A VEGAN/PLANT-BASED DIET HAS YOUR PERFORMANCE LEVEL GONE UP? WHAT IS YOUR ADVICE TO OTHER ATHLETES OR WOMEN WHO MAY BE INTERESTED IN TRYING A PLANT-BASED DIET?

I definitely feel like my recovery time is way better and in general, I just feel so much better. As an athlete, you have to make sure that you get all of your nutrients in, but that counts for any athlete, plant-based or not.

I do take extra vitamins (but in the end, all athletes do that) I also use a vegan protein powder.

I do recommend working with a vegan bodybuilder in the beginning, even if you're doing a totally different kind of sport. Nutrition is basically the same for all athletes, but bodybuilders really know everything the body needs.

AMY KATE

CONNECT WITH AMY:
INSTAGRAM: @AMYKATEFIT
jakdfitness.com.au

"What started as a journey to improving my health, quickly turned into finding out a lot more than I ever expected. Veganism has led me to find my passion and has completely changed my outlook on life. We all grow up thinking and being taught to live our lives ONE way... but it wasn't until I challenged myself and found my path, that I began to truly find out who I was and why I was put on this planet."

"Veganism has helped shape my life in my twenties and has opened my eyes in so many ways. I have learnt to make the connection between what is on my plate. I am ashamed to have ever contributed to the injustice and enslavement of innocent beings. Now that I am vegan, I am advocating for these beings – I now want to educate, motivate and inspire as many people as I can to make the connection too."

273

Amy Kate Perry is an online vegan health and fitness coach and social media influencer. Amy and her husband, Jesse, own Jakd Fitness, where they help clients train while simultaneously educating them on the principles of plant-based fitness.

WHAT IS ONE OF THE BEST OR MOST WORTHWHILE HEALTH-RELATED INVESTMENTS THAT YOU HAVE MADE?

100% my blender. I use my blender daily. Having a good quality blender is so handy for making all types of smoothies and recipes. Especially if you have young kids, because you can hide greens and veggies in their smoothies. You can make all sorts of meals using a blender, like sauces, soups, dips, smoothies and even healthy desserts. I would recommend anyone to purchase a good quality blender if you are wanting to go vegan or eat cleaner.

HOW IMPORTANT IS NUTRITION FOR A TOP-LEVEL ATHLETE? AT WHAT POINT DID YOU DECIDE THAT A PLANT-BASED DIET WAS THE BEST DIET FOR YOU?

It is very important. What we eat is the fuel to our performance. If we don't fuel our bodies correctly, we will not perform at our best. Your diet is important for not only your physical performance, but also controls your mood, hormones and mental abilities.

It was a gradual process for me. I went vegetarian first and felt the effects straight away. I continued to do my research and discover the benefits of this lifestyle. It soon became apparent that it was the best choice for me and my future.

What started as a journey to improving my health quickly turned into finding out a lot more than I ever expected. Veganism has led me to find my passion and has completely changed my outlook on life.

Veganism has helped shape my life in my twenties and has opened my eyes in so many ways. I have learned to make a connection with what is on my plate. Now that I am vegan, I am advocating for animals and I now want to educate and inspire as many people as I can to make the connection too.

DO YOU TAKE ANY SPECIAL SUPPLEMENTS OR POTIONS? MENTION ANY SPECIFIC BRANDS YOU USE AND WHY YOU THINK THESE HAVE BENEFITED YOU AND YOUR HEALTH.

I am a big believer in taking vitamins and supplements for optimal health unless you are eating mainly raw, organic and whole fruits and vegetables daily.

It is hard to know if you are getting enough vitamins and minerals into your diet daily. I get two blood tests per year to check my levels and they have always been perfect. My husband and I have both improved with our blood results since going vegan.

I take a B12 sublingual spray, vitamin C, iron and magnesium. I am also on a Pregnancy Multi as I am currently pregnant.

I don't take anything religiously as I am very in tune with my body. I like to just take vitamins and minerals based on how I am feeling. I also take a vegan protein powder daily, post-workout, to help with muscle recovery.

WHAT IS YOUR GREATEST STRENGTH? WHAT DRIVES YOU AND KEEPS YOU AT THE TOP OF YOUR GAME?

My greatest strength would be that I always want to be the best version of myself. I believe in always working on yourself, both mentally and physically. Life is busy and tough at times and we need to have the tools to handle any stressful situations that life may throw at us. I continue to build my confidence DAILY, and will always keep pushing myself outside of my comfort zone to continue to be the best version of myself for myself, my husband, my friends, my family and for our little one on the way.

HOW DO YOU HANDLE THE UPS AND DOWNS OF GOOD AND BAD DAYS? WHAT STRATEGIES DO YOU USE?

We all have good and bad days. That's LIFE!! But when bad days pass, they are what makes us grateful for the good days. Without bad days we wouldn't know what good days felt like.

I like to always remind myself of what I am grateful for and practice gratitude and mindfulness daily. I try to always be present and in the now, and to appreciate each day as it comes.

Some strategies I like to practice are:

1. *Write in a gratitude journal daily with ten things I am grateful for.*
2. *Create vision boards of my goals.*
3. *Remember to be present and not think too much of the future or past.*
4. *Meditate.*

WHAT KIND OF TIME COMMITMENT DOES YOUR TRAINING AND TRAVELING SCHEDULE DEMAND? HOW DO YOU BALANCE THAT WITH FAMILY, FRIENDS AND EATING HEALTHILY?

At the moment, my training hasn't been my number one commitment. My husband and I have been concentrating on setting up our future for our little one to arrive.

I am still training four or five days per week. But I am a very organized person, and I like to plan out my weeks ahead so I can have time to myself and get myself to the gym. I also get all my work done for the week with as little stress as possible.

Being organized and practicing time management is the key to running a successful business and life. I like to use Sundays as a prep day to write out what I need for the week, fill the cupboards and fridge with food and have some meals cooked, so my week is a lot more smooth.

WHAT KIND OF REACTION DID YOU RECEIVE WHEN YOU ANNOUNCED THAT YOU WERE GOING VEGAN? WHAT DID YOUR COACH, FAMILY, AND FRIENDS SAY? WHAT IMPACT HAS THIS HAD ON YOUR PERFORMANCE? RECOVERY?

It was a long process for me (I was vegetarian first and everyone kind of knew I was dabbling with going vegan) so they kind of expected it.

But yes, I would still get the odd comment here and there about how I would have to watch my iron levels and B12, etc. But, we should all watch our iron and B12 levels, vegan or not. We are not always eating a well-balanced diet and not always aware of any nutrients we may be lacking. So as I said earlier, I recommend taking supplements whether you're vegan or not.

SINCE TRANSITIONING TO A VEGAN/PLANT-BASED DIET HAS YOUR PERFORMANCE LEVEL GONE UP? WHAT IS YOUR ADVICE TO OTHER ATHLETES OR WOMEN WHO MAY BE INTERESTED IN TRYING A PLANT-BASED DIET?

I only started at the gym when I was a vegetarian, so I can't compare my performance to what I felt like before. That being said, my recovery has been amazing and every day fogginess and fatigue have definitely improved.

I was always having afternoon naps before becoming vegan and would have a coffee to start my day. Now I don't need stimulants to keep me going all day, and my mind is a lot clearer and more focused.

WHEN YOU SET A GOAL, HOW DO YOU STICK TO IT?

By setting small goals and stepping stones to my bigger goal. For example, I will set a goal like, "entering a body-building contest." Then I will have a plan for what I am going to do during my months of training and dieting to get to my end goal. Having those stepping stones helps to keep me motivated and on track.

Also, speaking my goals and making myself accountable by telling others about my goals. Get it out of your head onto paper and voice it to the world. It's scary, YES, but it will help keep you accountable along the way.

Creating a vision board will help you to stay motivated and on track. Place it somewhere you can see it as a daily reminder of your WHY.

Setting a "why" is also important. WHY are you doing this goal? WHAT do you want out of this goal?

Don't just set a goal because you just want to lose 20 kilograms. WHY do you want to lose weight? How will it make you feel? How will this impact your life? List all the reasons WHY you are setting this goal in the first place and write this on your vision board.

YOUR FONDEST MEMORY OF YOUR CAREER IN THIS SPORT?

So far, it has been finding my passion and helping people all around the world. The feedback of hearing that I have helped motivate and inspire someone to live a healthier and happier life is the best feeling in the world.

I feel I have been put on this earth to help people and make a difference, and any way I can help someone, I know I am fulfilling my life purpose.

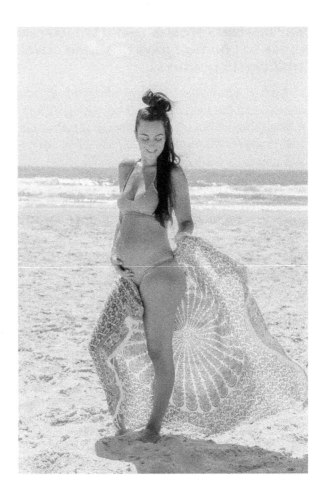

DO YOU NOW OR HAVE YOU HAD A MENTOR IN YOUR LIFE? IF SO, WHO WAS IT AND WHAT IMPACT HAVE THEY HAD ON YOU? ARE THEY STILL YOUR MENTOR TODAY?

I can't think of just ONE person who has been a mentor for me. My husband would have to be my number one since he is my best friend and soulmate. We have a connection that is so special and unique that I am so grateful for. He helps motivate me and always knows when I need lifting and to be put back on my path.

My other mentor would be my Dad. He passed away back in 2005 from a brain tumor, but I feel like he mentors me daily. He is a constant reminder to me to live each day and be grateful for life itself. We never know when our time is up, so I don't waste my time worrying about the little things. Instead, I live each day in the now and am grateful for what I have in my life at this current point.

Chapter 5 | ATHLETES

ANY INSPIRING STORIES THAT HAVE HAPPENED TO YOU OR PEOPLE CLOSE TO YOU THAT HAVE NOT BEEN COVERED ABOVE. STORIES THAT CAN HELP OTHERS.

I have had a past where I suffered from anxiety, depression and panic attacks, and this held me back from saying YES to so many opportunities. It stopped me from my own personal growth. I became a hermit and was always saying NO as I let my fear win every time. I was unhappy, depressed and unmotivated in ALL areas of my life.

What made me break out of my NO bubble?? SAYING YES and facing my fears. When I started to step outside my comfort zone, I started to break down my security walls and find my voice and also my life purpose. I had always wanted to help people, but I just thought I never had the confidence to do so. I also had no idea where to start. This was when YouTube gave me that voice and also the opportunity to help people all around the world.

Now, I LOVE WHAT I DO. And yes, I still have my down days, but hey, that's just life. I started entering bodybuilding competitions and really throwing myself into challenges that would scare me and help me build a thicker skin. I mean, what's scarier than training your butt off and standing on stage to be judged in front of hundreds of people, right? Best decision I ever made.

I did it without a coach as I wanted to add more pressure on myself, and to really know that I did it for me and all by myself. I placed in both my competitions and the feeling of accomplishing something I once doubted myself for was so empowering. It's what led me to do another competition only one year later.

Another saying I love is, "let your fear fuel you." See failure as a sign to change direction or try again. Don't ever see failure as a sign to give up. If I gave up every time I failed, I would not be where I am today. I have failed at so many things in my life and guess what? It is guaranteed I am going to fail a heck of a lot more in the future. But I am totally fine with that. As I said, I see it as a chance to change direction, and I see it as a sign from the universe telling me, "hey you're nearly there, but you just have to try another way. Keep going, you are so close." Please don't be afraid of failing as it's one thing that is always guaranteed in life.

Let the fear fuel you and grow and learn every time you do fail.

To find out who you are or what your life purpose is, you need to get comfortable with being uncomfortable. Say YES and just wing it and figure it out as you go, because in life we are all the same. We are just winging it and learning along the way.

LEILANI MÜNTER

CONNECT WITH LEILANI:
INSTAGRAM: @LEILANIMUNTER
FACEBOOK: LEILANI MUNTER
leilani.green

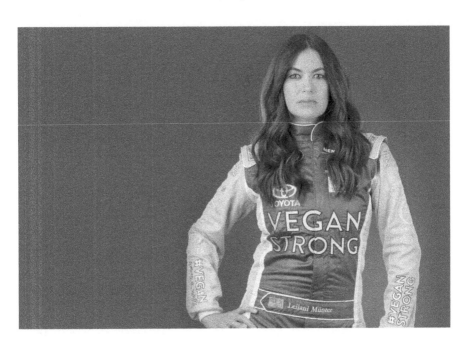

279

"In my personal life, I do everything I can to set a good example for the race fans by reducing my carbon footprint as much as possible. I compost my food scraps, have a veggie garden and a rainwater collection system, I have been driving an electric car since 2013, and my home and car have been solar powered since 2014. I have been vegan since 2011, and have been vegetarian almost my entire life...It's just better for our climate, the animals, our bodies — whatever reason they decide to look at that change, that's what I want to focus on."

Leilani Münter is a professional race car driver, environmental activist, and lobbies for causes such as solar power, electric cars, plant-based eating and animal rights. Discovery's Planet Green named her the #1 eco athlete in the world, ELLE Magazine awarded her their Genius Award, and Sports Illustrated named her one of the top ten female race car drivers in the world. Leilani has been a guest at The White House and the United Nations in Geneva. Since 2007, she has been adopting an acre of rainforest for every race she takes part in.

WHAT IS ONE OF THE BEST OR MOST WORTHWHILE HEALTH-RELATED INVESTMENTS THAT YOU HAVE MADE?

My juicer. At least once a year I do a ten to fourteen-day juice fast.

AT WHAT POINT IN YOUR LIFE DID YOU DECIDE TO CHANGE YOUR DIET? HOW HAS THAT DECISION IMPACTED YOUR LIFE? WHAT IS YOUR GO-TO FOOD TO FUEL YOUR BODY?

In the summer of 2011, I went vegan. I made the switch for ethical reasons: for the animals and our planet.

Eating a plant-based diet is easy once you try it. I think people who are just starting to go plant-based should start slow, like being meat-free on "Meatless Mondays." I think that asking for people to be perfect — whether it be their diet or anything else — is the quickest way to lose their interest altogether. Just work your way there slowly, and I think you will find that it's easy, it just takes practice and time.

WHAT IS YOUR GREATEST STRENGTH? WHAT DRIVES YOU AND KEEPS YOU AT THE TOP OF YOUR GAME?

My greatest strength is when I want to do something, I jump in and do it. I don't wait for the plan to be perfect before moving forward.

HOW DO YOU HANDLE THE UPS AND DOWNS OF GOOD AND BAD DAYS? WHAT STRATEGIES DO YOU USE?

I try to keep everything in perspective. There will always be someone out there who is having a worse day than I am. I do things to relax me, or I have a cocktail to take the edge off.

WHAT KIND OF REACTION DID YOU RECEIVE WHEN YOU ANNOUNCED THAT YOU WERE GOING VEGAN? WHAT DID YOUR COACH, FAMILY AND FRIENDS SAY? WHAT IMPACT HAS THIS HAD ON YOUR PERFORMANCE? RECOVERY?

I was already a vegetarian, so it didn't come as a big surprise. My health improved (I've only had one cold in nearly eight years), I have more energy, and I have better concentration.

SINCE TRANSITIONING TO A VEGAN/PLANT-BASED DIET HAS YOUR PERFORMANCE LEVEL GONE UP? WHAT IS YOUR ADVICE TO OTHER ATHLETES OR WOMEN WHO MAY BE INTERESTED IN TRYING A PLANT-BASED DIET?

Both my health and my focus have definitely gone up. My advice would be "Do it!" Be open to try lots of vegan products on the market, though it will take some time to find the ones you love. There are also free resources at TryVeg.com if you are looking for guidance.

Eating animal products is not just harmful to animals, but to the planet as well. Everyone is focused on fossil fuels, but more greenhouse gas emissions come from raising animals for food than all of the transportation emissions from planes, trains, cars, trucks, ships, etc combined. We need to help people understand that the food on their dinner plates has a big effect on their carbon footprint.

I have talked with several different groups that are working on electric race cars, and each time I race I adopt an area of the rainforest.

In my personal life, I do everything I can to set a good example for the race fans by reducing my carbon footprint as much as possible. I compost my food scraps, I have a veggie garden and a rainwater collection system, I use solar lighting and I am installing solar panels. Soon I will be buying an electric car as my personal vehicle (right now I don't have a personal car at all).

YOUR FONDEST MEMORY OF YOUR CAREER IN THIS SPORT?

Daytona. I have lots of memories from there. It's a magical place.

DO YOU NOW OR HAVE YOU HAD A MENTOR IN YOUR LIFE? IF SO, WHO WAS IT AND WHAT IMPACT HAVE THEY HAD ON YOU? ARE THEY STILL YOUR MENTOR TODAY?

Ric O' Barry. He is the most dedicated and humble activist I have ever known. He is an inspiration to so many people including me, and I am so thankful to have him as a friend.

ANY INSPIRING STORIES THAT HAVE HAPPENED TO YOU OR PEOPLE CLOSE TO YOU THAT HAVE NOT BEEN COVERED ABOVE. STORIES THAT CAN HELP OTHERS.

We are adding one billion people to our planet every twelve years. Every single environmental crisis we face, including climate change, ocean acidification, habitat loss, pollution and species extinction are accelerated by our rapidly growing population. The ultimate intelligence of our species will be determined by whether we face our population issue and get it under control, or continue to sweep it under the rug because it's an uncomfortable conversation. The future of life on Earth depends on us doing the former.

" "

I'M A VEGAN "MEATHEAD"
AND I EAT QUITE A HIGH
PROTEIN VEGAN DIET. MY GO-
TO MEALS ARE SUPER SIMPLE
BODYBUILDING MEALS, LIKE
TOFU, RICE, BROCCOLI, PROTEIN
OATS, FAKE MEATS, AND RICE
CAKES. MY DIET IS A PRETTY
TYPICAL "BODYBUILDING DIET,"
BUT INSTEAD OF MEAT AND
DAIRY, I USE THE PLANT-BASED
ALTERNATIVES.

EMMA SEITERI

EMMA SEITERI

CONNECT WITH EMMA:
INSTAGRAM: @EMMASEITERI
FACEBOOK: EMMA SEITERI FITNESS
YOUTUBE: EMMA SEITERI
emmaseiteri.com

Emma Seiteri is a vegan personal trainer, online coach, IFBB Bikini Athlete, award-winning bodybuilder, and owner of a line of activewear clothing called Flex Active Apparel. Emma is passionate about fitness, health and plant-based eating, and she uses her growing social media platforms to motivate others who are interested in plant-based fitness.

WHAT IS ONE OF THE BEST OR MOST WORTHWHILE HEALTH-RELATED INVESTMENTS THAT YOU HAVE MADE?

I think that investing in your health is like putting money into a bank. Health can't be bought, and that's why it is so important to invest in your health because that is making yourself a priority. The best investment in my health has been hiring a coach. Even coaches have coaches. For me, the most important part is to have someone else to do the "stressing" part. For example, a competition prep in itself is a highly stressful journey, and if I were to make all of my own adjustments, I would always be thinking "am I doing enough?" or "Is this the absolute optimal decision?." Having another pair of eyes looking at your progress and making those decisions for you is priceless. Having a coach also adds that accountability factor there, and having invested money in it makes you even more invested and willing to make those changes towards better health.

283

AT WHAT POINT IN YOUR LIFE DID YOU DECIDE TO CHANGE YOUR DIET? HOW HAS THAT DECISION IMPACTED YOUR LIFE? WHAT IS YOUR GO-TO FOOD TO FUEL YOUR BODY?

I went vegan overnight. I had done a lot of research before I went vegan, and at first it was because of environmental reasons. I studied biology at university, and I was friends with a lot of environmental scientists. They made me aware of the environmental issues of the meat and dairy industry. I finally went vegan when I made the ethical connection, and there was no turning back. After becoming vegan, I noticed all the health benefits, and that's what made me stay vegan. I felt so much better, more energized and recovered better from my workouts.

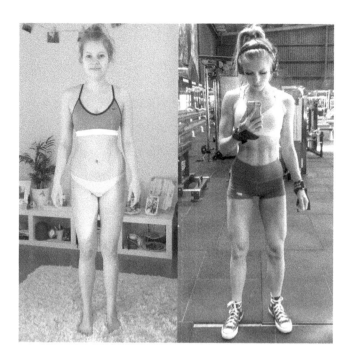

I'm a vegan "meathead," and I eat quite a high protein vegan diet. My go-to meals are super simple bodybuilding meals, like tofu, rice, broccoli, protein oats, fake meats and rice cakes. My diet is a pretty typical "bodybuilding diet," but instead of meat and dairy I use the plant-based alternatives. I don't cook too often. I meal prep in bulk and have meals prepped and ready to go in my fridge and freezer. That makes it so much easier to stay healthy because there are always healthy meals available when I get a craving.

WHAT IS YOUR GREATEST STRENGTH? WHAT DRIVES YOU AND KEEPS YOU AT THE TOP OF YOUR GAME?

My greatest strength is my attitude. The first step to success is to understand that you have to be willing to put in the hard work and stop making excuses. Life is meant to be the way it is. Your life can't always be rainbows and unicorns. You have to work hard to get where you want to be and to feel that accomplishment and true satisfaction. Being driven and disciplined is the highest level of self-love. You have to give up instant rewards and guilty pleasures to achieve something truly great.

I feel like what keeps me going when I feel unmotivated and "blah" is the fact that my reason and "why" is so much bigger than me. I want people to look at me and ask me, "wow, how did you achieve that?" That is always an opportunity for me to teach and educate about my lifestyle and how to live a more compassionate, cruelty-free life while still crushing your goals.

HOW DO YOU HANDLE THE UPS AND DOWNS OF GOOD AND BAD DAYS? WHAT STRATEGIES DO YOU USE?

I'm pretty down to earth with a no BS attitude. There are no shortcuts in life and to achieve something you need to put in the hard work and effort. That is just how it is. So if there are bad times you just need to rise above that. Remember why you started, suck it up and keep going. Sometimes things get hard and I know how it feels, but that's when the autopilot takes over. A common thing amongst champions is that they just never quit. That's what I repeat in my head when things get hard. I remember the feeling of satisfaction when I achieve something I've worked so hard for. That's what keeps me going.

WHAT KIND OF REACTION DID YOU RECEIVE WHEN YOU ANNOUNCED THAT YOU WERE GOING VEGAN? WHAT DID YOUR COACH, FAMILY AND FRIENDS SAY? WHAT IMPACT HAS THIS HAD ON YOUR PERFORMANCE? RECOVERY?

I'm really lucky to have a very supportive, close circle of people. Their reaction has almost always been positive. I do, however, feel like people make fun of me a lot more, especially acquaintances. I believe it's because I have the courage to stand out. When they hear what I lift or that I'm a competitive bodybuilder, their attitude often changes.

Being vegan has had so many benefits on my gym performance. I definitely notice that I recover much better, I never get sick or injured, and I'm always able to train. Back when I used to eat meat, I could never imagine training for at least three hours after a meal because I needed to digest longer, and I felt discomfort with digestion. But with a vegan diet I am fueled, and it leaves me energized to push my workouts.

SINCE TRANSITIONING TO A VEGAN/PLANT-BASED DIET HAS YOUR PERFORMANCE LEVEL GONE UP? WHAT IS YOUR ADVICE TO OTHER ATHLETES OR WOMEN WHO MAY BE INTERESTED IN TRYING A PLANT-BASED DIET?

Absolutely. I think the biggest thing is the feeling I have overall. Digesting food is never an issue, and I never have to sit down for hours to digest. Food fuels my body and keeps me going rather than stopping my day.

I think the best advice I have for someone interested in a plant-based diet is to find a mentor. Find someone who has transitioned to a vegan lifestyle with good results and ask them all your questions. I didn't have anyone around me who was vegan, so I had to make all the mistakes myself. You can skip that phase by finding someone who is thriving with a vegan lifestyle and ask/hire them. They have made those mistakes for you and can tell you what actually works and how to compose a balanced, fit, plant-based diet.

YOUR FONDEST MEMORY OF YOUR CAREER IN THIS SPORT?

Definitely placing second in Bikini Open in the prestigious Arnold Classic stage! The federation is not tested for drugs, so placing second as a natural vegan athlete was an amazing experience. It really showed that you don't need meat or drugs to succeed in this sport. One day I want to win Olympia as a natural vegan athlete, which is the most valued bodybuilding competition in the world!

DO YOU NOW OR HAVE YOU HAD A MENTOR IN YOUR LIFE? IF SO, WHO WAS IT AND WHAT IMPACT HAVE THEY HAD ON YOU? ARE THEY STILL YOUR MENTOR TODAY?

I always have a mentor: my coach. I have changed my coach a few times in my bodybuilding career because a specific coach can be perfect for that place and time. But as I evolve as an athlete, it also means that my current coach might not be able to serve my needs anymore. I always have a coach and take advantage of it. I ask all the questions! You are the one who is the paying client, so you have all the right to ask all the questions.

ANY INSPIRING STORIES THAT HAVE HAPPENED TO YOU OR PEOPLE CLOSE TO YOU THAT HAVE NOT BEEN COVERED ABOVE. STORIES THAT CAN HELP OTHERS.

You and only you are in charge of the direction of your life. You can't control everything in life, but you have full control over how you react and what decisions you make.

I wasn't content with my life, so I decided to save as much money as humanly possible, sell everything I own and go and look for my place. I travelled around the world trying to find my place, and that's how I ended up where I'm now – living in Australia, competing in bodybuilding, and having my dream fitness coaching business called Pro Plant Physique and my own activewear line called Flex Active Apparel.

If I hadn't hit that wall a few years ago where I was working on a job that didn't fulfill me by building somebody else's dream, only to realise that this was not the life I wanted, I wouldn't be where I am now. You are always one decision away from a totally different life. Change is scary and hard, but if you want something enough you will make it happen, regardless of how scary it is. You are just as capable as anyone else, don't let anyone tell you anything else. All the greatest people in this world were crushed over and over again by other people, but they listened to the fire inside them and went for it! Only you know what's best for yourself. Listen to that voice and go conquer whatever it tells you!

ELLA MAGERS

CONNECT WITH ELLA:
INSTAGRAM: @SEXYFITVEGAN
FACEBOOK: ELLA MAGERS, SEXY FIT VEGAN
YOUTUBE: SEXY FIT VEGAN
sexyfitvegan.com

"During my young adulthood, I went through a dark period where I struggled with a poor body image rooted in a lack of love and acceptance for myself. I became obsessed with having a super lean, toned, strong body. When I looked in the mirror, I saw all my "faults." I saw fat that was barely there and I soon dropped to a dangerously low weight. I started measuring my portions and counting macros. I found myself falling into a cycle of restricting and binging that caused me to suffer greatly behind closed doors. Discovering my love of Thai Boxing was a catalyst for me to start doing the work necessary to find unconditional love and acceptance for myself. My journey also involved unlearning the fear of carbs and obsession with protein (plant protein of course) that, to this day, is ingrained in the fitness community's culture. My own struggles fueled my desire to combine my passion for vegan fitness with a career helping people become strong and healthy through exercise, nutrition and a positive mindset."

From an unhealthy relationship with food and her body to a journey of self-love and empowerment, Ella Magers uses her personal story of growth to inspire people all over the world through her brand, Sexy Fit Vegan®. Ella created the Plant-Empowered Coaching Program to help clients align their actions with their values and build a plant-strong body and mind for life.

WHAT IS ONE OF THE BEST OR MOST WORTHWHILE HEALTH-RELATED INVESTMENTS THAT YOU HAVE MADE?

The book, Breaking the Habit of Being Yourself, by Dr. Joe Dispenza. This is such a powerful read because Dr. Dispenza explains how to use your mind to become the person you want to be and create the life you want to lead. He backs his words with science (in the fields of Quantum Physics, Epi-Genetics and Neuroscience) and gives specific steps on how to make the transformation so that you can reach your true potential!

AT WHAT POINT IN YOUR LIFE DID YOU DECIDE TO CHANGE YOUR DIET? HOW HAS THAT DECISION IMPACTED YOUR LIFE? WHAT IS YOUR GO-TO FOOD TO FUEL YOUR BODY?

It all started when I was seven years old. I got in the car after school. My mom had picked me up to take me to gymnastics practice and asked how my day was. I told her we had learned about Daniel Boone that day (for those of you who don't know, Daniel Boone was one of our first American folk heroes who carried a shotgun around and wore a raccoon hat). I was confused. "Daniel Boone was supposed to be a hero, but he was not mom," I said. "He was a mean man. He killed and ate animals."

My mom was honest with me. She said, "well Ella, we are just fortunate nowadays. We get to go to the grocery store to buy our meat." It was at that moment that I connected the food on my plate with the animal that it was. I was horrified! I told my mom, "I'm not going to do that anymore." That was it - I never ate meat again!

I was extremely fortunate to have such loving parents. They let me be me and gave me the autonomy to explore my place in the world.

Not only did I stop eating meat, but it was also like I knew my purpose in life. I recently looked back on the writing I did in school, and every chance I got I would write about how it made no sense for us to eat animals. Why would we kill another living being when we can easily live without causing suffering? I simply couldn't understand how anyone could love their dog and then turn around and eat a pig. I saw all creatures on this earth as equal in their right to live, and I saw us as humans, the only animals who have the ability to consciously choose whether or not we eat other animals.

As far as my go-to foods for fueling my body, I am admittedly a chickpea-a-holic, and I devour avocado and pineapple like they're disappearing from the earth! I even eat chickpeas for breakfast, with avocado, parsley, hearts of palm and grape tomatoes.

When I am craving comfort food, I often make mac 'n cheese with Banza chickpea pasta and Follow Your Heart Smoked Gouda vegan cheese. My go-to snack is Mary's Seed Crackers with Miyoko's cream cheese and cucumber slices.

WHAT IS YOUR GREATEST STRENGTH? WHAT DRIVES YOU AND KEEPS YOU AT THE TOP OF YOUR GAME?

I am one of the most determined human beings you'll ever meet. It's all about empowerment and growth. We have the power to write our own stories about who we are and how we move through the world.

I've had experiences in my lifetime that, although I would never wish those

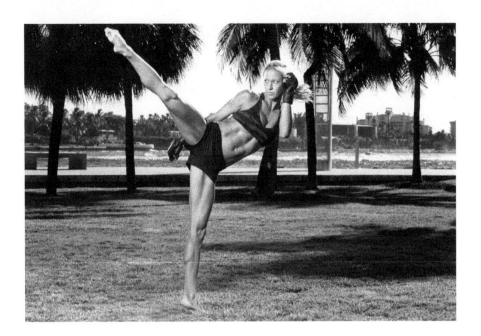

experiences on anyone else, I wouldn't take back (even the most painful parts). Every experience provided me with an opportunity to learn and grow. I look back and am able to see just how resilient I am!

I am driven mostly by my enduring commitment to my life's purpose of saving animals by empowering people to transition to a vegan lifestyle. Since I was a kid, I've always had the deep-rooted belief that we, as humans, have a responsibility to protect and care for animals, as opposed to exploiting them and causing suffering and death.

In part, I think my beliefs have never wavered because I always chose to believe that my voice mattered. For example, I led my first circus protest when I was 16-years-old. Fast forward over 20 years, and in 2017, the Ringling Brothers and Barnum and Bailey Circus have removed animals from their acts. Sure, it took two decades, but by believing that we could make a difference, countless animals will be saved a life of captivity and exploitation moving forward. That is something to celebrate!

HOW DO YOU HANDLE THE UPS AND DOWNS OF GOOD AND BAD DAYS? WHAT STRATEGIES DO YOU USE?

On those days where I feel "down," I remind myself that a full array of emotions, positive and negative, are a part of the human experience and that I want the full human experience! It's important to be able to sit with negative emotions, allowing them to be there without having to numb them or find a way to distract yourself from them. We need negative emotions in our lives! Without sadness we wouldn't know joy, and without fear we wouldn't have the opportunity to build courage. The place of discomfort that negative emotions put us in is the very place where growth happens!

WHAT KIND OF REACTION DID YOU RECEIVE WHEN YOU ANNOUNCED THAT YOU WERE GOING VEGAN? WHAT DID YOUR COACH, FAMILY AND FRIENDS SAY? WHAT IMPACT HAS THIS HAD ON YOUR PERFORMANCE? RECOVERY?

When I decided to stop eating animals at the age of seven, most people thought it would be a "phase." As I started to do my own research and discover the truth about what goes on behind the closed doors of factory farms, however, my deep-rooted compassion for animals quickly became my passion. It was no surprise when, at 15, I went totally vegan.

I started gymnastics and joined the swim team at five-years-old and remained active in sports throughout my entire childhood. I was full of energy and remember doing more pull-ups during our fitness test in fifth grade than any of the boys. My high performance seemed to keep people from questioning my dietary choices!

In my young adulthood, I was constantly being asked how I achieved my strong, lean physique. This gave me constant opportunities to share my lifestyle choices and educate people on the benefits of veganism. I broke the stereotypes most people had back then about vegans being scrawny and unhealthy. It was so gratifying being able to share my way of life with people who, because of my strength and athletic performance were open to learning.

SINCE TRANSITIONING TO A VEGAN/PLANT-BASED DIET HAS YOUR PERFORMANCE LEVEL GONE UP? WHAT IS YOUR ADVICE TO OTHER ATHLETES OR WOMEN WHO MAY BE INTERESTED IN TRYING A PLANT-BASED DIET?

Go for it! Start by simply increasing the amount of whole, plant foods on your plate so your gut bacteria can start adjusting. Eat as wide a variety of vegetables (the more dark greens, the better), legumes, nuts, seeds, fruits, and whole grains as possible. Experiment and explore. Have fun with it instead of seeing change as a source of stress.

Remember that what works best for one person, doesn't mean it will work best for you. For example, some athletes thrive on a diet high in complex carbs and low in plant-protein and fats (many endurance athletes eat this way). Other people feel their best and get the most energy from a diet containing lots of high-protein plant foods like edamame, tofu, tempeh, and other legumes and less whole grains. Find what works best for you by getting extremely in tune with your body and what it's telling you.

DO YOU NOW OR HAVE YOU HAD A MENTOR IN YOUR LIFE? IF SO, WHO WAS IT AND WHAT IMPACT HAVE THEY HAD ON YOU? ARE THEY STILL YOUR MENTOR TODAY?

Although I admire and have learned from countless people throughout my lifetime, I continue to give credit and gratitude to my parents for my continuous growth, development and success. From day one, they gave me the unconditional love and support I needed. They gave me space and freedom to be me! When I was just a kid leading protests and sitting in cages on sidewalks to demonstrate the horrific conditions on factory farms, they had my back. In fact, one-by-one, my family became vegan as well! When my Dad's cholesterol became a problem, he went from vegetarian to vegan and quickly regained healthy numbers. My mom made the full transition during her battle with cancer, which she won. My sister now has two beautiful, healthy vegan girls. When I met my life partner, he opened his mind and heart and went vegan too! I am beaming with love and gratitude.

ANY INSPIRING STORIES THAT HAVE HAPPENED TO YOU OR PEOPLE CLOSE TO YOU THAT HAVE NOT BEEN COVERED ABOVE. STORIES THAT CAN HELP OTHERS.

For most of my adult life, I put A LOT of pressure on myself to be a shining example of a fit, healthy (physically and emotionally) vegan. It's been my lifelong mission to bring veganism into the mainstream, and up until recently the misinformation about plant-based nutrition, and the stereotypes about vegans in general were so intense, I purposefully made it my job to focus on only positives.

I felt I needed to hide my imperfections in order to inspire people to open their minds about veganism. This self-imposed drive for perfection, however, led to a decade of body dysmorphia and disordered eating. I would restrict my food intake, count calories, track macronutrients and walk around hungry 95% of the time. The other 5% I was binging in secret and hiding in shame. At one point in my twenties, I played the, "how lean can I get" game, in a subconscious attempt to feel in control of my life. I am strong and lean at 120ish pounds, so can you imagine what I was like at 99 pounds? Looking back at photos is quite terrifying.

It was a long, agonizing journey for me to come to terms with and work through, my disordered eating and body image issues. It wasn't until 2016, many years after I had built a name for myself with my brand, Sexy Fit Vegan®, I made it my mission to change my story of being unworthy and not good enough and to heal myself.

I self-coached my way to self-love. The last piece involved ridding myself of the shame by getting vulnerable and sharing my story with the world, which I did in 2017, starting with a series of blog posts, called "My Journey from Disordered Eating to Plant-Empowered Living." Out of sharing came a sense of empowerment like I'd never experienced before. I finally felt free in my authenticity!

Don't get me wrong. The negative self-talk didn't just disappear all of a sudden. It's a process. A part of my journey that will take years and years to master, if ever. I still observe the self-destructive thoughts creeping in about my body and myself.

The difference is that I no longer let my feelings take my power away. I am no longer a victim or my own worst enemy. I started approaching myself with curiosity and compassion. I became confident in observing the defeating thoughts when they came up while introducing thoughts that align with my new story of worthiness and self-love and acting on THOSE healthy thoughts instead.

From there, I created and launched my online Plant-Empowered Coaching Program. The program is based on true transformation through empowerment and self-love. It's built on the basis of aligning your actions with your values. It teaches people to approach themselves with curiosity and compassion and to accept and respect themselves and their bodies. It coaches people down the path toward not only a healthy and happy life, but also a free and meaningful life. The program coaches people to a place where they become the inspiration for others and make a positive impact in the world.

This has lead me to where I am today! Continuing to spread my message of veganism through empowerment, aligning actions with values and rewriting your story with self-love as the foundation.

TORI BARRY

CONNECT WITH TORI:
INSTAGRAM: @TORIBARRY_
YOUTUBE: TORI BARRY

After years of struggling with an eating disorder and an unhealthy relationship with food, Tori Barry found two things that became her saving grace: cycling and plant-based eating. One informed the other, and slowly, she began to heal her body and mind through plant foods and the sport of cycling. Now a sponsored racing cyclist, model and popular YouTube vlogger, Tori uses her platforms to inspire her audiences through her story and living by example.

WHAT IS ONE OF THE BEST OR MOST WORTHWHILE HEALTH-RELATED INVESTMENTS THAT YOU HAVE MADE?

To be honest, I don't spend much money. Most of my money goes on food. Some of the best investments have been free!

If I had to choose, however, I would probably say that the best health-related investment I've made would be constantly having a good pantry and fridge. My fridge and pantry will always be filled with healthy, nourishing food.

As an athlete, you always have to think about what you are putting in your body. You have to think about if it is going to help with your training recovery or make you feel icky.

I am a big believer in balance as well! We all love our vegan donuts, pizza, etc. It's what you do the majority of the time that matters!

HOW IMPORTANT IS NUTRITION FOR A TOP LEVEL ATHLETE? AT WHAT POINT DID YOU DECIDE THAT A PLANT-BASED DIET IS THE BEST DIET FOR YOU?

Nutrition plays a huge role as an athlete. If eating a junk diet without getting enough carbohydrates, healthy fats, protein, sugar, etc, you can really suffer! Eating ENOUGH is also so important. I learned to listen to my body when I started cycling! If you don't eat enough, your energy will drop. It's as simple as that. It is impossible to be at the top of your game when your diet is poor. This is something I know from experience.

293

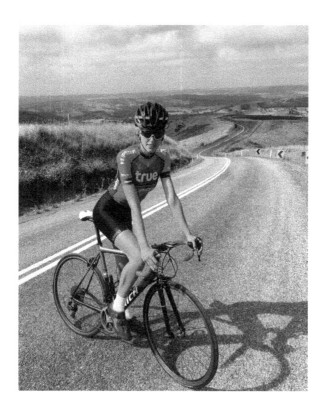

I used to compete at a national level for soccer and rowing when I was in school. Unfortunately, I became unwell with anorexia and I was simply too weak. I lost the love, the passion - everything. I couldn't keep up and I was dropped.

Eating enough is crucial, and it's all about eating the right foods! This is why I eat a high-carb vegan diet. On the bike, sugar is my best friend! It is so quick to digest and contains good calories. Same with carbohydrates as well.

In my diet, I focus on carbs the most! I burn a lot while cycling and can easily burn 2,000 calories in a ride. This is why it is so important to eat enough to replenish your body and to eat the right kind of foods.

I went vegan around the end of 2014, and at this point, I was still in the depths of my eating disorder. When I finally chose to recover, I started cycling (around the end of 2016) and learned that if I want to improve, I've got to eat.

I am such a competitive person and always want to improve. I found that eating all this food and nourishing my body made me strong and fit again. My fitness level has never been higher, and without a proper diet, I'd still be stuck in the depths of my eating disorder and unhappy. I've learned that nutrition is so important.

DO YOU TAKE ANY SPECIFIC SUPPLEMENTS? DO YOU RECOMMEND ANY SPECIFIC BRANDS? WHY DO YOU THINK THESE HAVE BENEFITED YOU AND YOUR HEALTH?

The only supplement I take is B12 and iron, and I only take them when I remember to! As a vegan, B12 is the only thing that is extremely difficult to get in plant-based food. It is important to make sure you are getting it in a supplement.

WHAT IS YOUR GREATEST STRENGTH? WHAT DRIVES YOU AND KEEPS YOU AT THE TOP OF YOUR GAME?

I think my greatest strength would be passion!!! I am so passionate about my cycling, and I only want to improve. When you are passionate, you will want to do that thing. You have the drive and it isn't a chore. Cycling, for me is a love. When you love the sport, you will always get better.

What keeps me at the top of my game is setting goals and keeping it fun!

HOW DO YOU HANDLE THE UPS AND DOWNS OF GOOD AND BAD DAYS? WHAT STRATEGIES DO YOU USE?

We are all living this thing called life, and we are always going to have amazing days as well as not so amazing days. In the end, we are only human. It can't always be perfect, and if you have a bad day you know it can only get better.

I don't like to focus too much on negative things, and I try to turn the bad into good. I think that when focusing more on positives, life will be much brighter.

Some days I realise that on the bike, I can't push as hard as the previous day and that is ok. My body is probably tired and needs rest. Instead of beating myself up, I look on ways to change it and improve!

WHAT KIND OF TIME COMMITMENT DOES YOUR TRAINING AND TRAVELING SCHEDULE DEMAND? HOW DO YOU BALANCE THAT WITH FAMILY, FRIENDS, AND EATING HEALTHILY?

For me, I am so lucky. My bike is pretty much my life and part of my career. Working online allows me a lot of time to ride every single day. Usually I ride in the morning and have the rest of the day to work, see friends and family and rest.

I take my training seriously and always have a spot for it in the morning. It's just like a routine! On average, I cycle about 14 hours per week, so it's not too much time! I usually go early in the morning. The most important thing when I'm done though, is making sure I have some recovery time

295

and have enough healthy foods.

I also am lucky enough to have a lot of friends to train with! That's a fun bonus.

WHAT KIND OF REACTION DID YOU RECEIVE WHEN YOU ANNOUNCED THAT YOU WERE GOING VEGAN? WHAT DID YOUR COACH, FAMILY AND FRIENDS SAY? WHAT IMPACT HAS THIS HAD ON YOUR PERFORMANCE? RECOVERY?

Truthfully, when I first went vegan, it was because it was a way to eliminate more food out of my diet because I was still struggling with my eating disorder. However, over time, ethics became a big role in my choice to stay vegan and because of how good I felt. I felt so good, and there was just no excuse to not be vegan!

My Mum just wanted me to be healthy again. She supported me and was the best Mum! She is so loving and supportive of me always! She also is the best vegan chef I've experienced.

My friends also support me. If they are your true friends, they will support you through anything, even though some of them aren't vegan!

SINCE TRANSITIONING TO A VEGAN/PLANT-BASED DIET HAS YOUR PERFORMANCE LEVEL GONE UP? WHAT IS YOUR ADVICE TO OTHER ATHLETES OR WOMEN WHO MAY BE INTERESTED IN TRYING A PLANT-BASED DIET?

100% yes. Going vegan isn't a diet for me, it's a lifestyle; I have become so passionate about it and have researched a lot because I want to feel my best and perform my best. At this point, I have read many articles about veganism, watched many documentaries and learnt so much!

My biggest tip to people who want to try out the vegan diet is to make sure you eat enough! Plant-based vegan foods digest so quickly and are naturally lower in calories. It may seem like you are eating a lot, but when looking at the calories, you need more than you think.

When people get hungry they crave what they are used to eating, so you might find yourself craving meat, dairy, etc. Don't bash yourself up and feel guilty. It is normal. It just means you haven't had enough nutrients.

Making sure you have enough carbs, fats, and protein is important.

WHEN YOU SET A GOAL HOW DO YOU STICK TO IT?

I like to set goals that are realistic and that I can achieve quickly. I think that when I set year-long goals, I lose motivation because they seem so unreachable. Having short-term goals and ticking them off regularly makes me so happy and motivated! It makes me want to go even harder and make even more goals!! Small and consistent successes keep me motivated and passionate to succeed!

YOUR FONDEST MEMORY OF YOUR CAREER IN THIS SPORT?

One of the most memorable rides I have done was Doi Inthanon. It was 223 kilometers and over 5,000 meters of elevation. I cried, I laughed, I cried again, I bonked, I was so angry and I was so happy. I felt EVERY emotion possible. It was one of the toughest things I've ever done!!!!

At the time I did this ride, I had only been riding for six months, and was still so new to the sport. This ride made me push my body so hard, but I loved it.

Setting challenges and doing them gives you such good memories. This was such an adventure for me.

I love that you can cycle alone and that you can do it socially. You can see the most amazing things. It makes me feel so calm and at peace, which for many years I didn't feel.

I never thought I'd be a cyclist and wearing lycra. I thought it was a Dad sport, haha! But I learned that until you try something in life, you don't know what you are missing out on.

297

DO YOU NOW OR HAVE YOU HAD A MENTOR IN YOUR LIFE? IF SO, WHO WAS IT AND WHAT IMPACT HAVE THEY HAD ON YOU? ARE THEY STILL YOUR MENTOR TODAY?

I look up to so many people and I am inspired by so many people around me. I love learning from people. I have many mentors in my life because I look up to many people. I always want to hear their stories and learn from their life experiences.

Riding with strong riders inspires me a lot as well.

I also have a coach (Paul) who has raced against Chris Froome and is super strong on the bike. He is very motivating to watch and is helping me reach my potential.

ANY INSPIRING STORIES THAT HAVE HAPPENED TO YOU OR PEOPLE CLOSE TO YOU THAT HAVE NOT BEEN COVERED ABOVE. STORIES THAT CAN HELP OTHERS.

Cycling is my greatest hobby right now! It is what gave me happiness again. It got me over my eating disorder. I love it!

When I was younger, I trained at very high levels for soccer and rowing.

I was training at a national level. The girls I rowed with and against went to the Olympics. I had to stop both sports. I got dropped. I lost all power and all motivation. When I had my eating disorder, I lost my greatest passions in life. Sports have always been my happy place. I love pushing barriers and taking it to the extreme! Seeing progress makes me thrive. When I lost it all I literally lost my life.

For a few years of my life I stopped all sports. I was living with no purpose. I was having weekly appointments, weigh-ins and monitored eating. It was not living. For those years, I missed sports so much. I wanted to do it again. I loved the feeling of success, however, I was scared. I had no energy to do anything. I had sky-high anxiety. At this point in my life, I never wanted to leave my bed. I was crying and screaming every day. I was not myself. I was scared of life.

My Dad was one of my biggest role models. He cycled. He had so much stamina and power. He rode over 200 km multiple times. I had no idea how he did it. But he did and loved it.

When I was getting over my eating disorder and recovering, I wanted to start a new sport. I wanted to cycle. I had many friends to help me along the way. I remember my first ride up Norton Summit. I was so nervous beforehand. I think it took me twenty-seven minutes. My friends Dolan and Shannon helped motivate me so much. I loved it. I felt alive and that was such a great feeling to feel again, I was hooked.

Cycling made me forget those stupid things going on in my head. I felt free! It also made me realise that we need to nourish ourselves if we want to succeed. Nourishment is important for anything in life. Without food, we die. Food is a celebration. Plus, it's delicious!

Cycling made me love food again. And cycling made me love life again.

When I started cycling, it ramped up my hunger and my metabolism. I got healthy again. I found love and passion for life again. I always ride my bike with passion. It isn't a chore - it isn't exercising to me. It's love.

CASSIE WARBECK

"Fighting is many different things for me, one of which is portraying what it can mean to be a plant-based athlete. I want to prove to the world that you can be strong and fierce and compassionate all at the same time. As every fighter knows, win or lose, stepping into the ring is a victory in itself. I like to think that it's also a victory for the vegan movement: the health of society, our planet and the animals."

Cassie Warbeck is a black belt in Goju Ryu karate, holds the WKA (World Kickboxing Association) North American Bantamweight Muay Thai Title, and will be fighting for the WKA World Flyweight Title this fall. She fuels her competitive and athletic spirit with a plant-based diet.

WHAT IS ONE OF THE BEST OR MOST WORTHWHILE HEALTH-RELATED INVESTMENTS THAT YOU HAVE MADE?

My Instant Pot. It's been life-changing. I love cooking my beans from dried (they are cheaper, and it avoids BPA-lined cans), and now I can do this in half an hour without having to plan ahead and soak them overnight.

A close second would be my sleep mask. Quality sleep is so essential; ensuring that I block out all outside light is key for me. Right now I'm using the YUNS Mulberry Silk Sleep Mask (found on Amazon for $12).

AT WHAT POINT IN YOUR LIFE DID YOU DECIDE TO CHANGE YOUR DIET? HOW HAS THAT DECISION IMPACTED YOUR LIFE?

I transitioned to a whole-food, plant-based diet in the Fall of 2013 after reading The China Study by T. Colin Campbell. It was a pretty gradual transition for me, until one day I realized I was completely vegan! It felt so natural and was fuelled by my desire to figure out how I could eat in the best way for my health. I need to mention the incredible organization, NutritionFacts.org, here as well. I spent countless hours watching the videos on this site, and the more I discovered, the more I knew I could never return to my old dietary habits.

My go-to food is fruit! Bananas are just so easy, and I eat several a day, especially during intense training weeks. Other staples include matcha tea, oatmeal, pumpkin seeds, sweet potatoes and all kinds of beans!

WHAT IS YOUR GREATEST STRENGTH? WHAT DRIVES YOU AND KEEPS YOU AT THE TOP OF YOUR GAME?

My greatest strength is that I never back down from a challenge! I want to live without regrets. I never want to look back and wish that I had taken advantage of a given opportunity. I try to always keep improving myself and reaching for my highest potential; it doesn't matter if it's in martial arts or my education. I never want to feel complacent with where I am at in my life.

HOW DO YOU HANDLE THE UPS AND DOWNS OF GOOD AND BAD DAYS? WHAT STRATEGIES DO YOU USE?

I'll be the first to admit that I'm not an expert at this. Sometimes I just can't keep the tears in (especially during a fight camp), but I try to remember that whatever emotion I happen to be feeling at the moment will pass. It's only a temporary state. When I'm extremely stressed/anxious, going for a walk outside in the sun usually helps put things into perspective. I also attribute my morning meditation practice to helping me be less reactive to upsetting situations throughout the day.

300

WHAT KIND OF REACTION DID YOU RECEIVE WHEN YOU ANNOUNCED THAT YOU WERE GOING VEGAN? WHAT DID YOUR COACH, FAMILY AND FRIENDS SAY? WHAT IMPACT HAS THIS HAD ON YOUR PERFORMANCE? RECOVERY?

I didn't really announce this at all! I was vegan before I even started training with my Coach (Paul Sukys), so that wasn't an issue. My teammates have never questioned my eating since it's apparent that this is working for me (although I do have to put up with a lot of vegan jokes!). I really try not to push my dietary choices on others and instead strive to set a positive example. I want my health and performance to speak for itself, although I welcome questions when they do come.

My fitness continues to improve, and I feel like my recovery has never been better. This diet also helps me maintain a consistent weight, even when I'm not training for an upcoming fight. I usually don't count calories, I just eat whole, plant foods. When I do need to drop weight, I simply decrease portion sizes and snacks. I've never had a difficult weight cut.

SINCE TRANSITIONING TO A VEGAN/PLANT-BASED DIET HAS YOUR PERFORMANCE LEVEL GONE UP? WHAT IS YOUR ADVICE TO OTHER ATHLETES OR WOMEN WHO MAY BE INTERESTED IN TRYING A PLANT-BASED DIET?

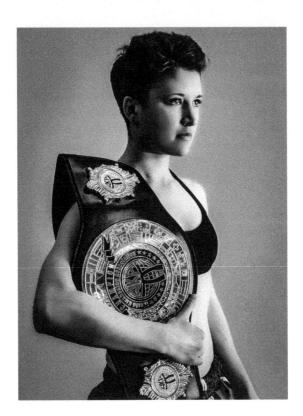

I've been vegan my entire amateur career, so I can't really say that it has improved my performance, but it definitely hasn't hindered it! My advice to other women is to just start!

A plant-based diet isn't nearly as complicated as some people make it out to be. Eat more plants; it's pretty simple. It's okay to transition gradually and ensure that you're getting enough calories, especially if you are an athlete, because the energy density of plants is usually less than animal products. Even though you might be physically full, you may find yourself eventually running a caloric deficit.

YOUR FONDEST MEMORY OF YOUR CAREER IN THIS SPORT?

My recent WKA North American Bantamweight Title win is one of my fondest memories. What made this so special was the amount of love and support I felt from all my teammates, friends and family leading up to the fight. My coach, Paul Sukys, secretly designed t-shirts with my nickname for everyone to wear to the venue. I didn't have a clue until literally an hour before! Muay Thai may seem like an individual sport, but I know without a doubt that I wouldn't be where I am without all the incredible people I'm surrounded by.

DO YOU NOW OR HAVE YOU HAD A MENTOR IN YOUR LIFE? IF SO, WHO WAS IT AND WHAT IMPACT HAVE THEY HAD ON YOU? ARE THEY STILL YOUR MENTOR TODAY?

My Sensei, Tammy Thankachen, first inspired my love for martial arts. I obtained my black belt in Goju Ryu karate under her excellent mentorship, and she instilled a sense of belief in me and what I am capable of achieving. Her authenticity, compassion and generosity are virtues I strive to practice every day. She is a testament to feminine strength and continues to be one of my strongest supporters.

ANY INSPIRING STORIES THAT HAVE HAPPENED TO YOU OR PEOPLE CLOSE TO YOU THAT HAVE NOT BEEN COVERED ABOVE. STORIES THAT CAN HELP OTHERS.

When I first stepped into the ring I was terrified. Not surprisingly, I lost that fight, and since then I've had a love-hate relationship with competition. I like to joke that I've "retired" multiple times, but something inside keeps bringing me back to the challenge that fighting offers. I still struggle with anxiety, but over the years it has improved immensely. I'm so grateful that I continued with this sport and for the opportunities and relationships it has given me. My point is, even though you might fear something, that doesn't mean this opportunity/goal/dream is not worth pursuing.

"

I HAVE NEVER HAD
A RUNNING-RELATED
INJURY IN MY TWO
DECADES OF MARATHON
RUNNING - HITTING
AROUND 150 KILOMETERS
A WEEK WHEN TRAINING
FOR AN EVENT - AND
MY RECOVERY IS QUITE
ASTONISHING, EVEN AS
I GET OLDER.

FIONA OAKES

SHANEVE SWIFT

CONNECT WITH SHANEVE:
INSTAGRAM: @SWIFTANDFIT
FACEBOOK: SWIFTANDFIT
swiftandfit.com

Shaneve Swift is a vegan bodybuilder, former NCAA Division 1 track and field athlete, online fitness coach, NFF Bikini Pro and plant-based eating advocate. She has combined a passion for nutrition and the power of weight training to form a unique online fitness course that educates students on the powerful connection between mind and body.

WHAT IS ONE OF THE BEST OR MOST WORTHWHILE HEALTH-RELATED INVESTMENTS THAT YOU HAVE MADE?

It would be hiring a nutrition and fitness coach.

AT WHAT POINT IN YOUR LIFE DID YOU DECIDE TO CHANGE YOUR DIET? HOW HAS THAT DECISION IMPACTED YOUR LIFE? WHAT IS YOUR GO-TO FOOD TO FUEL YOUR BODY?

It was when I first watched some documentaries about environmental effects, health effects and animal cruelty that comes from animal agriculture. It was after watching these as well as reading some books and studies that I knew I had to make the change to a vegan lifestyle. My go-to food to fuel my body would definitely be lots of green leafy vegetables such as spinach, kale and lettuce.

WHAT IS YOUR GREATEST STRENGTH? WHAT DRIVES YOU AND KEEPS YOU AT THE TOP OF YOUR GAME?

My greatest strength would be my discipline to continue to push forward towards a goal and stick with a plan of action. Focusing on the end goal keeps me motivated, and truly taking care of my mental and physical state keeps me at the top of my game.

HOW DO YOU HANDLE THE UPS AND DOWNS OF GOOD AND BAD DAYS? WHAT STRATEGIES DO YOU USE?

I sometimes give myself some time to relax, whether it be something as simple as taking a nice hot bath, taking a walk outside, heading to the mall, reading a good book, or listening to something motivational to get me out of a bad state.

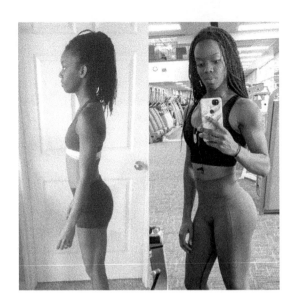

WHAT KIND OF REACTION DID YOU RECEIVE WHEN YOU ANNOUNCED THAT YOU WERE GOING VEGAN? WHAT DID YOUR COACH, FAMILY AND FRIENDS SAY? WHAT IMPACT HAS THIS HAD ON YOUR PERFORMANCE? RECOVERY?

My parents and friends thought I was crazy. My parents were definitely concerned about my health, but in time, I convinced them otherwise. It completely improved my performance overall.

I not only wanted to prove myself wrong, but I wanted to be an example for others who have their uncertainties about the vegan lifestyle. Even as a former NCAA Division 1 track and field athlete, I have more stamina, strength and energy now as a vegan bodybuilder.

SINCE TRANSITIONING TO A VEGAN/PLANT-BASED DIET HAS YOUR PERFORMANCE LEVEL GONE UP? WHAT IS YOUR ADVICE TO OTHER ATHLETES OR WOMEN WHO MAY BE INTERESTED IN TRYING A PLANT-BASED DIET?

Absolutely! I would let them know that it is best to find someone who has already done what they want to accomplish. By getting a coach all the guesswork is gone, and having a tailored nutrition plan is essential for an athlete.

YOUR FONDEST MEMORY OF YOUR CAREER IN THIS SPORT?

My fondest memory would be at my last bikini competition when I was crowned the winner in my bikini class and became a natural pro athlete.

It was an incredible experience, and I loved being able to represent the vegan community and be an example to others about what is possible.

DO YOU NOW OR HAVE YOU HAD A MENTOR IN YOUR LIFE? IF SO, WHO WAS IT AND WHAT IMPACT HAVE THEY HAD ON YOU? ARE THEY STILL YOUR MENTOR TODAY?

Yes. I would say my nutrition and fitness coach has been a huge mentor of mine: Korin Sutton. He has an incredible drive to help others, and he himself has a positive attitude. He believed in me even when I doubted myself. Having a mentor like him helps keep me striving to become the best version of myself.

ANY INSPIRING STORIES THAT HAVE HAPPENED TO YOU OR PEOPLE CLOSE TO YOU THAT HAVE NOT BEEN COVERED ABOVE. STORIES THAT CAN HELP OTHERS.

The biggest awakening I had for switching to a plant-based diet was my Dad. A few summers ago, he landed in the hospital because of a diabetic coma. He was completely delusional and had no idea where he was and was barely functioning properly.

During his stay in the hospital, while they were trying to bring down his blood sugar levels, I noticed the food that they were feeding him. It was generic, some high carb processed foods and some with dairy products. I was in shock about what they were feeding him and wondering who decided what he should be eating. It truly was a wake-up call not only for me to focus on making sure I never end up in that situation but to also help and inform others about the importance of taking control of one's health.

His past definitely brought him to that point because he didn't put his health first. Fortunately, he was able to come home after his blood sugar levels went down, but that was when I informed my parents they have to make a change in their diet.

After practicing a plant-based diet he got off of the diabetes drug Metformin after a few months. My mom used to have issues with her menopause, and those issues were gone as well.

Living the vegan and plant-based lifestyle is truly amazing, and I love to continue hearing the countless stories of people turning their lives around while eating this way.

FIONA OAKES

CONNECT WITH FIONA:
INSTAGRAM: @OAKES.FIONA
FACEBOOK: FIONA OAKES
fionaoakesfoundation.co.uk

Fiona Oakes lays claim to four Marathon World Records including a Guinness World Record for being the fastest woman to run a marathon on all seven continents (including the North Pole), with a personal best of 2 hours and 38 minutes. She is a patron of the Captive Animal Protection Society as well as an honorary patron of the Vegan Society. Currently, she runs the Tower Hill Stables Animal Sanctuary, a non-profit organization where she provides a home to over 400 rescued animals that have histories of abuse and exploitation.

WHAT IS ONE OF THE BEST OR MOST WORTHWHILE HEALTH-RELATED INVESTMENTS THAT YOU HAVE MADE?

My Raidlight Olmo 20 litre backpacks - not exactly health-related but probably one of the most important factors in staying healthy in an extreme running situation. I have used them in every stage race I have entered and never come away with any "pack related" problems, such as sores or muscular related injuries. Believe me, when you are cramming all your life's supplies for a whole week into a tiny pack and then attempting to run 250 kilometers across the toughest desert terrain in temperatures which can often exceed 50 degrees Celsius, you need to be as "comfortable" as you feasibly can be with the pack you are carrying. The only difficulty now is that they have stopped making them, so I am searching for a replacement!

AT WHAT POINT IN YOUR LIFE DID YOU DECIDE TO CHANGE YOUR DIET? HOW HAS THAT DECISION IMPACTED YOUR LIFE? WHAT IS YOUR GO-TO FOOD TO FUEL YOUR BODY?

I went vegan at age six. It was a totally self-inspired action born out of a simple love for animals. I always veer away from saying it was a "decision" because at that age, I think I was too young to make one. I wasn't familiar with the term vegan, just the principles. It was a reaction against the abhorrent cruelty and exploitation of animals. If you love something, you do not harm it or stand by and watch others cause harm on your behalf or for your supposed benefit.

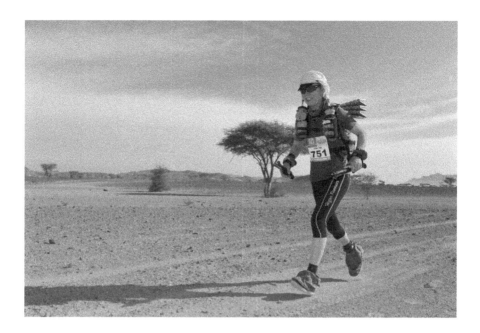

As for my go-to food, any food is a good food to me, so long as it is vegan! I do love anything made with potatoes though, and I think the potato is a vastly under-rated and versatile product which is so economical to use and so effective in filling, nourishing and fueling the body.

WHAT IS YOUR GREATEST STRENGTH? WHAT DRIVES YOU AND KEEPS YOU AT THE TOP OF YOUR GAME?

My mental capacity to endure pain and to self-motivate. I am extremely determined, dedicated and disciplined. I know my strengths and weaknesses and have learned to accept both and make one work for the other. The drive I have to remain at the top and to achieve and break new ground is the actual reason I am out there. It's all to benefit animals, too.

HOW DO YOU HANDLE THE UPS AND DOWNS OF GOOD AND BAD DAYS? WHAT STRATEGIES DO YOU USE?

When I am having a good day with training, it's great. It really lifts me and enforces my belief that anything is possible. The motivation to achieve more and do more is incredible, but the self-belief it generates is all-consuming.

Though the bad days are extremely tough to endure, I have learned to embrace them. I know that during races, I am going to be taken to some extremely difficult places, both mentally and physically. If life is a "bed of roses" in training and I never go to the edge of my ability, I won't be able to get there in races. I have learned that training isn't just about physical statistics and readouts; it's about something much more personal and unique to yourself. It's about how to cope with suffering, how to find a way to win, and this has to be done in training. So, although not enjoyable, I know the bad days are equally, if not more important than the good ones.

WHAT KIND OF REACTION DID YOU RECEIVE WHEN YOU ANNOUNCED THAT YOU WERE GOING VEGAN? WHAT DID YOUR COACH, FAMILY AND FRIENDS SAY? WHAT IMPACT HAS THIS HAD ON YOUR PERFORMANCE? RECOVERY?

I have been vegan so long that there has never really been a "before and after" or an announcement. Vegan is what I have always been. I have, however, noticed a lot of resistance to and suspicion of veganism among sports professionals. I do think that it is changing and that is due to the massive growth in awareness of veganism and what it means among all sections of society.

I have never had a running-related injury in my two decades of marathon running - hitting around 150 kilometers a week when training for an event - and my recovery is quite astonishing, even as I get older. I am still able to train twice a day easily (sometimes three times) and be recovered and ready to do it all again the next day.

The biggest impact I can say my veganism has had on my training is my mental wellbeing. It's something very often overlooked by sportspeople who tend to focus purely on physical results. I know that when I line up on the start line, no one else has suffered for my performance, and this is critically important to me and the very reason I am out there in the first place. I believe my results speak for themselves and are a testament to my lifestyle choices.

SINCE TRANSITIONING TO A VEGAN/PLANT-BASED DIET HAS YOUR PERFORMANCE LEVEL GONE UP? WHAT IS YOUR ADVICE TO OTHER ATHLETES OR WOMEN WHO MAY BE INTERESTED IN TRYING A PLANT-BASED DIET?

I honestly believe I have "punched way above my weight" when it comes to my running. I have a personal best of 2:38 in the marathon, and I've done it with a very severe and detrimental injury. I had my knee cap removed on my right leg when I was younger. I was told I would never walk properly again, let alone run. As a result of this, I can't run the bends of a track as my knee is just too unstable so I have to do all my speed work on a treadmill.

To be placing in the World's Major Marathons is something I never dreamed possible, and I attribute 100% of my success on my vegan diet in terms of physical ability, consistency, longevity, sustainability and recovery.

You are only as good on race day as the amount of training your body has allowed you to do in the run-up. I have always recovered well enough to endure very high and intense levels of training and this is what has enabled me to produce the results time after time, year in and year out.

From the mental side of things, my veganism has brought me strength, determination and purpose. Couple this with being able to do the miles in training and you have a winning combination.

My advice to other athletes (men or women) is to grab it and go for it and run with veganism all the way to the finish line - whatever and wherever that may be for you!

YOUR FONDEST MEMORY OF YOUR CAREER IN THIS SPORT?

My fondest memory is the lovely people I have met along the way that live across all the continents and corners of the earth. One in particular that stands out is when I was in running a marathon in Omsk - the biggest race in Russia - as part of my World Record attempt. All the school children were lining the streets excitedly and had drawn pictures of me and Percy Bear (my ever-present running "companion"), to cheer us along the route. It was lovely to see, very inspiring and motivating, a constant reminder that a smile translates in any and every language!

DO YOU NOW OR HAVE YOU HAD A MENTOR IN YOUR LIFE? IF SO, WHO WAS IT AND WHAT IMPACT HAVE THEY HAD ON YOU? ARE THEY STILL YOUR MENTOR TODAY?

When I started to ask my Mum questions as a very small child about where and why we ate animal products, it was very difficult for her because there was no information readily available (it was the 70s). It's easy for older people to forget a time before social media and younger ones don't have any memories of this life at all. We were lucky because even though I was brought up in a small town, my Mum knew a vegan lady. This was quite a phenomenon at the time because the word "vegetarian" was one which few were familiar with, so vegan was quite literally unheard of. My Mum was able to turn to her for advice and to articulate in adult terms what I was feeling and thinking as a child. Sadly, she is now passed, but her impact and influence live on!

ANY INSPIRING STORIES THAT HAVE HAPPENED TO YOU OR PEOPLE CLOSE TO YOU THAT HAVE NOT BEEN COVERED ABOVE. STORIES THAT CAN HELP OTHERS.

I have always been skeptical of doctors and hospitals after my involvement with them in my teenage years. At that time they likened my veganism to an eating disorder and my Mum's apparent acceptance of it as "child abuse." However, in order to run the multi-stage races that I now run, I have to get medical certificates and ECGs as part of the requirements of entry. This is to prove that you are medically fit to attempt them.

In 2012 (my first time in Marathon des Sables) I decided that my only option was to seek out the help of a private doctor to fill in the forms. This is when I met my now friend, Dr. Jossen. She acknowledged, embraced and accepted my "unusual" statistics (including a resting pulse of 36 bpm), but more than this, she was inspired and respectful of my vegan diet. This made going to her so much easier for me, especially because I couldn't bear the ridicule of something so important to me by a health professional who was supposed to be there for my well being.

A couple of years ago, Dr. Jossen wrote to me and told me she and her family had gone vegan due to seeing my performances and the obvious reasons behind them: my veganism. This was so inspiring to me. It was amazing to know that medical professionals who have such power to influence others are embracing and adopting veganism.

Then more recently, I was invited to speak at a conference organized by plant-based health professionals, a whole community of consultants, general practitioners, anesthetists and other health specialists who are actively engaged and committed to promoting veganism. To hear and be among such people speaking so positively and passionately about veganism was something I never even dreamed would, or could happen after the extremely negative experiences I had in the past with health professionals.

It is happening after so many years of ridicule and negativity. Veganism is being recognised by influencers in a medical capacity as the most viable way to a healthy future on an individual basis. By doing so, we are also advocating for an end to animal agriculture and abuse, a more positive and equal distribution of food and water resources for other humans, and a positive and prosperous future for all. As I said, veganism is a win-win situation and promoting it will continue to be my motivation for every new chapter in my life, however many there may be left to write.

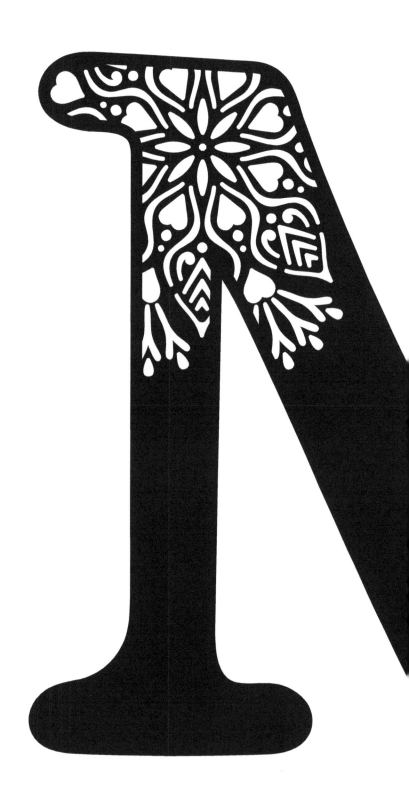

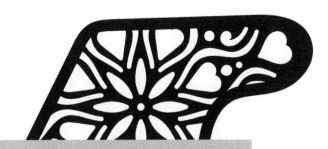

CHAPTER 6

MUMS

NIKKI BRAVATA

CONNECT WITH NIKKI:
FACEBOOK: NIKKI BRAVATA

"I went for an interview [at an alternative cancer treatment center], and I was given some documentary films to watch. That night, I watched them both. One was called Eating and the other was called Healing Cancer From the Inside Out. After watching these films, I got off my couch, dragged my garbage bin over to my freezer, and cleared out all of the frozen meat I had saved. Then, I opened the refrigerator and dumped out the whole milk that I was giving to Milana (she was 16 months old, and I had just stopped breastfeeding her). My husband looked at me in shock and said, 'what will you give the baby?' I said, 'I don't know, but NOT THIS!'"

After working at an alternative cancer treatment center for eight years as a nurse, Nikki Bravata began to understand the important link between diet and health. A plant-based advocate and Mum, Nikki endured questioning and concern from almost everybody in her life, but she persevered because the positive benefits from plant-based eating were too great to ignore.

WHAT IS ONE OF THE BEST OR MOST WORTHWHILE HEALTH-RELATED INVESTMENTS THAT YOU HAVE MADE?

By far, my Vitamix blender. I use it several times a day, whether it's for smoothies, salad dressings, soups, or raw pie filling - I get my money's worth from this investment. When my children were babies, I blended everything they ate and would freeze the leftover portions in ice cube trays or containers for future use.

AT WHAT POINT IN YOUR LIFE DID YOU DECIDE TO CHANGE YOUR DIET? HOW HAS THAT DECISION IMPACTED YOUR LIFE?

I NEVER thought that I would become a vegetarian, let alone vegan. I grew up in Michigan, where we consumed the standard American diet, of course. I always had intestinal issues, weight issues, acne, and I was constantly tired. I just thought this was normal.

I graduated from nursing school in 2003 and worked for five years in intensive care and moved to Arizona as a travel nurse. I finally became

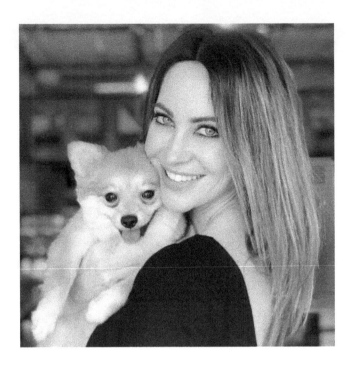

burnt out and quit my job halfway into my pregnancy in 2007. I just couldn't stay awake working nights. After I had Milana I wanted to go back to work, but not in the hospital. I felt that I wasn't helping people and questioned whether I should even be a nurse anymore. I looked and looked at jobs, and one kept popping up for an alternative cancer treatment center. At this time, my grandmother had just passed away from breast cancer, so I thought it might be too sad to work in this field. But the job kept coming up in my search, so I thought I'd see what it was all about.

I went for an interview and I was given some documentary films to watch. That night, I watched them both. One was called Eating and the other was called Healing Cancer From the Inside Out. After watching these films, I got off my couch, dragged my garbage bin over to my freezer, and cleared out all of the frozen meat I had saved. Then I opened the refrigerator and dumped out the whole milk that I was giving to Milana (she was 16 months old, and I had just stopped breastfeeding her). My husband looked at me in shock and said, "what will you give the baby?" I said, "I don't know, but NOT THIS! I'm going to bed; I'll figure it out tomorrow."

The next day, I drove to the book store and bought any book I could to find about vegan nutrition, and I dove in. I read and read and read. I interviewed every doctor, dietician and experienced vegan I could find. I wasn't just changing my lifestyle, I was changing the nutrition for my one-

" "

I ALSO WANTED TO MAKE IT EASY FOR
MY KIDS BY MAKING EVERYTHING IN
OUR HOUSE VEGAN SO THEY DIDN'T
EVEN HAVE TO THINK ABOUT IT. I NEVER
PUSHED OR INSISTED ON MY HUSBAND
CHANGING HIS DIET, BUT OF COURSE
SINCE I WAS COOKING DELICIOUS
VEGAN FOOD, HE WAS HAPPY TO EAT
IT, AND WHEN HIS ASTHMA SYMPTOMS
DISAPPEARED AND HE COULD SEE THE
DIFFERENCE IN THE HEALTH OF OUR KIDS
COMPARED TO OTHERS, HE COULD SEE
THAT THIS LIFESTYLE WAS POWERFUL.

NIKKI BRAVATA

year-old daughter too. Trust me when I say that in 2008, there were a lot of concerned people. I heard everything from, "where will you get your protein?" to people claiming "child abuse!!"

But despite this, I persevered. It took one year to completely get rid of all of the dairy and eggs in our diets. I realized that I was completely addicted to sugar, too. Strong cravings and desires for the things I was used to was a challenge at first. Giving up meat was not an issue - I never looked back - but the tastes I was use to with dairy, eggs and sugar was tough. I eventually learned how to make alternatives and I felt confident enough to tell all of the worried people that from now on, we would no longer take anything with any animal products.

The toughest part was dealing with the critics, but I didn't care. This was when the magic happened. All the stomach cramping, bloating, acne and fatigue disappeared. I felt ALIVE!

A few years later I had my second pregnancy - this time completely vegan- and what a difference. I didn't experience the weight gain, indigestion, constipation, or the acne I had experienced with my previous pregnancy. None of it. I delivered Gisella at home, in the water, naturally, and perfectly healthy. Even my breast milk was different. It was thick and not watery like when I was eating high animal protein (I was trying to eat only meat and vegetables to get rid of the 60 pounds I had gained). This time, I was eating a 90% raw diet.

Compared to when I had my first daughter, Gisella was thriving. She was healthy, slept well and didn't get ill. Milana, I am sorry to say, was a very uncomfortable baby who cried all the time, was underweight and got sick often. The good news is that with the change to a vegan lifestyle, I believe that Milana and I both detoxed from our previous lifestyle and over the course of a few years regained our health. Now, both myself and my children do not take sick days. We stay well and have vibrant health, even through stressful times, I attribute this to our vegan lifestyle.

WHAT WERE THE FIRST STEPS YOU TOOK IN MAKING YOUR NUTRITIONAL CHANGES AND WHY DID YOU START DOWN THIS PATH?

I stayed at my job in the cancer center for eight years. Every day I learned something from my patients and the experts I worked with. The first step was trusting my intuition. I knew that I could improve my health, but I had to be an active participant. I read and asked anyone I could for their advice. Once I started to see improvements in my health, it was the proof that I needed. I was not turning back because I had the armor I needed: knowledge.

As far as the husband thing - I was married for ten years to a man who was just happy to be fed! Although he never totally gave up meat (with an Italian mother who loved to feed her son, he would never say no to her chicken parmigiana or meatballs!) But at home he was respectful of our vegan kitchen.

I also wanted to make it easy for my kids by making everything in our house vegan, so they didn't even have to think about it. I never pushed or insisted on my husband changing his diet, but of course since I was cooking delicious vegan food, he was happy to eat it, and when his asthma symptoms disappeared, and he could see the difference in the health of our kids compared to others, he could see that this lifestyle was powerful.

DO YOU TAKE ANY SPECIFIC SUPPLEMENTS? DO YOU RECOMMEND ANY SPECIFIC BRANDS? WHY DO YOU THINK THESE HAVE BENEFITED YOU AND/OR YOUR CHILDREN'S HEALTH?

I give my kids vitamin D and B12 year-round. For vitamin D, I used the liquid drops when they were babies, and now I will give them 1000 milligrams once or twice a week. For B12, I always chose 500 -1000 micrograms of methylcobalamin a few times a week. At times that I felt that their immune systems were a little compromised, I gave them 1000 micrograms of vitamin C every three to four hours or so. Another immune booster I used in the U.S. is by a brand called Child's Life. They have a product called First Defense, which has helped to prevent sickness in the earlier years.

I certainly was never a germaphobe and felt it was important to be exposed to some germs. With a vegan lifestyle, my kids just never really got very sick. If they did get a little something, it would be a fever for one day with no other symptoms, and they would be fine the next day. When they had a fever, I would let them rest, stay hydrated, fast (if they didn't want to eat, I didn't push it, just keep hydrated) and sleep. There is no better medicine than sleep, and I am very serious about it. I ensure my kids get a minimum of ten hours of sleep each night. Same with myself. I try to get eight hours every night and be asleep by 10 pm.

WHAT HAS BEEN YOUR BIGGEST RESOURCE FOR COOKING RECIPES? WHO HAS BEEN YOUR BIGGEST INFLUENCER FOR YOUR VEGAN/ PLANT-BASED DIET CHANGE?

I was fortunate to have the guidance of a doctor that I worked for at the cancer center in Arizona named Dr. Thomas Lodi. He was my mentor and my inspiration, and I was lucky to have his support if I had concerns when my girls were little. Especially because many people in my life were convinced that a vegan lifestyle was wrong for a child. I am so glad that I listened to Dr. Lodi's advice and also that I had hundreds of patients who I saw first-hand survive cancer and find their best health.

During the time that I worked for Dr. Lodi, I learned so much from our talented raw chefs and nutrition educators about how to make raw food. This was the inspiration for my lifestyle. The closer that we eat to the way we find food in nature, the better. This means an emphasis on raw foods, vegetables, fruits, nuts, seeds, sprouts and fermented foods because they have the highest nutrient value. If consumed without heating, they can provide us with all the vitamins, minerals, enzymes and antioxidants for glowing, vibrant health. Of course, I do also consume cooked foods, but we have as much of our day around raw as possible.

WHAT ARE YOUR KIDS FAVORITE DISHES? CAN YOU SHARE A FAVORITE RECIPE?

My kids love Mexican food - beans, rice, guacamole, salsa. There is so much fiber and flavor in these foods and so many different ways to enjoy this combination. They also love smoothies and bowls - this is the secret weapon for moms!! We can hide so much nutrition in a smoothie, and the key is to let them get involved. My kids love to make their food and fresh juices. It's fun, and if they made it they wanted to eat it.

Kid-approved chocolate shake recipe:

1 cup alternative milk / 1 tbsp raw cacao powder / 1/2 avocado /
1 cup spinach / 1 frozen banana / chia seeds / water and ice

This can also be made as "nice cream," just freeze and thaw before serving.

IF YOU COULD GIVE A MUM WHO IS LOOKING AT CHANGING HER KIDS OVER TO A PLANT-BASED DIET THREE TIPS, WHAT WOULD THEY BE? DO YOU HAVE ANY STORIES RELATED TO YOUR KIDS NOT EATING MEAT AND DAIRY ANYMORE?

Don't wait! The sooner you can make the switch, the better. Kids are curious about food, and getting involved with making it is exciting and fun in the early ages. After kids are about three, they have their taste preferences pretty set.

Don't worry! I used to get so caught up about micronutrients and if they are getting enough. Considering that many parents feed their kids foods that are not so nourishing and nutrient-dense (burgers, mac and cheese, happy meals, etc.), they will get enough if you're feeding them fresh fruits, veggies, legumes and other plant proteins. If you do worry, get their levels tested. Educate and arm yourself with knowledge and find other supportive Mums who have had experience with it.

We do not need as much protein as people think either. Imagine that a baby triples its birth weight and height in the first year of life on mostly breast milk with about 1% calorie protein. This is a good indication that protein is not needed at such high levels in humans and also contributes to the formation of diseases like cancer.

Don't lie! Kids are pretty instinctual. They really don't want to eat animals, and we just condition them to do so. If we tell our kids that they are eating the dead body of a cow, I would bet they would become uninterested. But, if we are all eating a burger and Mum and Dad say it's ok, well then it's ok.

My kids didn't really resonate with the "it's not good for your health" thing when they were big enough to start to have more choice for themselves, particularly when they went to school. What they did understand was how this industry contributes to the pain and suffering of animals, and when we choose to eat these things, even if they taste good (cookies, ice cream, etc) we also support the industries that harm the animals to get the ingredients for that food. I even allowed my kids to see some of the parts of the movie documentary, Earthlings, which shows the awful torture and death of animals. This helped them to understand that they can be part of the solution.

Also getting sick on a cheese pizza (actually vomiting after eating it at a birthday party) helped! I reminded them that when we make these choices, and life is full of choices, we may have to deal with the consequences. The more you can avoid having the taste of these foods and offer healthier versions the more adverse your kids will be to those items. I occasionally have to remind my eight and eleven-year-old about this. The influence of peers and the conventional choices even in packaging and marketing messages, is strong. I've had to not only set the example, fight for support in schools, supply my kids with options, pre-plan vacations around food availability, explain myself until I am blue in the face and answer the protein question a million times, but it's all been worth it. Nothing tastes as good as healthy feels. I am beyond grateful for my choice.

WHAT HAS BEEN YOUR DOCTOR'S RESPONSE (OR NON VEGAN FAMILY AND FRIENDS) WHEN THEY FIND OUT YOUR CHILDREN ARE VEGAN/PLANT-BASED? HAVE YOU HAD ANY ISSUES?

I had so many issues. There has been so much negativity and concern from people with zero nutrition education, including doctors. Even as a nurse, I was never trained in-depth about nutrition besides a basic, conventional nutrition training. Even now, only some hospitals serve their patient's vegan diets.

We really are in an exciting time with the lifestyle becoming more accepted. Of course, there are still people who will disagree, but I don't let that bother me. In fact, I support anyone who will agree that we can improve our health with nutrition no matter the lifestyle you choose. It's a sure bet that removing the crap, sugar, processed foods and fried foods is a great way to begin to improve your health. My only advice is to try it for yourself and see how you feel. Keep in mind however, that you may feel worse before you feel better, and the reason for that is because when you remove that crap from your diet, you may experience a detox. Detox doesn't always feel good. You may be more fatigued, have headaches, have cravings and this is not a bad thing, it's a wonderful thing actually! It means that your body is processing all the years of old garbage in the body, and if you can keep going, you can experience health like never before!

ANY INSPIRING STORIES THAT HAVE HAPPENED TO YOU OR PEOPLE CLOSE TO YOU THAT HAVE NOT BEEN COVERED ABOVE. STORIES THAT CAN HELP OTHERS.

We need to remember that health is very individual, but the same factors are important for everyone and it goes beyond nutrition.

1. Sleep - If you don't get good sleep, you probably won't make the best choices about health. You might not exercise, you might be moody, your relationships may suffer and you might not feel like eating healthy food. Skipping out on sleep means that you're skipping out on the time that our bodies are meant to be repairing and restoring our hormones, which when imbalanced, leads to everything from weight gain to difficulty sleeping to infertility. Get your sleep right.

2. Don't put toxic substances in your body, including alcohol. It is not a healthy beverage. It's toxic to the body, and there are plenty of other ways to get antioxidants. If you are drinking it to relax, learn to meditate instead. Be careful about the products you put on your skin as well. They get absorbed easily and can be very toxic.

3. Exercise. Move your body frequently, whether it's walking, swimming, yoga, etc. These activities are especially great for any health condition. Add in resistance training a few days a week to keep your muscle and bone mass up as well.

4. Reduce your stress! Ok, this is easier said than done, but if you can get the other factors nailed down like great nutrition, sleep, movement, and avoiding toxins- even if things get tough in life - you will protect your health tremendously.

We need to constantly keep these factors in check for ourselves and our kids to protect our health and avoid disease. If there's one thing I learned after caring for cancer patients for nearly ten years, it's to protect your health like gold!

REBECCA FRITH
AUTHOR OF THIS BOOK

CONNECT WITH REBECCA:
INSTAGRAM: @LEGENDSOFCHANGE

"I initially chose to be vegan for health, though after learning just how detrimental the livestock industry is, my decision also became about the animals and the earth.

I had an aunt that died of breast cancer, and after seeing her try and fight this disease, and losing her, I decided that this was not going to happen to me. Through my research, it appeared that eating a plant-based diet was my best defense against cancer, and finally, it made total sense to me. I made the switch overnight. Since that day, my family and I have never been healthier.

I believe in nature and that nature is perfect, and it will supply us with everything we need. I just needed us all to eat as much food from the earth as possible and of course, organic when it is available.

I have wasted so many years thinking about food, restricting food and thinking bananas could make you fat (ridiculous, right?) Now, I totally get it. I eat from nature and if there is no label on it, I eat as much of it as I like because it's something that will nourish my body and not harm it. I look at my children and know that one day they will be so grateful they were taught the truth."

WHAT IS ONE OF THE BEST OR MOST WORTHWHILE HEALTH-RELATED INVESTMENTS THAT YOU HAVE MADE?

It would definitely be my Thermomix. I bought it before going vegan as I wanted to start to make more of my own sauces with vegetables rather than relying on store-bought products. I made my own stock, tomato sauce, jams, sauces, dressings. Before long, I was using my Thermomix about five times a day. We blended smoothies for breakfast in it, we cooked in it, made dressings and soups, and it is the master for making bliss balls and banana "nice" cream. I can highly recommend one of these. They are pricey, but I required no other utensils in the kitchen, and we certainly get our money's worth from it.

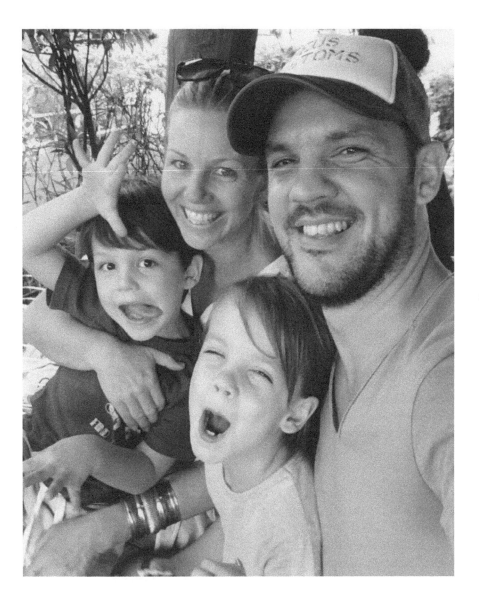

323

AT WHAT POINT IN YOUR LIFE DID YOU DECIDE TO CHANGE YOUR DIET? HOW HAS THAT DECISION IMPACTED YOUR LIFE?

I have always considered myself a healthy eater; it's what Mum taught me. Milk for calcium, lean meats for protein and salmon for good fats as well as avocado. I rarely ate junk food or chocolate and I was not a big eater in general. I have always been into health and exercise. I trained as a personal trainer when I was twenty, so I have been surrounded by the "protein myth" for years.

Then one day while I was training on my indoor trainer (I was starting to get into triathlon training), I was watching a YouTuber who was a triathlete. He was a fruitarian and I thought, "wow I could do that, I love fruit and he is a really good triathlete maybe there is something in this." So, off I went on my research crusade.

I also had an aunt who died of breast cancer only a few years earlier, which rocked my world. I always feared that this would happen to me. The more research I did, the more I started to realise that this was not just about being fitter and faster, it was about health. Through my research, it appeared that eating a plant-based diet was my best defense against cancer, and it made total sense to me. I thought really hard about being fruitarian at first, but I have two children and a husband, so I decided that going straight from omnivore to fruitarian might be a bit extreme. So, the next day, I announced to my husband I was going vegan.

WHAT WERE THE FIRST STEPS YOU TOOK IN MAKING YOUR NUTRITIONAL CHANGES AND WHY DID YOU START DOWN THIS PATH?

I cleared out my cupboards and fridge of all animal products and started to research recipes, products and alternatives to animal-based meals. I started by making the kids' favorite meals but making them plant-based. I'd make bolognese but instead of mince, I used lentils. The kids didn't even mind too much.

As for the hubby, I told him that he could eat whatever he liked when we were out, but I would not have animal products in the house, and he seemed ok with this. He was enjoying my new creativity in the kitchen. At first, however, he was a little reluctant and he would say things like, "well this would be really good if it had chicken in it." This got frustrating after a while so I sat down with him and we watched a few documentaries.

What The Health was probably the turning point for Sam. He felt angry that we had been lied to and that there was a lot we didn't know about with regards to what was on our plate. From that day on, Sam has also become plant-based. I remember the last meat meal he ate, which was duck, a dish that used to be his favorite. He ended up feeling physically sick afterwards and after that he said, "that's it, I'm done."

Sam has spent the past two years now researching nutrition and exercise. He has turned his knowledge into an online health and fitness business that helps other men and women, teaching them about plant-based diets and how to get a healthy and fit body with plants.

DO YOU TAKE ANY SPECIFIC SUPPLEMENTS? DO YOU RECOMMEND ANY SPECIFIC BRANDS? WHY DO YOU THINK THESE HAVE BENEFITED YOU AND/OR YOUR CHILDREN'S HEALTH?

I am not really a big believer in medication. We do however, as a family, supplement B12. I believe that nature provides us with all we need so it's more a case of making sure my family receives an adequate amount of balanced, real whole-foods. I also seek out organic where possible to guarantee higher levels of nutritional benefit.

WHAT HAS BEEN YOUR BIGGEST RESOURCE FOR COOKING RECIPES? WHO HAS BEEN YOUR BIGGEST INFLUENCER FOR YOUR VEGAN/ PLANT-BASED DIET CHANGE?

Oh, there have been so many. I am a big fan of @ohsheglows, @bosh.tv @Earthyandy, and of course @nutrition_facts_org. Dr. Greger is my go-to guy if I have any questions. His channel, nutritionfacts.org, is an absolute wealth of information, with extensive research to back-up his suggestions. I like to question things, so doing research is important to me. I also like to cross-reference, as I know there can always be arguments both ways. Dr. Greger is always a site that I like to cross-reference with.

325

WHAT ARE YOUR KIDS FAVORITE DISHES? CAN YOU SHARE A FAVORITE RECIPE?

My boys absolutely love Buddha bowls. We love to put corn, rice, edamame beans, lettuce, tomatoes, tofu with sesame seeds, broccoli, carrots, sweet potatoes and avocado in our bowls. We love them so much because you can put whatever you have into them, the color always looks so amazing, you always know it will nourish your body, and they are super easy to prepare. My kids love to eat deconstructed meals and like to have many choices, so Buddha bowls work perfectly for that.

IF YOU COULD GIVE A MUM WHO IS LOOKING AT CHANGING HER KIDS OVER TO A PLANT-BASED DIET THREE TIPS, WHAT WOULD THEY BE? DO YOU HAVE ANY STORIES RELATED TO YOUR KIDS NOT EATING MEAT AND DAIRY ANYMORE?

I have one child who didn't like meat at all when he was age two. My four-year-old on the other hand, was an absolute meat eater.

First, I recommend making their favorite dishes, but make them plant-based. I don't really like mock meats so I used grains, lentils etc. It is a bit of trial-and-error and finding what recipes you like. You will be amazed at how quickly your taste buds change. I think after two weeks you will see a different child who is eating so much more variety then they were before.

Second, give them lots of choices and opportunities to try new foods. Buddha bowls are so great for this and you can change up the ingredients and dressings that you use. My kids like to feel that they have some control over what they are eating and these bowls give them that.

Third, go to a great vegan restaurant. Let them experience how amazing plant-based food can be.

I also find that getting them involved in going to the market and helping prepare food is a great way for them to connect with it and enjoy eating it after.

I have also sat down with my boys and watched the introduction to the film Dominion, which shows the conditions that the animals live in and how sick these animals look. All kids love animals and seeing them living like this made them really sad. It is helping them make the connection that animals are not food. Kids totally get it.

WHAT HAS BEEN YOUR DOCTOR'S RESPONSE (OR NON VEGAN FAMILY AND FRIENDS) WHEN THEY FIND OUT YOUR CHILDREN ARE VEGAN/PLANT-BASED? HAVE YOU HAD ANY ISSUES?

We did get an awful lot of questions at the start, but mostly from family. Both Sam and my parents were worried and asked regularly if the kids were getting everything they needed. They'd ask things like, "are they growing?" or say "maybe you need to supplement." At the beginning, we were just feeling our way through. I felt healthier, so surely they must be as well.

I had watched every program possible including *What the Health*, *Eating to Live*, *Food Matters*, and *Prescription Thugs*, and I had read Dr. Greger's book, *How Not To Die*. In my heart, I knew that this was a healthy way of living and I totally believed that we were supposed to eat this way. Nature is perfect and it will supply us with everything we need. I just needed us all to eat as much food from the earth as possible and of course, organic when it is available.

Late last year Sam decided that he would do a 30-day challenge and started to calculate everything he was eating. We did a comparison with an old day of eating versus a new one for him, and we were shocked. We had really thought that previously we had been eating a healthy and balanced diet.

It turned out that all of Sam's nutrient targets were 100 - 300% better than they were with his previous diet. He was getting so many more nutrients including more protein and calcium through the plants we were eating. We knew we were healthier, but could not believe how much healthier we were. Once we produced this evidence to our parents, their minds were opened, both mine and Sam's mum are now eating plant-based diets and thriving. After switching to a plant-based diet, in just under a year my own Mum was able to stop taking her blood pressure meds she'd been taking for 25 years - the power of plants.

ANY INSPIRING STORIES THAT HAVE HAPPENED TO YOU OR PEOPLE CLOSE TO YOU THAT HAVE NOT BEEN COVERED ABOVE. STORIES THAT CAN HELP OTHERS.

There are so many things I could say, but after being vegan for almost four years at this point, I honestly just wish that I had found this sooner. I have wasted so many years thinking about food, restricting food and thinking bananas could make you fat (ridiculous, right?) Now, I totally get it. I eat from nature and if there is no label on it, I eat as much of it as I like because it's something that will nourish my body and not harm it. I look at my children and know that one day that they will be so grateful that they were taught the truth.

Kids are naturally animal lovers and yes, there are some times when they say to me that they don't care that the cake is not vegan, and I just remind them of the animals that might have been harmed to produce the cake. Generally they say they no longer want it anymore. I try to make them vegan cakes instead or "nice cream" each week so they don't feel like they miss out on any of that kind of food that they see their friends eating. We take them to vegan restaurants each week as well, so they can order anything they like off the menu and there is no need to say to them no sorry you can't have that because it's not vegan. I think it is great for them to be able to sit there and have whatever it is they want. I also make a point of saying to them, "yes everyone in here is vegan or likes to eat plant-based foods like us."

Sometimes for them, they only see what the kids are eating at school and feel like they are different and the only ones, so it's great to remind them that there are actually plenty of people eating this way and that have seen the truth and are standing up for what they believe in. I show them kids on YouTube and they often are featured in their Dad's videos for Instagram. They always just say to us, "hurry up guys, we need to turn more people VEGAN. Make another video."

HANA DEAVOLL

CONNECT WITH HANA:
INSTAGRAM: @MYVEGANCHILD, @VICECREAMNZ
FACEBOOK: MY VEGAN CHILD, VICE CREAM NZ
myveganchild.org, vicecream.co.nz

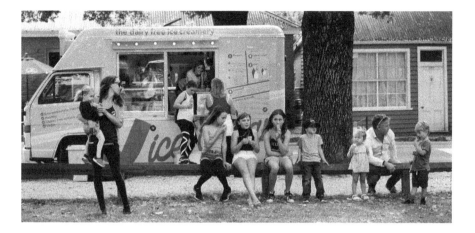

Business owner, Mum, and plant-based eating advocate, Hana Deavoll was initially inspired to switch her family to a plant-based diet after watching a friend heal their chronic disease by eating whole plant foods.

"Initially, we went plant-based for health reasons. A friend of ours had cancer and was fighting this with a plant-based diet. We watched the documentary Food Matters and A Delicate Balance. We thought, "if people can use a plant-based diet to cure cancer and heart disease, then why can't we use one to prevent it in the first place!?" So that was it for us, we made the change.

WHAT IS ONE OF THE BEST OR MOST WORTHWHILE HEALTH-RELATED INVESTMENTS THAT YOU HAVE MADE?

The book, World Peace Diet, by Will Tuttle, an Optimum 9400 blender (big) and a Tribest bullet blender (small).

WHAT WERE THE FIRST STEPS YOU TOOK IN MAKING YOUR HEALTH / NUTRITIONAL CHANGES AND WHY DID YOU START DOWN THIS PATH?

Watching documentaries! I watched all these life-changing documentaries with my husband, so it was easy for us to make the change together. He was especially open to it because his Dad had heart attacks at a young age,

"

I DIDN'T WANT MY KIDS TO
FEEL LIKE THEY WERE MISSING
OUT, AND THEY NEVER HAVE.
IN FACT, THIS CHANGE LED
TO US STARTING UP OUR
VERY OWN ICE CREAM TRUCK
CALLED *VICE CREAM*, WHICH
IS 100% DAIRY-FREE
AND VEGAN.

HANA DEAVOLL

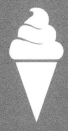

and he thought he would probably get heart disease too. It was watching documentaries like Forks Over Knives, What the Health and Food Matters, that really opened our eyes to the truth: you can control your health and your destiny by eating a whole-food, plant-based diet. This is what helped my husband, and I remain open to a diet change.

After years of eating plant-based, we became more open to learning about the horrors of the animal agriculture industry. It was easy to be vegan after seeing slaughterhouse footage and learning about the detrimental effects of animal agriculture on the environment. We just didn't want to contribute to that anymore.

DO YOU TAKE ANY SPECIFIC SUPPLEMENTS? DO YOU RECOMMEND ANY SPECIFIC BRANDS? WHY DO YOU THINK THESE HAVE BENEFITED YOU AND/OR YOUR CHILDREN'S HEALTH?

While I was pregnant and breastfeeding, I took a good quality natal supplement that included iron, B12 and folic acid. I got this from a naturopath on prescription, and the brand is called Bio Medica. I also use the Bio Medica b12 spray and add it to smoothies. In the winter we take Vitamin D (again, I add it to smoothies) since we don't get enough sunlight in Queenstown in the winter.

WHAT HAS BEEN YOUR BIGGEST RESOURCE FOR COOKING RECIPES? WHO HAS BEEN YOUR BIGGEST INFLUENCER FOR YOUR VEGAN/ PLANT-BASED DIET CHANGE?

Revive Cafe cookbooks were a great introduction to easy, plant-based cooking for me - lots of soups, stews, and curries. I also enjoy BOSH! and The Happy Pear cookbook.

As far as my biggest influencer, I credit vegan activists such as Earthling Ed, James Aspey, Joey Carbstrong, and Joshua Entis. They remind me why I am vegan and give me hope that the world is growing more and more vegan every year.

WHAT ARE YOUR KIDS FAVORITE DISHES? CAN YOU SHARE A FAVORITE RECIPE?

Bean nachos, lentil shepherd's pie, "chicken" nuggets, vegan sausages, pesto pasta, sushi bowl with tempeh and pizza. We pretty much do those meals on repeat all the time. The first three recipes are on the My Vegan Child website.

IF YOU COULD GIVE A MUM, WHO IS LOOKING AT CHANGING HER KIDS OVER TO A PLANT-BASED DIET THREE TIPS, WHAT WOULD THEY BE? DO YOU HAVE ANY STORIES RELATED TO YOUR KIDS NOT EATING MEAT AND DAIRY ANYMORE?

Explain to them the "why," then allow them to process this in their own time. Eventually, they will get it. If not straight away, give them a year or two, especially if they have been strongly socially conditioned.

When we were first going plant-based, the one thing that we slipped up on was allowing the kids to choose any ice cream they wanted while out at cafes/ice cream parlours. Of course, they chose the creamy dairy ice creams because they wanted something yummy, and there weren't many vegan choices at that time either. Over time, I began to feel increasingly uncomfortable with this, until one day, I decided I wasn't going to contribute one more dollar to the dairy industry. I explained to my kids why by saying that when we consume or buy milk products, it means that a mother cow has had her breast milk taken away and her baby has been taken away from her too. Surprisingly, my kids accepted this very quickly. Of course, they didn't want baby cows to suffer so they could have ice cream or chocolate! We came up with a solution to ensure they still got to have lots of yummy vegan treats, and I upped my baking skills too. I didn't want my kids to feel like they were missing out, and they never have. In fact, it was this that led to us this year, starting up our very own ice cream truck called Vice Cream, which is 100% dairy-free and vegan.

WHAT HAS BEEN YOUR DOCTOR'S RESPONSE (OR NON VEGAN FAMILY AND FRIENDS) WHEN THEY FIND OUT YOUR CHILDREN ARE VEGAN/PLANT-BASED? HAVE YOU HAD ANY ISSUES?

Everyone has been very supportive. They know I research things and they respect our decision. My bloods were always good throughout my pregnancies so my doctor and midwife were happy. My kids are incredibly healthy and strong, which is a justification in itself.

ANY INSPIRING STORIES THAT HAVE HAPPENED TO YOU OR PEOPLE CLOSE TO YOU THAT HAVE NOT BEEN COVERED ABOVE. STORIES THAT CAN HELP OTHERS.

Veganism is so important, but it really is the least we can do. As vegans, we need to be active in some way so as to further the movement, normalize veganism, and save more animals. There are all types of activism, and you can find whatever suits your personality.

It might be baking yummy vegan treats to share with others, attending protests and cubes, sharing articles on social media, or starting a vegan/plant-based business. Every little bit counts towards creating a kinder, more compassionate and sustainable world. Let's do this!

KATE THOMPSON-READE

Within a month of switching to a plant-based diet, Kate Thompson-Reade was off her previous medications for a pregnancy-related autoimmune condition called pemphigoid gestationis. Within a month, Kate found herself pregnant again, continued her plant-based diet, and remained completely healthy and pemphigoid-free for her entire fourth pregnancy.

WHAT IS ONE OF THE BEST OR MOST WORTHWHILE HEALTH-RELATED INVESTMENTS THAT YOU HAVE MADE?

Good quality vegan ingredients! Marinated tofu, nutritional yeast, vegan seasonings and other things to make our plant-based meals pop.

AT WHAT POINT IN YOUR LIFE DID YOU DECIDE TO CHANGE YOUR DIET? HOW HAS THAT DECISION IMPACTED YOUR LIFE?

I was pregnant with my third child and suffering from a pregnancy-related autoimmune condition called pemphigoid gestationis. This is a rare autoimmune skin disease that is characterised by an itchy rash that develops into blisters. It is most common during the second and third trimesters of pregnancy. My condition started at fourteen weeks and was continuing at five months postpartum. At this point, I researched a lot about the role of diet (particularly a vegan diet) in helping autoimmune conditions. I was already mostly vegetarian for ethical reasons, so I thought it was worth a try.

I started with a full, plant-based diet, eating nothing pre-made, just lots of whole-foods. Within a month, I was off all my medications, and my rash was clearing. I could not believe that changing my diet could have such an impact on my health. I continued to eat the same way, and despite having PCOS, I got pregnant again a month later. Despite only being in remission for a short time and therefore at high risk of contracting my autoimmune condition again, I remained completely pemphigoid-free and healthy for my entire fourth pregnancy!

WHAT WERE THE FIRST STEPS YOU TOOK IN MAKING YOUR NUTRITIONAL CHANGES AND WHY DID YOU START DOWN THIS PATH?

I was vegan for nearly a year while continuing to cook omnivore food for my family. My husband was starting to enjoy vegan food with me, mostly as a side dish though. One day he came into the room while I was watching the documentary, Dominion. Since that day, to my delight and probably to the credit of that documentary, he and our four children are all vegans. This documentary is available to watch free on YouTube, and I recommend that everyone should watch it. It is real and raw, but it is the truth.

WHAT HAS BEEN YOUR BIGGEST RESOURCE FOR COOKING RECIPES? WHO HAS BEEN YOUR BIGGEST INFLUENCER FOR YOUR VEGAN/PLANT-BASED DIET CHANGE?

I love Forks Over Knives: The Cookbook, and "Bosh" on Facebook. I follow a lot of different pages on Instagram, which is where I pick up some inspiration. In general, though, we just make it up as we go.

WHAT ARE YOUR KIDS FAVORITE DISHES? CAN YOU SHARE A FAVORITE RECIPE?

I love making bowls with some crumbled tofu, brown rice and salad. I usually top it with nuts and some hummus. These are so great for the whole family.

IF YOU COULD GIVE A MUM WHO IS LOOKING AT CHANGING HER KIDS OVER TO A PLANT-BASED DIET THREE TIPS, WHAT WOULD THEY BE? DO YOU HAVE ANY STORIES RELATED TO YOUR KIDS NOT EATING MEAT AND DAIRY ANYMORE?

Teach your kid's about kindness to animals in an age-appropriate way. We visit lots of animal sanctuaries and read books on the topic as well. *Dave Loves Chickens* is fabulous!

Always remember that it's a marathon, not a sprint. I'd rather my kids make their own informed choices to be vegan than to force it on them against their will.

WHAT HAS BEEN YOUR DOCTOR'S RESPONSE (OR NON VEGAN FAMILY AND FRIENDS) WHEN THEY FIND OUT YOUR CHILDREN ARE VEGAN/PLANT-BASED? HAVE YOU HAD ANY ISSUES?

Only positive! But I do think we are well-researched and well-informed when any questions are asked, which helps.

ANY INSPIRING STORIES THAT HAVE HAPPENED TO YOU OR PEOPLE CLOSE TO YOU THAT HAVE NOT BEEN COVERED ABOVE. STORIES THAT CAN HELP OTHERS.

Being vegan and raising my family vegan has been one of the most positive and life-changing things I have ever done. I feel proud to be teaching my kids about compassion to all beings and at the same time about caring for their bodies with nourishing food. My only regret is not doing it sooner!

NICOLA NEAL

CONNECT WITH NICOLA:
INSTAGRAM: @NICOLAMNEAL
FACEBOOK: NICOLA NEAL (NICOLA BANKS)

"I have always called myself an animal lover, but I had also always been a meat-eater. Like so many others, I just had not made the connection or seen the duplicity in my morality. Ironically my journey to veganism came about through rescuing a Romanian puppy. I became Facebook friends with a lady who also had a dog from the same rescue organisation as me. This inspirational lady had been super morbidly obese, with a BMI of over 80 and many associated health problems such as diabetes, high blood pressure, hyperthyroidism and even had a brain tumor. Whilst in the hospital with sepsis, she decided one day to take her health into her own hands and overnight became a raw vegan. I followed her journey of incredible weight loss, reversal of diabetes, lowered blood pressure, normal thyroid function and the shrinking of her brain tumor and it made me realise that WE are responsible for what we put in our bodies and if we want to be healthy then we need to eat the fuel that our body craves; natural, raw foods like fruits, vegetables, nuts and seeds."

Nicola Neal was always an animal lover but only made the connection between the animals on her plate and the animals she called her pets within the past few years. Now she and her family enjoy plant-based eating, and she continues to share her passion for this lifestyle and the simplicity of meal preparation via recipes and mouthwatering food photography through her Instagram page.

AT WHAT POINT IN YOUR LIFE DID YOU DECIDE TO CHANGE YOUR DIET? HOW HAS THAT DECISION IMPACTED YOUR LIFE?

My son (now aged nine) always hated meat. I used to think he needed meat for protein and insisted he ate some. It was a battle! Quite ironically, I have always been an animal lover but had never really made "the connection." You know, that moment when you realize that you are actually eating the dead flesh of a beautiful animal that is really no different to the pet dog you have draped across your knee while you watch TV and pet it.

I started to become more aware of the cruelty of the industry and at the same time, became friends with a lady on Facebook (by chance, really).

334

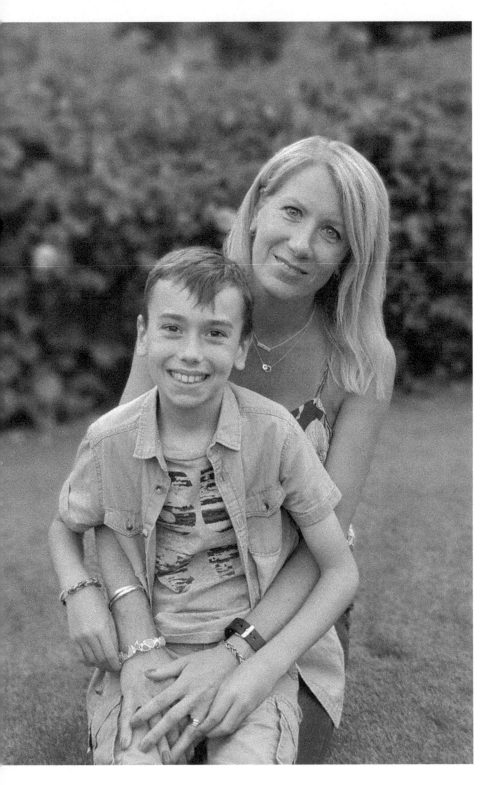

Our only connection was that we had both adopted rescue dogs from Romania, but I saw her asking about dog food in a Romanian rescue Facebook group, so I gave her some advice.

We "friended" each other and I began to see her life. I was amazed. This lady had been super morbidly obese with a BMI of over 80 and suffered from numerous health problems related to that. She also had a brain tumor. She was not in a good way, and she decided overnight to go almost exclusively raw vegan. I saw the difference it made to her. The weight dropped off and she changed. She reversed her diabetes, hyperthyroidism, high blood pressure, and her tumor stopped growing. I was in awe, and I began to realize that food is medicine. It is the first line of defense against disease, and what we put inside our bodies determines, to a massive degree, our health.

So with the increased awareness of the cruelty involved in meat production and the glaringly obvious health benefits of eating the fruit of the earth, I went vegetarian overnight in September 2017. I did not find it hard and I started to educate myself about the food I was eating. I joined a vegan group on Facebook and then became aware of the cruelty of the dairy and egg industries. I decided to try Veganuary on January 1st, 2018. I have not looked back since.

WHAT WERE THE FIRST STEPS YOU TOOK IN MAKING YOUR NUTRITIONAL CHANGES AND WHY DID YOU START DOWN THIS PATH?

Like I said, on January 1st, 2018, I became fully vegan overnight. In preparation for this, I started to follow vegans on Instagram looking for inspiration for things to cook. I wanted to see real food cooked by real people, so I followed normal everyday people who posted pictures of what they ate and most importantly, gave recipes for the dishes! My absolute favorite Instagram page was @vegan_meals_made_easy.

I took screenshots of all his meals and studied them until I was confident I could cook like that. I was looking for food that my husband would eat since he was not intending to be vegan at all! My plan was to cook hearty family meals that he would eat, and I could add a meat substitute to if he really insisted!

My husband, whilst totally supportive of my choice to be vegan, was adamant that he was not changing and would not be going vegan or even vegetarian. He wanted me to continue to buy meat products for him, which caused a lot of issues between us. I tried to show him the cruelty and the health benefits, but he is a stubborn man, and he dug his heels in. The more I tried to force it on him, the more he insisted that he wanted meat. It was a battle of wills.

I just continued to cook beautiful vegan dinners for myself and added meat to his. Gradually, I started not adding meat to his meals and he agreed that the food I served him was good. I carried on cooking good, tasty, filling meals for him, and he could see that I was not missing anything by leaving the meat off my plate.

One day he announced out of the blue, that he was now vegetarian. I was overjoyed. In effect, this meant he was practically vegan because I did not use any dairy or eggs in my cooking. Once he ditched the meat, his meals were 100% vegan.

I guess I learned that men like to feel they have made their own decisions, and the more we try and push them the harder they pull back. The way to win is to cook awesome food and wait for them to make the decision for themselves.

My son, who I now see had always been a natural vegan, was delighted that I no longer forced meat on him, but he still ate eggs and cheese. Eventually, he asked if he could be vegan too when he knew I was doing Veganuary.

I agreed immediately and he has been vegan ever since. He is totally committed and has educated himself on the realities of the meat, dairy, and egg industries, and I know now he will be vegan for life. He had been trying to be vegan his whole life, and I had forced him to eat meat and eggs "for protein!"

DO YOU TAKE ANY SPECIFIC SUPPLEMENTS? DO YOU RECOMMEND ANY SPECIFIC BRANDS? WHY DO YOU THINK THESE HAVE BENEFITED YOU AND/OR YOUR CHILDREN'S HEALTH?

I take a VEG1 supplement from The Vegan Society, and my son takes Nature's Plus Animal Parade chewable tablets (he didn't like the Veg1 tablets).

I think it's important to recognize that as vegans, we often do not get enough vitamin B12, and by taking a supplement, I do not need to worry about me or my son being deficient in anything.

James (my son) actually eats a good variety of beautiful fruits and vegetables, but taking a supplement means I can rest assured he is covered in any event.

WHAT HAS BEEN YOUR BIGGEST RESOURCE FOR COOKING RECIPES? WHO HAS BEEN YOUR BIGGEST INFLUENCER FOR YOUR VEGAN/ PLANT-BASED DIET CHANGE?

As mentioned above, my initial biggest influencer was a lady I met through our mutual love of rescue dogs. Seeing her health turnaround awakened me to the health benefits of real food.

My initial resource for recipes was Instagram. Following people who cooked real food and not the kind that looks like it was photographed in a studio or picture-perfect. I wanted to see what normal vegans ate.

I have since joined Veganuary and other Facebook groups where people share their food ideas and have invested in several vegan cookbooks. My favorite cookbooks are BOSH! and The Vegan100 by Gaz Oakley.

I also search the internet for vegan recipes, and absolutely love "The Minimalist Baker" and "It Doesn't Taste Like Chicken" websites.

WHAT ARE YOUR SONS FAVORITE DISHES? CAN YOU SHARE A FAVORITE RECIPE?

My son is actually incredibly fussy, but I'm lucky that he eats a good variety of food. He just hates what I would call "proper family meals." He would not eat anything saucy or anything tomato-based. He would not touch a meal like spaghetti bolognese, lasagne, or curry of any kind. He likes a good variety of fruits and vegetables, so I gave up trying to make meals for him. Now he eats a lot of what we call "picnic dinners." These are basically platters of food, some fruits, some vegetables, some carbs, some protein, some cooked, some raw, some hot, some cold, all on one plate. It's basically a kaleidoscope of foods that I know he will eat all served together. Some would say, "that doesn't go with that" or "how can you have fruit and pasta on the same plate?"

I say, "I don't care about what goes with what but I care that my son eats a good variety." He is happy, so why not put it all on one plate? You can see many examples of my picnic platters on my Instagram page. I always try and make it look pretty for him too.

It only takes a minute to plate up the food in an attractive way, and I really think that we eat with our eyes. If it looks good, it makes you want to eat it. James is always so appreciative of the food I present to him. He always says thank you, and he often says "wow"!

James also likes pasta, so one of our easiest (and one of the only "normal meals" he will eat) is whole wheat pasta (no sauce - he HATES sauce) with broccoli, baby corn, spinach, broad beans, peas and some grated vegan cheese (Violife grated) mixed in. He always has ground black pepper on it too. It's so simple because it can all be cooked in one pot. When your pasta is almost done, just throw in the broccoli florets, baby corn, peas and broad beans, and cook for just two more minutes. Drain and then stir through some grated vegan cheese so it melts, and then serve with a grind of black pepper! Sometimes I will serve this with accidentally vegan garlic bread (most supermarkets basic/value range will be vegan as they do not use real butter in the cheap version).

IF YOU COULD GIVE A MUM, WHO IS LOOKING AT CHANGING HER KIDS OVER TO A PLANT-BASED DIET THREE TIPS, WHAT WOULD THEY BE? DO YOU HAVE ANY STORIES RELATED TO YOUR KIDS NOT EATING MEAT AND DAIRY ANYMORE?

1) Don't stress about what they won't eat. Focus on the healthy things they WILL eat and put them all on one plate. Don't worry about what food goes with what, just serve it all together. Let them pick at it. Make it fun and make it look nice on the plate.

2) Follow me on Instagram. I post pictures of pretty much everything James eats. You can be inspired.

3) My third tip is a secret way to get extra goodness into your kids. If they like Weetabix, serve them Weetabix for breakfast with some fresh raspberries or other berries and then top the Weetabix with some milled flax/sunflower/pumpkin seeds - it looks just like Weetabix crumbs, they'll never know! I use Linwoods milled flax products. They have a lot of varieties and are virtually undetectable on top of Weetabix!

If your kids are old enough to understand, educate them about where food comes from. If they know the truth, they may decide for themselves that they want to be vegan. The truth is the truth, and we owe it to our children to tell them the truth about their chicken nuggets and their McDonald's hamburger. Tell them in an age-appropriate way but tell them the truth.

WHAT HAS BEEN YOUR DOCTOR'S RESPONSE (OR NON-VEGAN FAMILY AND FRIENDS) WHEN THEY FIND OUT YOUR CHILDREN ARE VEGAN/PLANT-BASED? HAVE YOU HAD ANY ISSUES?

Since I became vegan, I have made it my mission to show people how easy it is and how good the food is because so many people just say "I could never be vegan, it's too hard." I understand this because I used to think about it too. I want to help people see that it is EASY. I photograph and post pictures of pretty much everything I cook and eat, and I also bombard the internet vegan groups with pictures of James and the food he eats. I want people to be inspired to change. I want them to see how well I eat and how the food I cook is as filling and satisfying as any meaty dish. I love veganising traditional meaty meals like sausage and mash and showing people that they won't miss out on anything by being vegan.

I cook cakes and show that vegan cake looks and tastes as good as a traditional cake. I am passionate about showing people how easy it is.

My Instagram following has gone from 80 real friends a year ago to 1300+

now, just by posting pics of real vegan food. I feel proud to be part of the vegan awakening. I have had other Mums come up to me in the school playground to tell me how good my food looks on Facebook and I have had James's school teacher tell me that James always has the best-packed lunch. She says that she wishes all the children brought in a lunch like his and asked if I wouldn't mind making one for her every day also.

As a direct result of my vocal veganism and constant posting of food (and some activism) on my Facebook page, I have lost some friends, but I have also made so many new friends. I have also had some amazing turnarounds with my own friends and family.

My oldest son (27) is now vegetarian and almost vegan. My father, aged 70, eats very little meat now as he has been very receptive to my "educational chats." My best friend owns a small holding and up until last year, raised pigs and lambs in small numbers. She has stopped doing this now. Her sheep are now pets, and she will not be getting any more pigs. She and her husband eat a predominantly vegetarian diet now, and she always has plant milk and vegan cheese for when James goes round for a playdate.

ANY INSPIRING STORIES THAT HAVE HAPPENED TO YOU OR PEOPLE CLOSE TO YOU THAT HAVE NOT BEEN COVERED ABOVE. STORIES THAT CAN HELP OTHERS.

I think I've pretty much said it all above. I am proud to be raising a beautiful vegan child with a kind soul who knows the reality that is hidden from so many children. I believe that children are naturally vegan and if they were completely aware of what they were being fed when they are given meat/dairy/eggs, they would reject it. If you put a lamb in front of a child, there is not a child alive who would see food; they would see a beautiful baby that they want to stroke and cuddle.

" "

DON'T STRESS ABOUT WHAT
YOUR KIDS WON'T EAT. FOCUS
ON THE HEALTHY THINGS THEY
WILL EAT AND PUT THEM ALL
ON ONE PLATE. DON'T WORRY
ABOUT WHAT FOOD GOES
WITH WHAT, JUST SERVE IT ALL
TOGETHER. LET THEM PICK AT
IT. MAKE IT FUN AND MAKE IT
LOOK NICE ON THE PLATE.

NICOLA NEAL

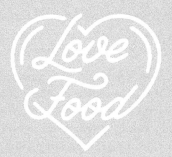

VICTORIA CONDE

CONNECT WITH VICTORIA:
INSTAGRAM: @VEGANVIXEN68

At 50 years young, Victoria Conde can now say that she's been vegan as long as she's been an animal-eater.

"First I was a vegetarian, then no red meat. Eventually, the dairy and eggs stopped, then finally the chicken. I saw a video then another. My heart broke and I am still traumatized. I was not physically ill when I went vegan; I didn't do it for my health… But it can be said that I did. I became vegan for the animals and for my mental health. I just could not be a part of the insanity I saw in videos of animal slaughter. I have always been physically active, I ran numerous marathons and even the Boston Marathon vegan. I have been a fitness instructor, a weightlifter, and a cardio queen vegan. I've been a Phys Ed teacher for the last 20 years. I got pregnant and maintained my veganism without the doctor's support. I raised my daughter vegan, again without the doctor's support. I walked out on her pediatrician when I was told she must have milk. I had no fear. I just fed her and knew from the depths of my being that she would be ok. She's 19 this year, and she's still vegan, beautiful, strong, smart and super talented as an artist"

WHAT IS ONE OF THE BEST OR MOST WORTHWHILE HEALTH-RELATED INVESTMENTS THAT YOU HAVE MADE?

I love my Vitamix!! I use it almost every day. To make ice cream; frozen bananas + water + any fruit you like. You must freeze the banana because that's what makes it thick and creamy like ice cream.

Smoothies - please go to my Instagram, @veganvixen68, and scroll down to summer 2018. I have TONS of simple smoothie ideas and beautiful pics. The base of them is bananas because it keeps them creamy, but you can also add any fruit to this. I buy tons of different frozen berries from Costco and use whatever I'm in the mood for. I buy bananas by the box - most grocery stores will sell you a forty-pound box of bananas. I do end up freezing if any are left over. Make sure to peel them and put them in a freezer-safe bag if you're gonna freeze them. Make sure they are VERY ripe and VERY spotted before you start to use them. I drink a smoothie every day in the summer!

342

Salad dressing - my favorite and go to is sunflower seeds, soy sauce, or coconut aminos and lemon, or apple cider vinegar and enough water to make it as thick or runny as you like. There are tons of recipes online and the sunflower seeds here can be exchanged for any nut or seed. I have a huge salad every day in the winter!!

With the Vitamix, you do not have to soak any nut or seed because the motor is so powerful it turns them very creamy. It also makes incredible cashew cheese - just Google for recipes.

AT WHAT POINT IN YOUR LIFE DID YOU DECIDE TO CHANGE YOUR DIET? HOW HAS THAT DECISION IMPACTED YOUR LIFE?

I've been vegan for 25 years. I can't pinpoint my defining moment, but there were many moments. When I was I young I moved from a city in Canada to a farm in Europe. I was lucky enough to see these animals up close and in person, as opposed to seeing their body parts all nicely wrapped up at the store. We are so disconnected. I made the connection then, but I kept eating them without question.

In the fall it is customary for each family to kill their own pig and bring it home. My father had been doing this in Canada since I was little. I remember going into the laundry room and almost crashing into a dead pig that was hanging upside down with all its organs removed. It was awful. But this time I was living surrounded by farms and on the day of the "pig kill" I was in my bedroom, and it sounded like a horror movie. I could hear screams from every corner of my room. I had to cover my ears, my stomach felt so sick, I was crying and helpless. This was one major awakening for me.

Another moment was at my neighbor's house. She had a beautiful cow that we would walk to the creek so she could drink. I remember walking right beside her eye, and how beautiful it was, how gentle she was and curious too.

I stopped eating pigs the day I saw a video of a man standing on top of a pig and smashing a cinder block onto its head. It traumatized me, and I have that image seared into my brain even today, over 25 years later. I stopped eating cows soon after. But I still ate chickens, eggs and cheese.

We had chickens and ducks and one of the ducks used to lay a mint green egg a few times a week. That was always my egg. I loved those ducks and taught them some tricks too!

At 18, I came back to Canada. My excuse to eat chickens was that "they're dumb." It was just an excuse to keep eating them because they tasted good. This lasted until I was about 23. One evening I was watching the news with my partner, and they showed the process of chicken slaughter. It was a video where they were getting de-feathered and hung upside down with some sort of machine. When I saw that it hit me right away, it was then that I said, "I'm never eating chicken again." A week later, I was at my favorite restaurant, Swiss Chalet, eating a chicken breast. My partner commented, "I thought you weren't gonna eat chicken anymore." It was like a bomb dropped. At that moment, I pushed the plate away and never had chicken again!! I wish I remembered the date, but I don't.

I was a vegetarian for a couple of years. I loved Havarti cheese and eggs. I made the best omelet with onion and sliced potatoes. It was delicious!! One day the cable man came to my house and we got talking. He saw a book on my table and asked if I had read it. I had. He asked me if I wanted to trade books. I said, sure. He gave me a book called something like, The Total Health Makeover. There was a chapter in there about dairy and she described it as sludge moving through our body. I am very visual. She challenged readers to go dairy-free for three months I think it was, and see how we feel. I love a challenge, so I did it! My energy soared, I felt amazing!! It was then that I looked into the industry. There wasn't much online back then that was public information, but there was enough for me. Soon after I looked into the egg industry and saw babies being ground up alive.

I was done with it all and never looked back. I went vegan 25 years ago. As of today, I have been vegan for half of my life. I am grateful that I was able to live with and get to know these animals while living on a farm. I think that if we all had exposure to animals there would be way more vegans.

Rayven is my daughter, and I made sure to take her to farm sanctuaries so that she could see, touch and feel these beings as beings and not as things. I made sure to do this when she was still a baby. We walked by the "graveyard" aisle at the grocery store, and I would point out the pieces of animals and say to her "look there's a cow, do we eat cows?" and she would reply "no" and I would reinforce that over and over. The pieces of neatly cut body parts were identified to her as animals. She has been vegan her entire life and has never had the urge to eat any animal product.

WHO HAS BEEN THE BIGGEST PLANT-BASED INFLUENCER IN YOUR LIFE AND HOW HAVE THEY HELPED YOU?

I've been vegan for a long time and to be honest, there was no one who influenced me. It was being exposed to the animals, getting to know them, playing with them and spending lots of time with them that influenced me.

We had a ram and a sheep who were siblings. My Dad would tie up the ram to let them graze, that way, his sister wouldn't go far. This field was about 400 meters from the house.

One day I heard her baying at the window in a panic. I looked, and she was walking in circles and speaking very loudly and agitated. I went outside, and she started to run to where her brother was, so I followed her. Her brother was on the ground, suffocating!! The rope wasn't tied properly and he was almost dead!! He was on his side with his tongue out. I never shook so much in my life! I ran home and grabbed the biggest knife I could find out of the kitchen. My heart was beating out of my chest, I was so scared! I ran back and all I remember was my hand shaking so much I could barely get under the rope. We were lucky. I had saved him, thanks to his sister.

They both trusted me; I used to play with them a lot, especially the ram who would come and head butt me in the butt after I would pretend to come at him.

I betrayed them though. When we returned to Canada, my Dad gave them to his brother. I guess he couldn't kill them himself. They became two of a flock of about ten that were destined to be killed one day. I am so sorry.

More recently, I would say Doug Graham has been a big influencer. I learned about him a couple of years before The 80/10/10 Diet book came out. I started adding lots and lots of fruit to my diet and at times, being completely raw for months. Fruit is my main food during the summer months.

In Toronto, Canada, winters are cold, so I move to a diet full of stews, soups and hot heavy foods. Theoretically, I love the 80/10/10 concept, but realistically, I like cooked foods and need them to keep warm in the winter. But his book and attending the Woodstock Fruit Festival in New York helped me to understand that eating a diet of fruit only was not only possible, it was also healthy!

345

HOW DO YOU THINK WE CAN ALL HAVE A BIGGER IMPACT ON INFLUENCING PEOPLE AND HELPING THEM MAKE THE CONNECTION TO HEALTH AND EATING A PLANT-BASED DIET?

I think we need to be in relationships with animals - to be able to physically touch them and feel their warmth and innocence. To see them as living beings with personalities, families and feelings. We are too removed from the source of our food - disconnected as to who it is we are actually eating. We've even changed the names from who they were, to something it is not. Cows are called steaks or burgers. Pigs are sausages or ribs. Chickens are poultry or drum sticks. I was blind too once. I did not see that they are one and the same!!

I think the movement is gaining a lot of speed now because of the internet, YouTube and Netflix. There are endless documentaries to watch. I have always said that if someone can sit through Earthlings (on YouTube) and still eat animals, they have no heart.

I want to believe that the human species is a compassionate and loving species, but we have been programmed and brainwashed into believing that these animals are only tools for our taste sensation. We need to plug into the source of our food to understand what it is, where it comes from and how.

I think the one thing that would have mass influence is to air these documentaries on national television. Yes, we do rallies, marches and have festivals, but to have the biggest impact, the masses need to be reached.

Adding to that by simply living the vegan lifestyle and putting it out there, we have influence. We are healthy, strong, intelligent, talented individuals who are living inspired lives. People are curious and they ask questions, which makes new thought patterns begin to grow inside their minds and hearts.

It's wonderful that we have very competent vegan speakers sharing their stories and challenging the "norm." I think we need more of this. We need a bigger platform. We have wonderful, scientific, peer-reviewed books, lectures and videos. There really is no excuse in today's age for not knowing. I do, however, know a few people who do not want to know because it would require that they change. Most would rather die than change and they do, from all the illness and disease that eating dead bodies brings them.

My biggest accomplishment in life has been raising my 18 year old, Rayven, vegan since birth. Too many people have deeply held beliefs that we need to eat animals and animal products to grow up healthy and strong. I love to tell them about Rayven's story. They usually don't know what to say.

IF YOU COULD HAVE A GIGANTIC BILLBOARD ANYWHERE WITH ANYTHING ON IT, WHAT WOULD IT SAY?

LOVE ANIMALS, DON'T EAT THEM

So many people say they love animals, but they don't understand their own speciesism. They love "pets," not animals. Let's try to group all animals under one umbrella and not separate specific ones to lose their lives for a snack. I don't even think people understand that they are eating what once was a living being who had their throats slit while they were kicking and screaming.

HOW HAS A FAILURE, OR APPARENT FAILURE, SET YOU UP FOR LATER SUCCESS? DO YOU HAVE A "FAVORITE FAILURE" OF YOURS?

In 25 years of being vegan, I've cheated twice.

The first time was about one year into this lifestyle. It was Christmas and my mom made her crab in garlic sauce. This was my absolute favorite dish. As she set it on the table, I said "stuff it" in my head and took the thickest claw I could. I remember biting into it and feeling my teeth go through layer and layer of flesh. I heard it in my head. I put it down and couldn't eat any.

The second time I cheated, was about two or three years into veganism.

I had four male family members working on my basement for a major renovation. I was home on a Saturday, and my Dad asked me to make them lunch. He told me to go buy cold cuts and beer. Instead, I bought Havarti, fresh buns and toppings. When I was making their sandwiches, I had a couple of bites of the cheese sandwich. Did it taste good? Not as good as I remembered it. It seems our memories lie to us.

Neither the crab or the cheese tasted as good as I remember, and the crab actually repulsed me. Since then, I have not knowingly cheated once. Of course, there may be cross-contamination at restaurants and such.

WHAT VEGAN RESOURCE COULD YOU NOT LIVE WITHOUT AND WHY?

I LOVE Gary Yourofsky. He was the original, and no one has come close to him for me. His charisma, knowledge, and the creative way he presents his findings are magical to me. I heard he retired because he got burned out - such a shame. Please do watch his "Greatest Speech Ever" on YouTube.

Today there are SO MANY vegan influencers, it's AMAZING!! I love to look at bodybuilders, especially Crissi Carvalho. She's definitely a huge inspiration to me.

WHAT ADVICE WOULD YOU GIVE A SMART AND DRIVEN 18-YEAR-OLD TODAY? WHAT ADVICE SHOULD THEY IGNORE?

My daughter is 18. I work with teenagers as well, because I teach high school.

I do talk about my lifestyle and why I do it. I do tell them to watch Earthlings. I do refer to their lunches as birds, cows and pigs. I do talk about speciesism and make them aware of the word and that it's the biggest social rights movement of their lives. I tell my students that I am vegan. We actually talk a lot about it, even though I'm not supposed to and have been called to the office a few times because of it.

I tell them that the choices they make today are not their choices. Their values and beliefs are not theirs. They have been passed down from their parents. I ask them to look at what's true for them and for them to educate themselves with documentaries like Earthlings, Cowspiracy, Forks Over Knives, Dominion and What the Health.

They ask me if my daughter is vegan, and I say yes. Their reply is, "you didn't give her a choice." I turn this around and say, "your parents didn't give you a choice. They made you eat animals because that is what they knew."

I encourage them to learn the truth. I show them my daughter's first place trophy from when she won a 15 kilometer race when she was 14. She won in the "19 and under" category. I show them my physical accomplishments, as well. They see me, 50 years old, full of energy, slim and healthy. My age brings a shock to their faces. I just say, "go vegan." I tell them, "you want to rebel? To be different? To break away from your parents' influence? Go vegan." The advice is not just given in words, it is shown to them in actions.

I tell them to avoid the fear, the doubts and the need to be accepted by their peers. To be their own individual self and to learn about the impact they have on the other beings we share this planet with.

I have been teaching at the same school for 25 years. I have many former students on my Facebook, and my biggest joy is when they reach out to me and tell me they are vegan and want to share recipes with me.

ANY INSPIRING STORIES YOU CAN SHARE?

When my father was 78 years old, I hadn't spoken to him in 20. Eventually, we reconciled and I introduced him to veganism. I forced him to watch slaughterhouse documentaries. He was in shock. This was a man who had killed his own chickens, rabbits, pigs and cows with his own hands, but the video got to him. It was not the animals' death that bothered him, but it was the way the animals were treated and the amount of death, pain and suffering he saw. Of course, I got on his case to not eat animals. I raided his fridge one day and threw out all the dairy. He almost killed me. He has a mentality of lack. He grew up poor, so throwing out food was seen as totally wrong. I replaced it all with vegan versions. My Dad always had a stuffy nose for as long as I can remember. He'd always be blowing it at the kitchen table. Once he was off all the dairy, his mucus stopped. No more blowing his nose. He was happy and surprised.

I bought him veggie burgers, veggie sausages, fake chicken and fish. He kinda didn't have a choice. I just kept filling his fridge with vegan things and showing him how to cook them. He still ate chicken and fish though.

In 2013, I rented a house in Costa Rica for four months. He and my daughter joined me for two months. While he was there, he ate only vegan food. He lost weight and felt great. At the age of 79, he was vegan!! This lasted until 83 when he started to eat fish once a week.

He has a very overweight man who was his friend and would laugh at his food choices. He said he would never give up meat. This man is my age and about 100 pounds overweight. He started to bring my Dad farmed chickens for him to eat! I was outraged. He was sabotaging my Dad's new eating style. I warned my Dad that one day soon his friend was going to die of a heart attack or get cancer. The chicken soon stopped because I confronted him.

Today, my Dad is 85 and on no medication and has never been on medication. Last week that same friend of my Dad's told him that he has Lymphoma. I was with my Dad when he found out. He said that Roger was sick, and I replied with, "told you so." To this, he started to smile and said that he's not eating meat now because it will allow him to live longer. I just had to laugh.

Why is it that something horrible has to happen to wake us up? I spoke to Roger and he is open to researching, but said that he will never give up meat completely, to which I replied: "some people choose to die instead of changing their diet, and they do."

The following weekend, my Dad was on the phone with his brother (who lives in Europe) when I arrive at his house. I heard him say, "eat less meat" to him. At that moment I said, "don't eat any meat!" and my Dad REPEATED what I said to his brother. That was music to my ears!!! It's just a shame that tragedy has to happen for people to see!!

I think my biggest contribution to the vegan movement is my daughter Rayven. Upon learning I was pregnant, raising her vegan wasn't even a question. I knew that was what I was going to do. Remember, she was born in 2000, so the products and the items available today were not available then. I remember looking for a pediatrician. I told her Rayven was vegan. She stopped attending to my daughter, and turned to me and exclaimed, "it's ok if she doesn't eat meat, but she needs to drink milk." This brought on a heated conversation. I left her office and never went back. From then on, I have chosen to stay far away from doctors unless needed. Rayven was the easiest baby. She had a fever twice that I treated with Tempra. She slept right through the night as soon as she was five months old. I never feared that she wasn't getting enough of anything. I just fed her healthy vegan food.

Something else to note is that protein deficiency is virtually unheard of in the West. I knew that if she ate enough calories, she would get enough protein.

She's an extremely talented visual artist and she blows my mind with her work. She graduated high school with honors. She has taken a gap year to travel with me, and in September, she will be attending university and majoring in psychology. She is my pride and joy, and living proof that causing suffering and death to others is not necessary for humans to thrive.

I believe most of our decisions are ruled by fear and that animal agriculture has us very fearful. They have us believe that we need milk for strong bones and flesh for muscles. I got so tired of answering people when they asked me where I got my protein, my reply was, "from puppies. I eat puppies." At other times I would say, "I don't get enough protein. I should be dead but instead, I'm running marathons. Go figure!"

This is a wonderful time to be alive. When I went vegan in 1993, the only options I had was bad soy milk and tofu. I remember when almond milk made its debut. It was so expensive that I didn't buy it for quite some time. It's been a pleasure seeing every kind of product like turkey, cheesecake, ice cream, and cheese being offered. It is a joy to see so many vegan restaurants popping up. Toronto has its own area called Vegandale now, with retail outlets, restaurants and pubs that are all vegan. My hope is that if I do not live long enough to see a vegan world, my daughter will.

Let our food choices be made with our hearts, not with our stomachs.

RAYVEN RIGATO-CONDE
(VICTORIA'S DAUGHTER)

CONNECT WITH RAYVEN:
INSTAGRAM: @RAYYVVEN

"Most people are absolutely shocked when I tell them I've been vegan since birth. It's as if the concept of someone never eating meat or dairy seems so impossible to society. I've been receiving the same reactions from people my entire life, but I am proud of being able to say that I've never consumed animal products."

Born in 2000 and vegan since birth, Rayven Rigato-Conde knows first-hand what it's like to be surrounded by peers who do not understand her personal food choices.

WHAT IS ONE OF THE BEST OR MOST WORTHWHILE HEALTH-RELATED INVESTMENTS THAT YOU HAVE MADE?

I am personally a big fan of the Yonanas machine; it basically makes ice cream out of frozen fruit. Now, at first, I know this doesn't sound anywhere near as satisfying as soy ice cream or whatever you enjoy, but trust me, it is honestly delicious. I usually use frozen bananas and strawberries, but plain frozen bananas also makes good ice cream! You can honestly use any fruit you want with bananas as the main base. Also, Hershey's chocolate sauce is vegan, and that drizzled on top is super good.

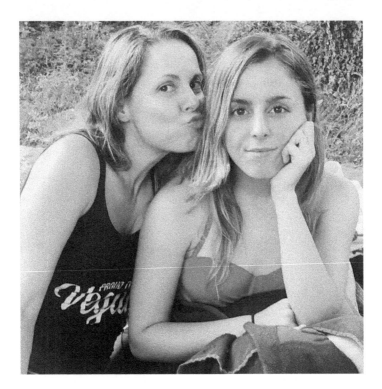

AT WHAT POINT IN YOUR LIFE DID YOU DECIDE TO CHANGE YOUR DIET? HOW HAS THAT DECISION IMPACTED YOUR LIFE?

I never made a transition into veganism, because I was born into it. I was born in the summer of 2000, and all I've ever known is a vegan lifestyle. When I was a little girl, my mother showed me slaughterhouse footage and told me about the cruelties of the meat and dairy industry. In all honesty, I do not remember much of my upbringing regarding being vegan, because it was my norm and still is. I always thought it was odd or illogical to consume animal products. In the mind of someone who never got accustomed or addicted to it, it always just seemed like a weird thing to do.

However, the moments I do remember the most from my childhood are all of the criticisms and feeling like an outcast. When I was in elementary school and middle school, most people had no idea what the word vegan even meant. I remember having to explain what it was very often. My friends did not really understand why I did not eat like them or like everybody else, and the only reasoning my younger self ever knew, was simply that I did not want to eat dead animals. But that reason on its own was and is, enough.

Of course, as I grew older I was able to understand why my mother raised me like this and why I wanted to continue for myself. In school, I found myself feeling like I needed to explain myself and defend why I eat the way I do to avoid judgment. I even felt awkward or out of place when my friends would share their snacks or when someone brought in homemade sweets for their birthday for the class to eat because I could never join in. It would make any kid sad to see the whole class eat cake without you. It did bother me and upset me a little, but at the same time, I knew my own morals, and I knew that those desserts were made possible by the suffering of animals.

On the other hand, my family has been making jabs and jokes about me being vegan for as long as I can remember. That is just what comes with this lifestyle; people are going to judge you, question you and make fun of you, maybe even be rude to you. I try to avoid conflict with people so I don't really even mention veganism unless someone asks me or I'm in a situation where I feel inclined to speak up.

Over the years, I've learned that most people do not want to hear about being vegan, or where their food comes from, or how it's killing our planet. Calling someone's actions wrong or suggesting change makes people uncomfortable and quite often hostile as well, which is a pretty expected reaction. But you can honestly tell a lot about a person's character based on their reaction to telling them you are vegan. It really shows who is open-minded and willing to educate themselves on the impact of their actions versus who's not, in my opinion.

WHO HAS BEEN THE BIGGEST VEGAN INFLUENCER IN YOUR LIFE AND HOW HAVE THEY HELPED YOU?

The biggest influencer as a vegan has been, of course, my mother, since she raised me into this lifestyle. She's educated me on it and spoken up for me when needed. When I was younger, a lot of adults in my mother's life would criticize her for raising me vegan and how it's not healthy. She would always defend me and her choices. She's shown me a lot of documentaries and videos that have solidified my opinions on being vegan and have further allowed me to understand why I want to continue this lifestyle forever. Most notable is the documentary Cowspiracy, which is available on Netflix. Also, as I was emerging into my teen years, she has introduced me to a lot of recipes and foods to make on my own.

HOW DO YOU THINK WE CAN ALL HAVE A BIGGER IMPACT ON INFLUENCING PEOPLE AND HELPING THEM MAKE THE CONNECTION TO HEALTH AND EATING A PLANT-BASED DIET?

As much as we want to start shooting information and facts out of our mouth about the meat and dairy industry when speaking to a non-vegan, I really think having a patient, mature and classy method of communication is what will get us the furthest in terms of educating others. So when it comes to talking to someone, first of all they need to already be open-minded or else the conversation will not go anywhere. Instead of telling people what they're doing is wrong, I think the smartest approach is to tell them what is happening to these animals, all the cruelties and horrors explained. Tell people our demand for meat and dairy is bad for our planet, how it is completely unsustainable and depleting our resources and our personal health. Offer resources and other places to learn about it, whether it is through YouTube, documentaries, articles or a book. Once we share this information, then we can ask people what they're going to do about it. Ask them what choice they are going to make every day for the rest of their lives when they pick up their forks and knives.

Other than a one-on-one conversation with people, other ways to share the awareness is, of course, through being an advocate. Posting about it on social media, suggesting things for people to try or watch. Going to public talks about it, participating in protests and events. I truly believe as time continues to pass veganism is just going to keep flourishing and growing in popularity, because that is already what's been happening over the last decade.

WHAT WAS THE REACTION YOU RECEIVED FROM PEOPLE WHEN YOU ANNOUNCED THAT YOU WERE GOING VEGAN? WHO WAS YOUR BEST AND WORST SUPPORTER?

Most people are absolutely shocked when I tell them I've been vegan since birth. It's as if the concept of someone never eating meat or dairy seems so impossible to society. I've been receiving the same reactions from people my entire life, but I am proud of being able to say that I've never consumed animal products. I'd say the most negative reactions have come from conversations with classmates or my family at dinner.

Throughout elementary and middle school, people did not harshly criticize me, which was probably because my peers and I were still fairly young and they did not have premeditated opinions about veganism. Throughout high school was when I experienced the most teasing in the cafeteria, usually through classmates or mutual friends. People would taunt me with their meat by waving it in front of me or make remarks like, "you don't know what you're missing." Or, they would really emphasize words like "yum" or "mmmm." Or I'd get lots of comments about how my food was "fake" or wasn't healthy, or how it was just a copy of their foods, and they'd argue that veganism isn't original. I know they'd only do it to get a reaction out of me, but it kind of came to the point where I was numb to those things because people have been making small jabs like that at me all my life.

A lot of people like to find any reason they can to be against veganism and tend to forget the main reason people actually go vegan: to reduce the suffering of animals and to reduce their environmental footprint. At family dinners, I also found my uncles and aunts trying to pressure me into eating meat when they knew I had no interest. People often discuss the stereotype with me that vegans push their views onto others, however, in my experience, I've been in plenty of situations where people judge me or tease me without seeing any harm done. But the instant I say something to defend myself, suddenly I'm the pushy one and no one wants to hear my "vegan propaganda."

I don't really judge others when they get personally offended because how else would you react when someone tells you something you've been doing all your life is wrong? But when my friends or anyone else is literally shown the truth, or I tell them about it and they are completely opposed to learning about what they are contributing to within their diets, I just find it sad and disappointing. I feel the reason some vegans can be "pushy" really has to do with their passion for animal welfare and promoting positive change. We know there is something very ethically and environmentally wrong with dairy farms and factory farms, and we know as humans that we have a moral responsibility to do better when we can. When our planet is facing this massive issue in which each individual could make a huge difference by simply changing their eating habit, we feel inclined to tell people about it and hope they'll want to go vegan too.

354

HOW HAS A FAILURE, OR APPARENT FAILURE, SET YOU UP FOR LATER SUCCESS? DO YOU HAVE A "FAVORITE FAILURE" OF YOURS?

When it comes to being vegan, I think it's normal for anyone to have slip-ups. For example, you may accidentally eat something with dairy, eat that piece of chocolate every once in a while, or buy that nice pair of leather shoes. We are not perfect, after all. That isn't to say that we should be excusing these mistakes or thinking they aren't a big deal either. I know in my personal experience, instances like these only lead to guilt building up until I really digest what I am doing and stop.

For example, when I was a child, one of the main things I struggled with was candy. Gelatin is in nearly everything that isn't chocolate, and this only made my Halloween earnings even smaller. As a child, it's sad enough seeing your candy split in half because of the chocolate, but when a third of the gummies have gelatin, it really sucks. Back then, I knew a lot of the chewy candy I was eating had gelatin like the classic gummy worms or teddy bears, starburst, and the gummy burgers/fries. I still ate it and felt guilty, but I still did it.

Thankfully, the majority of Maynard's candies, the biggest gummy company I know, are vegan! Also, my grandmother used to make me an apple cake, and she used eggs, and I would still eat it because I loved it so much. Of course, around the time I was in middle school, I would have instances where I'd refuse to eat gelatin candy, and then other times I'd find myself caving in. It really just was a progression of time, guilt and regret until I made the decision to stop eating things for my taste buds and to stop going against what I preach. Around the time I was about 12, I fully stopped consuming those products, and now I enjoy my Maynard's in peace and my grandma hasn't baked that cake in years.

WHAT ADVICE WOULD YOU GIVE A SMART AND DRIVEN 18-YEAR-OLD TODAY? WHAT ADVICE SHOULD THEY IGNORE?

I'm not sure I'm in the position to answer this because frankly, I am also an 18-year-old that appreciates some good advice. Everyone needs guidance and feels a little lost at times. I would tell somebody my age to be open-minded, to stop judging before actually knowing the reality. To have the heart and courage to look at yourself in the mirror and look for ways to improve your character. To not be afraid of trying new things or taking risks sometimes. Show yourself for who you really are and be as authentic as possible, because having authenticity makes you proud of who you are and makes you a genuine person. I also think people in general, are quick to jump to conclusions about other people based on their behavior or brief encounters, but we never really know what anyone else is going through. That is why we should be kind and supportive of one another. It sounds cheesy, but it is true. If one of my friends or peers wanted to go vegan and was afraid of judgment or had unsupportive parents, I'd say all you can do is be confident and passionate in what you believe in and try your best to follow through.

Sometimes teens that are living with their parents struggle to transition because their parents are so against veganism. In that case, I'd recommend trying to reach a compromise or offering to cook for yourself when you can. Perhaps taking the meat off your plate as a first step. Work towards it and don't get discouraged by your parents, because eventually you will have the complete freedom to decide what you eat and they will have to accept it. When it comes to friends, if your friends are insulting you or questioning your decisions, you need to either put them in their place or distance yourself from them. Friends should be supportive of your lifestyle and should be able to come from a place of understanding. It's tough being young in our society where there is so much pressure to be "good enough," to be liked, or pretty, or original, or smart or talented. All I can say is being yourself is enough, and stay true to your morals.

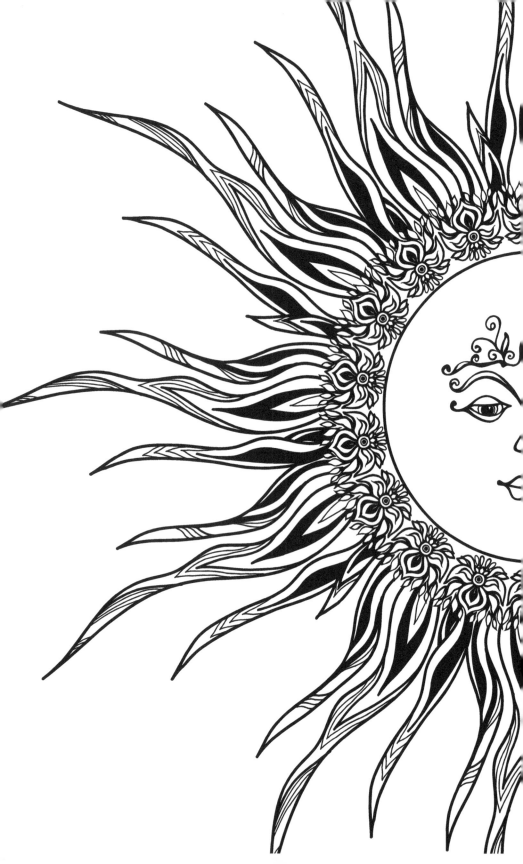

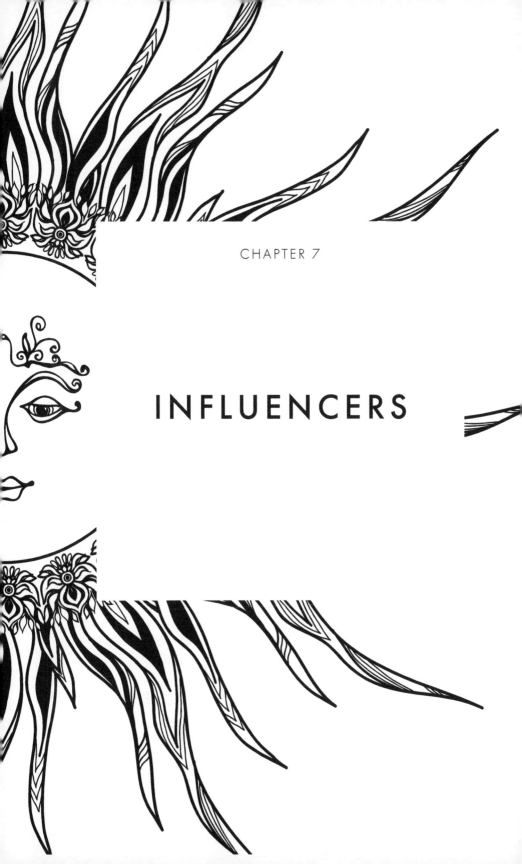

CHAPTER 7

INFLUENCERS

BLUE OLLIS

CONNECT WITH BLUE:
INSTAGRAM: @BLUEOLLIS
FACEBOOK: BLUEOLLISBLOG
YOUTUBE: BLUE OLLIS
BlueOllis.com

Blue Ollis is an animal rights activist and plant-based eating social media influencer, who inspires her audience by sharing how making the switch to veganism has positively impacted her life.

"I have been vegan for seven years now, and when I announced I was going vegan my brother automatically said he would follow suit and do it too and it wasn't long after that, that my Mum decided to join us. This has been life-changing for our family.

Self-education, alongside a support system, is the best thing you can do. Also, do what you love to do to make your activism sustainable. Find what you're good at and make it your unique form of outreach."

358

WHAT IS ONE OF THE BEST OR MOST WORTHWHILE HEALTH-RELATED INVESTMENTS THAT YOU HAVE MADE?

Definitely my food processor! I can make anything with that bad boy, from pesto and hummus to bliss balls and ice cream (you can find all of these recipes in my recipe ebook available for download on my blog).

AT WHAT POINT IN YOUR LIFE DID YOU DECIDE TO CHANGE YOUR DIET? HOW HAS THAT DECISION IMPACTED YOUR LIFE?

I have always been a keen questioner so inevitably, I began questioning my food more, and questioning where it came from. Learning about the dairy industry was life-changing and completely eye-opening. I have never been able to look at dairy in the same way. I enjoy my food now more than ever, knowing exactly how it got to me and what good it does my body.

WHO HAS BEEN THE BIGGEST PLANT-BASED INFLUENCER IN YOUR LIFE AND HOW HAVE THEY HELPED YOU?

Definitely vegan activists who take to the streets and to the slaughterhouses to expose the atrocities and exploitation that go on behind closed doors. They have taught me how important it is to be active as a vegan and to help spread the knowledge while empowering people to make healthier and more compassionate choices for themselves and others. These people are truly selfless and inspire me every day to do more for the movement.

HOW DO YOU THINK WE CAN ALL HAVE A BIGGER IMPACT ON INFLUENCING PEOPLE AND HELPING THEM MAKE THE CONNECTION TO HEALTH AND EATING A PLANT-BASED DIET?

There are so many ways we can help the movement grow. Do what you're good at and what you love, whether it's vegan art, poetry, public speaking, recipe creation, baking or music. There's something for everyone to get involved in and a way for all to impact others.

WHAT WAS THE REACTION YOU RECEIVED FROM PEOPLE WHEN YOU ANNOUNCED THAT YOU WERE GOING VEGAN? WHO WAS YOUR BEST AND WORST SUPPORTER?

When I announced I was going vegan, my brother automatically said he would follow suit and do it too. Then my Mum wanted to join us, and we created a Facebook page where we shared recipes and information we found along the way. It was outside of my family that I received the most judgment, which was mostly from strangers. People often respond defensively because they feel the guilt inside of them coming to the surface. This is more motivation to keep educating so that these people can find peace and harmony with their morals and align them with their actions.

HOW HAS A FAILURE, OR APPARENT FAILURE, SET YOU UP FOR LATER SUCCESS? DO YOU HAVE A "FAVORITE FAILURE" OF YOURS?

My favorite "failure" is my highly-sensitive nature. I'm incredibly empathic and this often leads to heightened emotions, especially surrounding injustices. I used to think this was a weakness and something to hide from others, but I've recently learned to embrace it and use it as a tool to share impactful messages about veganism through written word, art and video content. My sensitive nature is my strength and a true gift.

WHICH VEGAN RESOURCE COULD YOU NOT LIVE WITHOUT AND WHY?

There are so many powerful resources around veganism, so it's difficult to pick just one. *The China Study* and *How Not To Die* alongside the website *NutritionFacts.org*, are fantastic for health and wellness facts from a collation of the largest scientific studies. Truly fantastic if you're wanting to up your health game! Jonathan Safran Foer's, *Eating Animals*, and Peter Singer's, *Animal Liberation*, are important books surrounding ethics and our choices surrounding eating animals.

" "

USE YOUR GIFTS

TO INSPIRE OTHERS
AND LIFT OTHERS UP.
WHEN WE USE OUR
GIFTS IN THIS WAY,
WE HEAL THE WORLD,
AND WE HEAL
OURSELVES.

EMMA FRETTS

CAROLINE DEISLER

CONNECT WITH CAROLINE:
INSTAGRAM:@CAROLINEDEISLER
FACEBOOK: CAROLINE'S CHOICE
YOUTUBE: CAROLINE DEISLER
carolineschoice.com

"Being a full-time model in NYC, I was close to a mental breakdown due to the pressure of being extremely skinny. I needed a lifestyle and diet change to find balance again, and I thought I would find that by choosing to go plant-based, which was totally the case. No more calorie counting and no more emotional eating. Instead, I am celebrating the power of whole, fresh fruits and vegetables every single day."

Caroline Deisler is a certified nutritionist, former model, blogger, and popular plant-based social media influencer. Caroline uses her platform to inspire her audience to discover the healthful benefits of choosing to eat plant-based and the importance of focusing on "how you feel" instead of "how to lose weight."

361

WHO HAS BEEN THE BIGGEST PLANT-BASED INFLUENCER IN YOUR LIFE AND HOW HAVE THEY HELPED YOU?

I must say I have always followed my own journey and didn't follow any exact diet from other influencers. However, some of my favorite Instagrammers are @Earthyandy, @fullyrawkristina, @medicalmedium, @elsas_wholesomelife, @deliciouslyella, and @therawboy.

HOW DO YOU THINK WE CAN ALL HAVE A BIGGER IMPACT ON INFLUENCING PEOPLE AND HELPING THEM MAKE THE CONNECTION TO HEALTH AND EATING A PLANT-BASED DIET?

I think being a shining example is the way to go. Don't preach or criticize people; just live your life the way you believe is the best and others will be inspired by seeing how happy and healthy it makes you.

IF YOU COULD HAVE A GIGANTIC BILLBOARD ANYWHERE WITH ANYTHING ON IT, WHAT WOULD IT SAY?

Start NOW! It's never too late.

HOW HAS A FAILURE, OR APPARENT FAILURE, SET YOU UP FOR LATER SUCCESS? DO YOU HAVE A "FAVORITE FAILURE" OF YOURS?

To be honest, I think my success is pretty much based on my failures. I grew up feeling like I wanted to prove to everyone around me what I was capable of doing, since I felt like I never had people believing in me.

WHAT VEGAN RESOURCE COULD YOU NOT LIVE WITHOUT AND WHY?

I love the books, *The China Study*, *Medical Medium*, and the podcast *Plant Proof*.

WHAT ADVICE WOULD YOU GIVE A SMART AND DRIVEN 18-YEAR-OLD TODAY? WHAT ADVICE SHOULD THEY IGNORE?

1.) Only seek advice from successful people.
2.) Eat healthy, workout and meditate. The earlier you start taking care of yourself, the better.
3.) Surround yourself with honest, authentic, passionate people who bring out the best in you.
4.) Focus on what makes you happy, don't be afraid to follow whatever that is.

ANY INSPIRING STORIES THAT HAVE HAPPENED TO YOU OR PEOPLE CLOSE TO YOU THAT HAVE NOT BEEN COVERED ABOVE. STORIES THAT CAN HELP OTHERS.

When I was 19 and had just finished high school, my dream was to move to New York. I worked everywhere I could to save money to book a flight and survive the first few months. I found an apartment online, had no idea which area it was in, and didn't know anybody, but I was so determined to fulfill my dream. I went to every single modeling agency in New York with the hope of finding one that believed in me. That journey opened so many doors for me even though I'm not modeling anymore. I learned so much from just following my dream, not being scared of failure and proving to myself that I could do anything I wanted to do. Never be afraid of failure!! Whatever you think you can do, you can!

EMMA FRETTS

CONNECT WITH EMMA:
INSTAGRAM: @EMMA FRETTS

Emma Fretts is a musician, social media influencer, and plant-based eating advocate who inspires her followers through her music, plant-based recipes and downloadable content, such as her "Inspiration E-Journal."

"I'd begun living a plant-based lifestyle around the age of 18, but at the time it was only a facade for a restrictive diet. As we all know by now, restrictive diets never last, and I ended up reverting back to the standard American diet until I was 21. At that point, similar to so many others, I made the ethical connection by watching a few documentaries about the brutal truth behind the animal agriculture industry, and I went vegan overnight. I haven't looked back since. The more plants I eat the happier I am. Every day just gets better!"

WHAT IS ONE OF THE BEST OR MOST WORTHWHILE HEALTH-RELATED INVESTMENTS THAT YOU HAVE MADE?

Hiring a life coach has been one of the greatest health investments and gifts that I have ever given myself. Having someone to help me shift and rewire my mindset from one of self-sabotage to one of self-love in a way that made me feel celebrated and empowered, opened the doors for me to experience not only positive mental health, but physical health as well.

WHO HAS BEEN THE BIGGEST PLANT-BASED INFLUENCER IN YOUR LIFE AND HOW HAVE THEY HELPED YOU?

Claire Michelle (@plantifulsoul) was the main YouTuber I was watching when I went vegan. She and her friends in the vegan community were very outspoken about going vegan, how easy and fun it can be, and all of the beautiful benefits to be received by the lifestyle. She made me feel less alone every time I watched her videos. Even when my family or friends argued with me about it, rejected the idea, tried to prove me wrong, or told me not to talk about it openly, I felt like I always had someone I could connect with online who understood, even if I didn't know her personally.

HOW DO YOU THINK WE CAN ALL HAVE A BIGGER IMPACT ON INFLUENCING PEOPLE AND HELPING THEM MAKE THE CONNECTION

TO HEALTH AND EATING A PLANT-BASED DIET?

I think there are many different ways to make an impact. Some people are in the position to talk openly about it because their family or friends are receptive to the idea. Some people are better off modeling the plant-based lifestyle (rather than persuading others) if they are surrounded by people who reject the idea and attack their beliefs. And some influencers have a platform or an audience on whom they can have a great effect by powerfully sharing their choice to be plant-based and educating their audience.
It's all about feeling out your situation and being compassionate towards the opinions and beliefs of others as well, even in the face of resistance.

WHAT WAS THE REACTION YOU RECEIVED FROM PEOPLE WHEN YOU ANNOUNCED THAT YOU WERE EATING A PLANT-BASED DIET?

Initially, I received a lot of judgment because it was so radically opposed to the lifestyle of the people closest to me. My family made fun of me, rejected me, argued with me and tried to prove me wrong. My boss at the time told me I could not talk about it publicly online because she taught against it and it could look bad to the potential clients of hers who knew I worked for her. My sister always supported me and had my back when others attacked me. It took years of me patiently educating those closest to me and modeling how beneficial it is. Now everyone in my life has accepted my lifestyle - my sister has even gone vegetarian!

THERE ARE SOME PEOPLE WHO DON'T LIKE TO USE THE WORD VEGAN. DO YOU USE BOTH THE TERM "VEGAN" AND "PLANT-BASED," OR ARE YOU STRICTLY ONE OR THE OTHER AND WHY?

I use both. I know that they are different, but in my experience, it can be beneficial to use one over the other depending on the audience.

My extended family are hunters, so to hear the word "vegan" sounds radical and foreign to them. The majority of things they've heard about veganism probably has something to do with negatively-viewed PETA demonstrations in the news. Around them, it's best to use the term "plant-based," because it has no preconceived notions attached.

Other times, it's beneficial to use the term "vegan" because there's strength in numbers. The movement is growing, and people identify with it positively these days!

IF YOU COULD DO ONE THING DIFFERENTLY FROM YOUR PAST FIVE YEARS, WHAT WOULD IT BE?

I would stop putting my heart in everyone else's hands and understand that

I am worthy of giving myself the love that I so desperately gave to everyone else in hopes of being loved in return. I've always had the love inside of me; I just never gave it to myself.

WHAT VEGAN RESOURCE COULD YOU NOT LIVE WITHOUT AND WHY?

My journal. It is the ultimate source of self-growth for me. Every day for six months I wrote down everything I was proud of myself for, everything I accomplished, proof that I was getting closer to the life I wanted for myself, and one person I forgave and why. At the end of the six months, I was a completely changed person for the better. There's no book that I've read yet that has had this profound effect on me.

WHAT ADVICE WOULD YOU GIVE A SMART AND DRIVEN 18-YEAR-OLD TODAY? WHAT ADVICE SHOULD THEY IGNORE?

Listen to your intuition and go for it, even if you don't know how it's going to work out. Even if you're terrified. Even if you aren't the most talented or the most beautiful. Even if you have zero followers and no experience. Even if no one else believes in you. None of that matters because you are in charge of your life and if you truly understand that and put yourself out there, you will get where you want to be.

Learn from people who are already doing what you want to do. You can truly do anything as long as you believe in yourself and push past your comfort zone because that's where your greatness lies and it's waiting to see how high you'll jump to reach it.

ANY INSPIRING STORIES THAT HAVE HAPPENED TO YOU OR PEOPLE CLOSE TO YOU THAT HAVE NOT BEEN COVERED ABOVE. STORIES THAT CAN HELP OTHERS.

You only have 90 (give or take) years to play on this Earth. If you have a dream, do not give up on it. When I was 18, I was so afraid to chase my dream of being a singer/songwriter that I stopped singing, hid out, and gave up for four years. In that time, I was plagued with so much disappointment, self-hatred, and self-sabotage that my body began to physically give out - to the point of me being rushed to the hospital, minutes away from dying. It took all of that for me to realize that if I didn't chase my dream, the pain of regret would literally kill me. The fear of going for it is scary, but the anxiety and regret of not going for it is infinitely worse. This life can be magical and beautiful and insane if you are willing to say yes to your calling, even if you are trembling while living it out! Use your gifts to inspire others and lift them up. When we use our gifts in this way, we heal the world, and we heal ourselves.

DANIELLE ARSENAULT

CONNECT WITH DANIELLE:
INSTAGRAM: @PACHAVEGA
FACEBOOK: @RAWVEGANCHEF / @PACHAVEGALIVING
YOUTUBE: PACHAVEGA LIVING FOODS EDUCATION
pachavega.com

Danielle Arsenault is a raw food chef, Spanish teacher, world traveler, author, environmentalist, plant-based nutrition expert and lifestyle coach. A near-death rock climbing experience forever changed Danielle's relationship with the world as she knew it, and is what inspired Danielle to begin to take control of her health, not take it for granted and share her discoveries of the benefits of plant-based eating with the rest of the world.

"When I arrived at the hospital after a grueling ride in an ambulance on a bumpy country road, I was rushed into emergency pneumo-thoracic surgery to repair the hole in my lung. 40 minutes later, success. I was breathing oxygen and fluid was draining through a tube inserted into my lungs. In the days that followed, I began to heal. I had a lot of time to contemplate life and all the "what if's." What if I didn't cover my head, would I have died? What if I didn't have a climbing partner who caught the fall so well? What if I had gone to climb in a different area that day? Regardless of these questions, I was given another chance. The universe gave me a little reminder... PS, you are ALIVE. You have the opportunity to follow your dreams. There is no time like the present, and there may not be a tomorrow. What are you waiting for? The rest, as they say, is history."

WHAT IS ONE OF THE BEST OR MOST WORTHWHILE HEALTH-RELATED INVESTMENTS THAT YOU HAVE MADE?

The best health-related investment I've ever made was deciding that after ten years of traveling the world, exploring different cultures and teaching English, to shift my focus towards my real passion and go study at the Ann Wigmore Institute in Puerto Rico. That decision forever changed the trajectory of my life towards a life of abundance in health and happiness. The day that I learned that we have the power to heal our bodies with food was the day that everything changed.

AT WHAT POINT IN YOUR LIFE DID YOU DECIDE TO CHANGE YOUR DIET? HOW HAS THAT DECISION IMPACTED YOUR LIFE?

The defining moment for me was over 12 years ago while living in Mexico, rock climbing every weekend, and teaching English. I attended a PETA conference in Monterrey, Nuevo León, one of which exposed me to the violence within the animal industry. The unspoken cruelty that I had seen was something that I could never unsee. For me, ending the life of a sentient creature - especially in the horrible ways that large food companies do - just for the pleasure of my taste buds really wasn't worth it. The impact it left on me was profound. In the twelve years that followed, including today, I still feel a deeper sense of connection to the planet and all of the living things on it. This sense of harmony in the community gives me a greater sense of ease as my life unfolds.

WHO HAS BEEN THE BIGGEST PLANT-BASED INFLUENCER IN YOUR LIFE AND HOW HAVE THEY HELPED YOU?

I have met many people throughout my journey towards a plant-based lifestyle. I've also walked the path alone for many years. My belief in the peacefulness of a plant-based diet and how it has the power of positivity fused into the living cells of the living plants we eat has carried me through uncomfortable conversations and inspired others. Those whom I've looked up to from a distance include the late and great Ann Wigmore, especially the way in which she gave hope to all those she met and served her unbiased love, and how she strived to help the people of the world with their illnesses through the consumption of wheatgrass, sprouts and fermented foods. I have also been inspired by Vesanto Melina and Brenda Davis who co-wrote the books "Becoming Vegan" and "Becoming Raw." They really shine a light on the nutrition behind the food. Rich Roll and his amazing podcast and all the inspirational plant-based athletes he has as guests have also been such huge inspirations. I love Rich's continual deep dive into self-actualization and how plants can fuel us as athletes. These people and their messages match mine. We all share the same vision: to improve the lives of individuals by empowering them to become the best versions of themselves with love and with delicious, whole, plant-based foods.

367

IF YOU COULD HAVE A GIGANTIC BILLBOARD ANYWHERE WITH ANYTHING ON IT, WHAT WOULD IT SAY?

I would write two things: "It's not about what you do occasionally, it's about what you do consistently" and, to quote Ann Wigmore herself, "the food you eat can be either the slowest poison or the most powerful medicine." At the bottom of that billboard would be a call to action: to make the move and come meet me in Nicaragua to learn how easy it is to shift your life towards a plant-powered inspired lifestyle that will elevate your stoke and offer motivation to feel amazing!

HOW HAS A FAILURE, OR APPARENT FAILURE, SET YOU UP FOR LATER SUCCESS? DO YOU HAVE A "FAVORITE FAILURE" OF YOURS?

Haha! Good question. What is failure really? I see failures as opportunities to improve, learn and keep going. Failures are the zest of life. If everything always went according to plan and was perfectly executed, how could you ever really know if you are doing it right? In order to know if you are following your path, you inevitably have to make mistakes that keep you on your toes. I think it's not about the failure itself, but the aftermath. When you fall, do you get up? And how fast? Are you resilient? Can you see the lesson in the mistake and then grow from it? I think when you know you are on the right path, failures are just stepping stones to greater success. Looking back, those stepping stones only make us stronger. They are there to challenge us, to make us question our path.

A VEGAN RESOURCE YOU COULD NOT LIVE WITHOUT AND WHY?

In the literal sense of it, I could live without anything. I'm a minimalist. However, in the metaphorical sense of the term, the most influential books I have come across include the I Ching, Paul Pitchford's, Healing with Whole-Foods, Rebecca Wood's The New Whole-Foods Encyclopedia, Rich Roll's podcast, Tim Ferriss's, Tools for Titans, Gretchen Rubin's, The Four Tendencies, Dr. Wayne Dyer's, Change Your Thoughts, Change Your Life, Heather Ash Amara's, Warrior Goddess Training, and The Four Agreements by Don Miguel Ruiz. Why? Well, as diverse as I am, I could not just choose one book or influencer. Each of these books has a continual influence on my life. The messages within are my collective mantra. They all have something to teach me.

WHAT ADVICE WOULD YOU GIVE A SMART AND DRIVEN 18-YEAR-OLD TODAY? WHAT ADVICE SHOULD THEY IGNORE?

Follow your heart. Listen to your intuition and if you ever have the choice to be right or to be kind, choose to be kind (as per Dr. Wayne Dyer's orders). Avoid what you know to be wrong, and say a firm, yet respectful, "no." Be kind to those who need it most and live to serve. The meaning and purpose of life will be much more fulfilling when you do things for others without a need for anything in return.

ANY INSPIRING STORIES THAT HAVE HAPPENED TO YOU OR PEOPLE CLOSE TO YOU THAT HAVE NOT BEEN COVERED ABOVE. STORIES THAT CAN HELP OTHERS.

Rock climbing is a big passion of mine, just as much as a plant-based lifestyle. In 2011, I had a very traumatic climbing accident that left me breathing through a tube in a Turkish hospital. Trying to climb along a traverse, I found myself exhausted and decided to fall deliberately rather than lose control. It was going to be the biggest fall I had ever taken on a rope, but I trusted my climbing partner whom I had just met four days prior. It was terrifying. I took a deep breath and let go; my body was falling for 20 feet before the rope went taut, wrapped behind my leg and then flipped me upside down, smashing my upper back against the rock.

I wasn't wearing a helmet (and I know that you should always wear a helmet) so I put my hands up to protect my head. It was my ribs that received the impact and cracked like dry twigs. My lung had punctured and collapsed. As I was lowered down to the ground, I was faced with the reality that my partner and I had to self-rescue and get ourselves down the mountain as my lungs filled with blood and body fluids.

When I arrived at the hospital after a grueling ride in an ambulance on a bumpy country road, I was rushed into emergency pneumo-thoracic surgery to repair the hole in my lung. 40 minutes later, success. I was breathing oxygen and fluid was draining through a tube inserted into my lungs. In the days that followed, I began to heal. I had a lot of time to contemplate life and all the "what if's." What if I didn't cover my head, would I have died? What if I didn't have a climbing partner who caught the fall so well? What if I had gone to climb in a different area that day? Regardless of these questions, I was given another chance. The universe gave me a little reminder... PS, you are ALIVE. You have the opportunity to follow your dreams. There is no time like the present, and there may not be a tomorrow. What are you waiting for? The rest, as they say, is history.

I'm so happy to be alive. Many people don't even realize they are alive and that their life is what they make of it. It's the choices we make and the thoughts we think and the company we keep. It's the work we put in and the struggles we endure and the love that we give. This is the one chance we've got in this life. What is the legacy that you want to leave behind? What is the purpose that drives you?

369

VALERIA REY

CONNECT WITH VALERIA:
INSTAGRAM: @VALERIA.REY
YOUTUBE: VALERIA
blissfulval.com

Valeria is a plant-based social media influencer with a quarter of a million followers on Instagram. She's worked with brands such as Four Sigmatics, Uber Eats, Starbucks and Nature's Way and is the author of a plant-based cookbook *Blissful Val: A Journey Through Food*, featuring recipes, tips and motivation for transitioning to a plant-based lifestyle.

WHAT IS ONE OF THE BEST OR MOST WORTHWHILE HEALTH-RELATED INVESTMENTS THAT YOU HAVE MADE?

Definitely my Vitamix and my Hurom Juicer. They're a big investment, but they will last you forever, plus they are things that you will be able to use every day. I use it for things like smoothies, juices and banana ice cream. I highly recommend these items to everyone looking to get healthier or wanting to make more at-home meals.

AT WHAT POINT IN YOUR LIFE DID YOU DECIDE TO CHANGE YOUR DIET? HOW HAS THAT DECISION IMPACTED YOUR LIFE?

The defining moment was while I was watching the movie Okja on Netflix. It just clicked for me then, and I told my partner that tomorrow I was going to be vegan. I have never looked back since.

WHO HAS BEEN THE BIGGEST PLANT-BASED INFLUENCER IN YOUR LIFE AND HOW HAVE THEY HELPED YOU?

Honestly, I don't follow or take advice from any plant-based influencers. The people that were really game-changers for me made me realize that veganism is not so much about me, but actually about the animals. Vegan activists such as James Aspey, Gary Yourofsky and Earthling Ed really inspired me. Their YouTube videos were so educating and mind-blowing

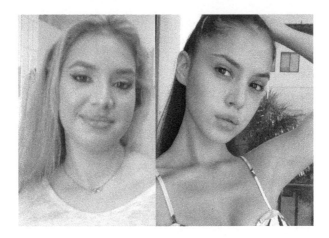

because you really start to see the world from a different perspective: one of compassion for ALL living beings, not just for humans.

HOW DO YOU THINK WE CAN ALL HAVE A BIGGER IMPACT ON INFLUENCING PEOPLE AND HELPING THEM MAKE THE CONNECTION TO HEALTH AND EATING A PLANT-BASED DIET?

I believe that everyone can influence someone; you don't have to be an influencer or a celebrity. I have experienced this with my own family as well. They're not vegan yet, but I can feel that they're more aware of what they're actually putting into their bodies than they were before, and this was influenced partly by me showing up and explicitly asking for a vegan meal or even bringing my own vegan meals to a family gathering. You gotta take baby steps and plant seeds along the way, but I believe that all the hard work and the difficult discussions about veganism will be worth it one day.

IF YOU COULD HAVE A GIGANTIC BILLBOARD ANYWHERE WITH ANYTHING ON IT, WHAT WOULD IT SAY?

Your body is a garden, not a graveyard.

HOW HAS A FAILURE, OR APPARENT FAILURE, SET YOU UP FOR LATER SUCCESS? DO YOU HAVE A "FAVORITE FAILURE" OF YOURS?

When I first went vegan and was starting to watch videos from these vegan activists, I was trying to make everyone go vegan (including my partner and my parents), and it did not work at all. It mostly just caused me pain because I set something in my mind that wasn't possible. Of course I was getting disappointed. In the end I learned that I should just lead by being an example, meaning cooking vegan meals and sharing with my family and friends and talking positively about how veganism has changed my life. After a year, my boyfriend has now turned vegan!

A VEGAN RESOURCE YOU COULD YOU NOT LIVE WITHOUT AND WHY?

I don't have a particular book or person I couldn't live without and I honestly don't think that we should have someone or something we could not live without. People change, and things lose meaning and value throughout the years. I am constantly educating myself and reminding myself why I'm living this lifestyle. It's ultimately for the animals, but the great thing is that you get a lot of bonuses from it, like helping the environment and getting healthier!

WHAT ADVICE WOULD YOU GIVE A SMART AND DRIVEN 18-YEAR-OLD TODAY? WHAT ADVICE SHOULD THEY IGNORE?

Follow the advice that makes sense to you. Around that age, I heard about so many different diets (like the keto or paleo diet) and honestly, there just wasn't anything about these that made sense to me. However, once I came across the vegan documentaries on Netflix like Cowspiracy, What the Health and Forks Over Knives, I immediately knew that this was the right thing to do.

Since I was a kid, I felt like there was something wrong with eating eggs or animals in general, but I could never justify it because society told us that it was the normal thing to do. Eventually, I stopped questioning. As I got older, I started to ignore these childhood feelings that I had and started following what everyone else was doing. But please, don't ignore these feelings but question everything. Just because we've done something for thousands of years doesn't mean it's humane or the right thing to do.

ANY INSPIRING STORIES YOU CAN SHARE?

If you're reading this, I hope you know what a big difference YOU make! I think a lot of people believe that they won't make a difference by changing their diet or lifestyle, but that is wrong. You vote with your money, meaning that whenever you choose a plant-based product over an animal product, you're telling these companies what you want! So in our case, we're demanding more plant-based products and fewer animal products and trust me, companies hear you! Well, they might not care about what you have to say, but they care about your money, so when they see that the money is going into plant-based milk or vegan "mock meat," they will invest into these products! At the same time, they will have to reduce their supply for dairy, meat, eggs, cheese etc because the people do not want to buy this. That means that fewer animals will be bred into existence only to be slaughtered for food. That's how we can change the world! So next time you're grocery shopping, remember that every single one of your food decisions matters. YOU MATTER.

JILL DALTON

CONNECT WITH JILL:
YOUTUBE: THE WHOLEFOOD PLANT-BASED COOKING SHOW
INSTAGRAM: @WHOLEFOODPLANTBASEDCOOKINGSHOW

Jill Dalton is the creator of the popular vegan YouTube channel, *The Whole-Food Plant-Based Cooking Show*. Jill's show offers a step-by-step guide to cooking delicious and healthy plant-based recipes from your home. Her recipes are based on nutritional research from experts like Dr. Joel Fuhrman, T. Colin Campbell, and Dr. Michael Klaper, and is based on eating for maximum nutritional density with a focus on whole, plant-based foods.

AT WHAT POINT IN YOUR LIFE DID YOU DECIDE TO CHANGE YOUR DIET? HOW HAS THAT DECISION IMPACTED YOUR LIFE?

I had just turned 40 and was having regular heart palpitations and generally just felt terrible every day. I knew that I was way too young to feel old.

WHO HAS BEEN THE BIGGEST PLANT-BASED INFLUENCER IN YOUR LIFE AND HOW HAVE THEY HELPED YOU?

I would have to say, Dr. Greger. His research and books are very thorough, and he gives the information with a great sense of humor. Whenever I have a question about plant-based foods or ailments that can be helped by eating a plant-based diet, I turn to his website first: nutritionfacts.org.

HOW DO YOU THINK WE CAN ALL HAVE A BIGGER IMPACT ON INFLUENCING PEOPLE AND HELPING THEM MAKE THE CONNECTION TO HEALTH AND EATING A PLANT-BASED DIET?

Be a good example rather than preaching. Whenever I get together with friends, vegan or not, I always ask if we can meet at a local vegan restaurant so that they can try new foods.

IF YOU COULD HAVE A GIGANTIC BILLBOARD ANYWHERE WITH ANYTHING ON IT, WHAT WOULD IT SAY?

Eat Plants; They will save your life!

HOW HAS A FAILURE, OR APPARENT FAILURE, SET YOU UP FOR LATER SUCCESS? DO YOU HAVE A "FAVORITE FAILURE" OF YOURS?

Raising chickens and ducks for food and eating only grass-fed beef as well as drinking lots of raw milk when we lived on our farm was a huge mistake. We really thought we were doing the right thing. It led to our mounting health problems, which led us to find the books Eat To Live and How Not to Die.

WHAT ADVICE WOULD YOU GIVE A SMART AND DRIVEN 18-YEAR-OLD TODAY? WHAT ADVICE SHOULD THEY IGNORE?

Stop worrying about what other people think of you. Think of what you can do to make a positive influence in this world. Eat plant-based vegan because that is the only thing that is going to save this planet.

ANY INSPIRING STORIES THAT HAVE HAPPENED TO YOU OR PEOPLE CLOSE TO YOU THAT HAVE NOT BEEN COVERED ABOVE. STORIES THAT CAN HELP OTHERS.

We have a 45-year-old friend that came to stay with us for five days last year. We hadn't seen him for about ten years, but when we picked him up from the airport, he was in pretty bad shape. He was over 300 pounds, completely stressed out and had dangerously high blood pressure. We fed him as much delicious plant-based food that we could, went on daily walks and spent a lot of time relaxing and talking together. After that five days were over, he had lost 15 pounds, was feeling great and felt really positive and refreshed. He went home and continued to eat this way and cooks healthy plant-based meals for his wife and two teenage sons.

RAOUM ALSUHAIBANI

CONNECT WITH RAOUM:
INSTAGRAM:@SUKKARILIFE
FACEBOOK: SUKKARI LIFE
YOUTUBE: SUKKARI LIFE
sukkarilife.com

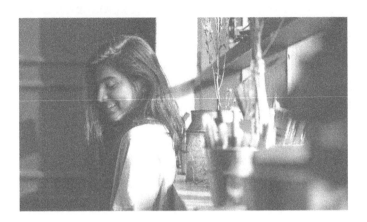

A popular plant-based eating social media influencer, Raoum Alsuhaibani was not always the biggest vegetable-lover! With time and continued education, Raoum began to rewire her taste buds, enjoy the taste of foods that nourished her body and experienced the innumerable positive benefits that coincide with eating solely plant-based foods.

AT WHAT POINT IN YOUR LIFE DID YOU DECIDE TO CHANGE YOUR DIET? HOW HAS THAT DECISION IMPACTED YOUR LIFE?

I slowly started switching to a plant-based diet. The first year of college I went vegetarian, and it made me feel better and made me try new dishes. I loved it and at the same time, it didn't make sense to me to eat animals when we have so many other options.

After I graduated, I had time to think about dairy and eggs, and how it doesn't make sense to eat them. I did my research. I read articles and studies that support eating those items and others that articulated the negative impacts they have on our health. The latter resonated with me more and it made sense. Most importantly for me as a vegetarian at the time, I didn't understand why vegans considered eggs and dairy inhumane until I watched the process of bringing these products to the market. Then I had no reason to consume these items.

WHO HAS BEEN THE BIGGEST PLANT-BASED INFLUENCER IN YOUR LIFE AND HOW HAVE THEY HELPED YOU?

I would say, Dr. Micheal Greger. The number of studies he provides on his platform helped me immensely. Nina Montange has also been a big influence in my life. Her outlook on life is very inspiring, as well as her lifestyle videos.

HOW DO YOU THINK WE CAN ALL HAVE A BIGGER IMPACT ON INFLUENCING PEOPLE AND HELPING THEM MAKE THE CONNECTION TO HEALTH AND EATING A PLANT-BASED DIET?

Simply by showing them how it's done and encouraging people to do their own research.

IF YOU COULD HAVE A GIGANTIC BILLBOARD ANYWHERE WITH ANYTHING ON IT, WHAT WOULD IT SAY?

"Everything is connected."

HOW HAS A FAILURE, OR APPARENT FAILURE, SET YOU UP FOR LATER SUCCESS? DO YOU HAVE A "FAVORITE FAILURE" OF YOURS?

One of my favorite ones is when I gained ten pounds in my senior year of high school. It was when I moved to the US as an exchange student. That weight gain is what made me take charge of my health and change my habits.

I went through a period of trial and error and now, after a few years I can say that I'm really happy with my overall health, but I still strive to learn more.

A VEGAN RESOURCE YOU COULD YOU NOT LIVE WITHOUT AND WHY?

I would say I couldn't live without the book, How Not to Die. It's filled with information and is organized in a way that makes it easy to look things up.

WHAT ADVICE WOULD YOU GIVE A SMART AND DRIVEN 18-YEAR-OLD TODAY? WHAT ADVICE SHOULD THEY IGNORE?

Avoid taking things to the extreme. Do your research before you jump on to something and be patient. Focus on what you can do rather than the end goal.

ANY INSPIRING STORIES THAT HAVE HAPPENED TO YOU OR PEOPLE CLOSE TO YOU THAT HAVE NOT BEEN COVERED ABOVE. STORIES THAT CAN HELP OTHERS.

We view weight gain, heart disease, diabetes, depression and sickness in general as bad things, but sometimes we need to go through that before we can understand what being healthy means.

SILKE DEWULF

CONNECT WITH SILKE:
INSTAGRAM:@THE_PLANTBASED_YOGATEACHER
YOUTUBE: SILKE DEWULF
silkedewulf.com

"Changing a habit takes time and courage. There will be days that you fall back into your old ways. But find the courage to always get back onto your feet. Like I said, it took me three years of falling and rising to get to where I am now. It is an on-going process and falling is part of it. The more you rise back up, the easier it gets. Each time you rebound, the period in between will become shorter and shorter.

Silke Dewulf struggled with disordered eating habits for years, restricting herself from food, binge-eating and over-exercising. Through the healing powers of yoga and mindful living, Silke began the journey of self-healing. Soon she discovered the benefits of plant-based eating and her life was forever changed. Now Silke shares her story through her popular social media accounts, along with tips on how to live a life of wellness.

377

AT WHAT POINT IN YOUR LIFE DID YOU DECIDE TO CHANGE YOUR DIET? HOW HAS THAT DECISION IMPACTED YOUR LIFE?

I went vegan in 2013, purely out of intuition. I hadn't seen any documentaries, and there wasn't really much of a vegan community on YouTube yet. I just realized that every time I had a meal with meat in it, I felt extremely tired and lethargic. So I decided to experiment by cutting out all animal products from my diet. After being vegan for six months, I stumbled upon the documentary Earthlings and that sealed the deal for me.

Ever since being a kid I had always suffered with chronic constipation, and switching to a vegan diet has helped me heal from that. I still have some underlying gut issues (such as histamine reactions and fatigue), but I am currently treating these with the help of a vegan nutritionist. I don't believe the vegan diet is a magic pill and can cure you from anything, but it surely is the best diet to prevent and reverse the most common lifestyle-related diseases.

WHO HAS BEEN THE BIGGEST VEGAN INFLUENCER IN YOUR LIFE AND HOW HAVE THEY HELPED YOU?

I have drawn inspiration from multiple people online. Some of my favorite

YouTubers are: Ellen Fisher, Jinti Fell, Maddie Lymburner and Tess Begg. These ladies have mainly helped me with inspiration for new recipes. Of course, there is also Dr. Greger from Nutritionfacts.org for anything diet or science-related. I've also been into Gojiman recently for gut health on a vegan diet.

HOW DO YOU THINK WE CAN ALL HAVE A BIGGER IMPACT ON INFLUENCING PEOPLE AND HELPING THEM MAKE THE CONNECTION TO HEALTH AND EATING A PLANT-BASED DIET?

I think that there are many different ways to influence someone and be a voice for veganism. Some people really resonate with activism and going to the streets to inform people. Others prefer to share recipes and show how yummy a vegan diet can be. I am one of those people who feels intimidated to go out on the street and participate in activism. I much prefer influencing the people around me by simply sharing my yummy dishes with them. Also, most people around you will inevitably notice the positive changes a vegan lifestyle does for you and ask you what you have been doing lately to achieve those changes (whether it's clearer skin, weight-loss, more energy and so forth).

WHAT WAS THE REACTION YOU RECEIVED FROM PEOPLE WHEN YOU ANNOUNCED THAT YOU WERE GOING VEGAN? WHO WAS YOUR BEST AND WORST SUPPORTER?

My parents were supportive but initially very worried about getting adequate amounts of protein, iron and B12. The first three years of being vegan I got a blood test every six months to prove to my parents and myself that it is absolutely possible to be healthy on a vegan diet. My grandpa, on the other hand, was really worried and decided to throw an almost fully carnivore Christmas dinner that year. The only things I could eat were the roast potatoes and veggies. I was not happy about that, haha! But the year after, he made a turn and was very accommodating to my diet change. Every time I visit him now, he has a selection of vegan goodies waiting for me.

HOW HAS A FAILURE, OR APPARENT FAILURE, SET YOU UP FOR LATER SUCCESS? DO YOU HAVE A "FAVORITE FAILURE" OF YOURS?

Let me paint you a picture of my high school self: really into my science classes, introverted, socially awkward, closed off and kind of a loner. I didn't want to be this girl. I wanted to fit in and be liked by others. Every day I was confronted with the fact that I didn't fit in. And as a teenager, you want nothing more than to fit in. I didn't know how to deal with these feelings, I didn't know I had the power within me to change my situation, so I just numbed the emotional pain with one of the fastest working, most socially acceptable drugs: food. From the peak in my binge-eating disorder, it took

" "

MAKE SURE YOUR 'WHY' IS POWERFUL ENOUGH, AND THAT IT'S COMING FROM WITHIN YOU. NOT OUTSIDE OF YOU.

SILKE DEWULF

me a solid three years to ditch this coping mechanism.

HERE'S WHAT I DID TO OVERCOME IT:

1. Know your triggers

What emotions trigger you the most? In what situations do you find yourself reaching for food to numb the existing pain or discomfort?

Mine are stress, overwhelm, worry and not feeling good enough about myself. The number one trigger for me during high school was low self-esteem. I was constantly beating myself up about not fitting in and being loved by others. Little did I realize how amazing I am, how worthy I am and all the talents that I have. This might sound like bragging to some, but I think it's so important to realize how powerful you are as an individual and how amazingly beautiful, talented and worthy you are. The triggers that still linger up to date are stress, worry and overwhelm. In those scenarios, my ego still tempts me with the justification to eat more than I physically need. It's in these moments that it's really important to figure out your 'why'.

2. Why do you want to change?

Binge eating is a habit. There's no baby in this world that binge eats. A baby cries when it's hungry and stops eating when it's satisfied. It's that simple. Emotional eating is something that you have taught yourself or something that you've seen other people do and are mirroring it. This is amazing news because it means you can unlearn it! Is it easy? Heck no, especially when you've been doing it for years like I had. Is it possible to unlearn? Heck yeah! So try to figure out why you want to change this habit. For me, I wanted to change because I was tired of feeling disgusting after eating so much. I wanted to feel good within my own body. I wanted to feel healthy and energized. Not drowsy and weighed down by all the food. Make sure your 'Why' is powerful enough and that it's something that is coming from within you. Not outside of you. Don't do it because your parents or boyfriend tells you to. Do it for you, because you want to feel amazing. Do it because you are worthy of feeling amazing.

3. Allow yourself to feel the emotions

For me, this was one of the scariest parts. I was afraid that if I'd allowed myself to feel anger or sadness there was going to be no end to it; I would get swallowed by the emotions. Emotions are like waves of the ocean. They come as quickly as they go as long as you allow the emotions to move through you. So next time you feel like emotional eating, stop and set a timer for five minutes. That's all I am asking for, five minutes. Go sit somewhere quiet and safe and close your eyes. Just sit. Allow yourself to feel what you are feeling without labelling it. Don't call it anger or sadness or whatever it is you're feeling. Labelling and judging is the ego at work. Just sit with it and feel it. What I even like to say out loud is "I'm ready to whole-heartedly feel you." Then slowly start focussing on your breath. Deepen your breath with every inhale. If you feel awkward sitting in silence, put on some calming background music. After those five minutes are done, you'll notice that you feel so much more at peace and centered. Feel free to journal about what came up if that helps you process your emotions.

4. Look for the deeper message

Our emotions usually hold a deeper message for us. Coming back to my high school experience, I wasn't conscious yet of how much I was hating on myself, how much I was giving away my power to my ego and actually believing it. Why are you overeating?? Do you hate your job, your relationship, yourself?? Emotions can guide us to a better version of us, but only if we allow them to. So get really honest with yourself on what is causing you to feel a certain way and take inspired action to change it. You have the power to change and redirect your life! Don't wait for Monday or a new year to better your life. You are so powerful. I don't think we as humans understand how much power we have over our life. How deeply we can guide it and manifest our desires. Start believing in your own power. Quit your shitty job, go find a new boyfriend if he's treating you like shit. Make your dreams come true.

5. Take it day by day

Changing a habit takes time and courage. There will be days that you fall back into your old ways. But find the courage to always get back onto you feet. Like I said, it took me three years of falling and rising to get to where I am now. It is an on-going process and falling is part of it. The more you raise back up, the easier it gets. Each time you rebound, the period in between will become shorter and shorter.

WHAT ADVICE WOULD YOU GIVE A SMART AND DRIVEN 18-YEAR-OLD TODAY? WHAT ADVICE SHOULD THEY IGNORE?

I would say do your research, but also know that your body is a smart vessel that will give you clues on where to look. Say you are a few months into your vegan diet and crave salmon. Look up what nutrients salmon is high in, and it'll give you an indication of where your diet is out of balance. Maybe you aren't getting enough omega 3's, so try adding more flaxseeds, chia seeds, or even algae oil. As long as you eat a balanced diet with a lot of variety, you will be absolutely fine! Avoid trying to restrict certain macronutrients and avoid going on any extreme diet. Just eat what makes you feel good and eat as much of it as you want. Eating a vegan diet is fun and so delicious!

EKATERINA SKY

Ekaterina Sky Antonova is a visual wildlife artist who has studied fine arts around the world, mastering traditional and modern techniques, she currently resides in Montreal and is highly regarded as one of Canada's most promising emerging artists. As a plant-based diet advocate, Ekaterina uses her artistic gifts and animal paintings to raise awareness about the conservation of wildlife.

WHAT IS ONE OF THE BEST OR MOST WORTHWHILE HEALTH-RELATED INVESTMENTS THAT YOU HAVE MADE?

The best health-related investment I have made is my Ninja blender. It makes cooking so much easier. Its motor is strong enough for making my favorite vegan ice cream from frozen bananas. It helps me start my day with my favorite, health-conscious, green smoothie.

AT WHAT POINT IN YOUR LIFE DID YOU DECIDE TO CHANGE YOUR DIET? HOW HAS THAT DECISION IMPACTED YOUR LIFE?

I've been vegetarian since I was a teenager because I did not want to cause harm to animals. The decision to go vegan was inspired by my husband Jonathan, who is a doctor. We were discussing diet and health, and we both agreed a vegan diet is the best for health and for animals.

I used to suffer from irritable bowel syndrome. Since becoming vegan, my IBS symptoms are gone, and I believe that is because I have less inflammation that was caused by dairy products.

WHO HAS BEEN THE BIGGEST VEGAN INFLUENCER IN YOUR LIFE AND HOW HAVE THEY HELPED YOU?

My Dad played a large role in my decision to stop eating meat. He once said a phrase that changed my perspective on food. He said, "why would you kill with your mouth when there is other food to eat?" As a teenager, this took me by surprise because I never thought I was causing harm to anyone. I never thought about the lives being harmed and sacrificed. I am very grateful to my Dad for his guidance and for opening my eyes to the cruelty that is happening in the world.

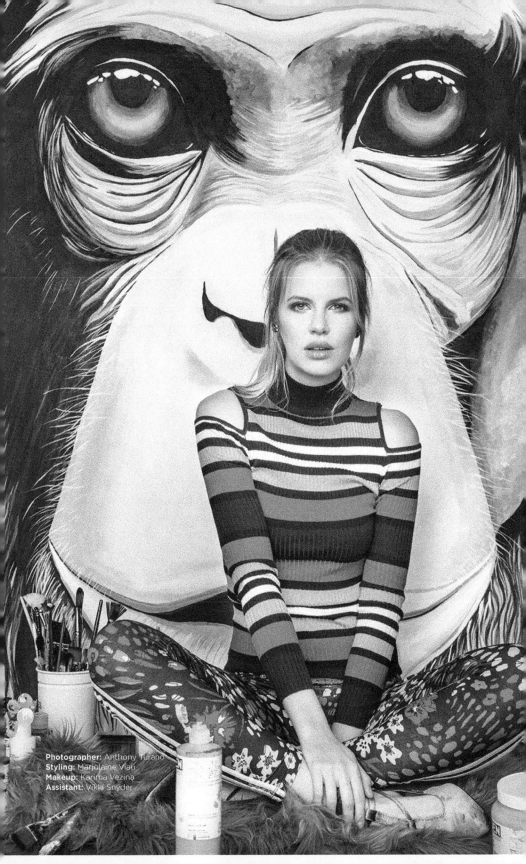

Photographer: Anthony Turano
Styling: Marjolaine Viau
Makeup: Karima Vezina
Assistant: Vikki Snyder

HOW DO YOU THINK WE CAN ALL HAVE A BIGGER IMPACT ON INFLUENCING PEOPLE AND HELPING THEM MAKE THE CONNECTION TO HEALTH AND EATING A PLANT-BASED DIET?

Influencing people towards living with more compassion and kindness is a surprisingly controversial topic. It is important to not make others feel like they need to defend their way of life or actions. If somebody asks me why I am vegan, I say it is because it makes me happy and that I feel good when I eat a plant-based diet. This way, no one can judge me based on my feelings.

Many people are on the hunt for more activities and lifestyle choices that will bring them happiness, therefore they may show interest in knowing more about why a vegan diet brings me joy. This leads to questions, and I believe it is much better to explore this topic because of the curiosity rather than imposing my views.

Another thing that I try to keep in mind is to lead the conversation with love and compassion instead of pointing fingers at what is wrong with the world. The best way to have an impact on somebody is through their heart.

WHAT WAS THE REACTION YOU RECEIVED FROM PEOPLE WHEN YOU ANNOUNCED THAT YOU WERE GOING VEGAN? WHO WAS YOUR BEST AND WORST SUPPORTER?

My husband and I became vegan together, so of course, we are each other's best supporters. It made things much easier knowing that we are a team and that we are doing it for a greater purpose.

Many people around us questioned our decision, and we often were asked: "where will you get your protein from?" Some people would be very defensive without me even saying anything because they felt offended, as if my dietary choices were suggesting that their lifestyle is unethical. Yes, it was hurtful at times because that was not my intention at all.

The purpose of my lifestyle change was to foster more kindness, compassion and love, while some saw it otherwise. Every day my beliefs and love for animals are strengthening, so there is no chance that I could ever go back to eating meat.

HOW HAS A FAILURE, OR APPARENT FAILURE, SET YOU UP FOR LATER SUCCESS? DO YOU HAVE A "FAVORITE FAILURE" OF YOURS?

Throughout my lifetime, I have been told that I am iron deficient. When I was vegetarian, this was the case too. So at one time because of health issues, I started eating meat out of fear of being anemic. It did not last long, however, and after one month I had a dream where I was punished for every single soul I've killed. After this experience I couldn't consider eating a piece of flesh again. Shortly after this experience I became vegan and believe it or not, my iron levels improved and I am no longer anemic.

WHAT VEGAN RESOURCE COULD YOU NOT LIVE WITHOUT AND WHY?

The person who I look up to the most is Jane Goodall. Her love and dedication to animals mesmerizes me. I remember watching her documentary and thinking to myself that hopefully one day, I can have as much positive impact on the world as she does. Jane is very upfront about how we affect the environment and other species. She stands strong for those who are speechless, and even today at her age when she could just sit back and relax, she still tours around the world to bring kindness and compassion into peoples' hearts.

WHAT ADVICE WOULD YOU GIVE A SMART AND DRIVEN 18-YEAR-OLD TODAY? WHAT ADVICE SHOULD THEY IGNORE?

What other people think about you is none of your business because you cannot frame how you see yourself based on other peoples' perceptions of you. Perception is only an illusion, never the truth. Believe in yourself, do things for a greater purpose, and it will elevate your spirit and bring fulfillment into your life. Keep on following your dreams and every single day, do something that brings you closer to that goal.

385

ANY INSPIRING STORIES THAT HAVE HAPPENED TO YOU OR PEOPLE CLOSE TO YOU THAT HAVE NOT BEEN COVERED ABOVE. STORIES THAT CAN HELP OTHERS.

Becoming a visual artist was always my dream, a dream that I thought could never come true. I have done three immigrations in my life in search of a better life. My family was not very thrilled with my dream as they wanted me to have a stable job where they would know that I would be financially stable. While I was studying international business in university, I was lacking creativity, and I felt down.

It was then that I realized, I can build my art career while studying business. With the support of my boyfriend at the time who is now my husband Jonathan, as well as my dear friend Julia Fata, I started moving towards my vision. Their belief in me gave me wings. They made me feel that I was capable of anything my heart desires.

As I started working on my first collection I was tired and lacking sleep, but I still felt like I was the happiest person in the world. Not only was I creating art, but I was also painting to speak for those who are speechless. My every brush stroke is a moment dedicated to my love of animals.

" "

YOU DON'T NEED TO BE
A CELEBRITY OR
INFLUENCER TO CREATE
CHANGE. SOME OF THE
LARGEST CHANGES HAPPEN
TO BE A SMALL RIPPLE IN
THE BEGINNING. GENTLY
EDUCATING OUR FRIENDS,
PEERS, COLLEAGUES AND
FAMILY IS VITAL.

FREYA HAYLEY

ELAINA SYDNEY

CONNECT WITH ELAINA:
INSTAGRAM: @ELAINASYDNEY
YOUTUBE: ELAINA SYDNEY
thekindlife.co.uk

Elaina Sydney is the voice behind the popular blog, thekindlife.co.uk. Interested in all things cruelty-free and vegan, Elaina writes about a variety of topics including fashion, beauty, food, travel and lifestyle.

WHAT IS ONE OF THE BEST OR MOST WORTHWHILE HEALTH-RELATED INVESTMENTS THAT YOU HAVE MADE?

Amongst the various gadgets out there, without a doubt, my most used pieces of technology are my juicer and Vitamix. These gadgets have enabled me to create delicious smoothies and juices, true powerhouses of nutrients that bring vitality to my everyday life! I've been able to create many recipes with the use of these two gadgets, from banana nice cream to homemade guacamole and even chocolate mousse. Creating these recipes is so easy!

387

AT WHAT POINT IN YOUR LIFE DID YOU DECIDE TO CHANGE YOUR DIET? HOW HAS THAT DECISION IMPACTED YOUR LIFE?

Growing up, I was always an avid animal lover. However, it took many years for me to realize my morals did not align with my actions. Despite many years of struggling with thyroid issues and endometriosis, I never made the link that perhaps the food I was eating was affecting my health!

Fuelled by habits and tradition, it wasn't until I heard of the documentary Earthlings, that I changed. I watched this documentary with tears rolling down my face, ashamed to have played my own part in fuelling the torture and abuse of innocent animals. The documentary changed my mindset. You can't eat animals and love them too. I decided to be vegan for them mostly, secondly for my health.

It's been three years now, and I'm forever learning about the environmental impact that the choices we make have on our mother earth. I wouldn't wish an animal to experience cruelty, especially not on my behalf. Eating plants has provided me with a newfound sensitivity to view animals in this world as equals. Living a life where I am avoiding inflicting suffering on others reinforces my daily habits of this lifestyle. I only wish I went vegan sooner!

WHO HAS BEEN THE BIGGEST VEGAN INFLUENCER IN YOUR LIFE AND HOW HAVE THEY HELPED YOU?

Thankfully, we live in an age with incredible activists fuelled to make a change and bring awareness to the plight of animals, the environment and our health.

Gary Yourofsky and Earthling Ed inspired me most to start understanding my previous mindset as to why I ate animals and why I didn't challenge myself earlier to change. Although I wish I had gone vegan earlier, I find it just as important to understand the psychology and thought processes of the human mind. Watching the videos of these two inspirational people has encouraged me to empathize with others and remember that I too, once thought that being vegan wouldn't make a difference. For the record, it's so much more than that, and I only hug trees part-time!

HOW DO YOU THINK WE CAN ALL HAVE A BIGGER IMPACT ON INFLUENCING PEOPLE AND HELPING THEM MAKE THE CONNECTION TO HEALTH AND EATING A PLANT-BASED DIET?

Everyone will have their own preferred way to influence people and bridge the gap to understanding veganism. I remember when I first went vegan I was fuelled by all the new information I had learned, and I wanted to tell everyone. I wanted them to see and feel how good I felt! At the beginning of my journey, learning about the injustice that animals face only to be brought to a dinner plate left me angry and fuelled to inform others. However, I realized for myself that being angry only created a further divide between people living a vegan lifestyle and those who weren't vegan but, may be curious.

Being vegan for a few years now, I've learned a lot. I've inspired others by encouraging them to make small changes and educating them along the way. Not everyone is willing to watch an animal documentary because they know the footage may upset them. This is why education, encouragement and leading by example is a great way to influence and spread the vegan message.

I wasn't born vegan, but I wish I had met someone earlier who had the time to show me amazing recipes and open my eyes to a new way of living. Encouragement and education are vital to promoting change.

WHAT WAS THE REACTION YOU RECEIVED FROM PEOPLE WHEN YOU ANNOUNCED THAT YOU WERE GOING VEGAN? WHO WAS YOUR BEST AND WORST SUPPORTER?

When I told my friends and family I was going vegan, they were shocked. My friends all asked me the same question. "what will you eat?!" This actually encouraged me further because it reinforced to me how distant we as humans have become to our food. People can feel lost when cutting animal products from their diet.

Anyone who knows me well knows that when I say I'm going to do something, I don't go back on my word. Although some people assumed it was a phase that I was trying and would soon grow out of, some knew I was being serious. It was a relief to finally match my actions to my morals.

Originally when I became vegan, I felt most unsupported by family members. They didn't understand veganism. I would be offered to have family meals and encouraged to eat their meals even when they contained only "a little dairy." Scenarios like that can be tough to deal with as all you want is their understanding and respect. However, over time this situation has changed, and I've since influenced them to stop eating animals.

My biggest supporter has been my husband. We decided to go vegan together, and now I'm his sidekick in the kitchen! Gone are the days where I became a fixture on the recliner and let him make the food. Being vegan has reignited a love of being in the kitchen for me. Making new recipes and experimenting with herbs and spices is a joy. There are endless dishes you can make using plants. Living and breathing this amazing lifestyle with my best friend has allowed me to fuel my passion for a life full of love and compassion for all beings. It has also increased what I didn't think was possible: my love for animals!

389

HOW HAS A FAILURE, OR APPARENT FAILURE, SET YOU UP FOR LATER SUCCESS? DO YOU HAVE A "FAVORITE FAILURE" OF YOURS?

After watching Earthlings, I went vegan overnight. However, over three months of trying the lifestyle, I succumbed to having a massive whipped cream chocolate cake, which wasn't vegan. The reality was, I knew I didn't want to eat animals, but I was lacking in understanding what my body needed to thrive and be healthy.

Understanding nutritionally what bodies require to function and thrive is vital for your own well being despite dietary choices. I stayed vegetarian for a few months after my slip up and built my knowledge by watching documentaries like Cowspiracy, Forks Over Knives, and Vegucated. I then decided it was time to go vegan for good this time! I've never looked back since.

My mentality when I tried veganism for three months was desperately wanting certain foods, but knowing I couldn't have them. I felt deprived and like I was missing out on tasty food, however, I know this was due to my lack of knowledge. After learning about factory farming, the environment and what animal products do to our health, I no longer felt deprived. I simply no longer desired those foods anymore. Now I see the foods that people eat daily around me in a completely different way.

WHAT VEGAN RESOURCE COULD YOU NOT LIVE WITHOUT AND WHY?

The best vegan book I've read is *How Not To Die* by Dr. Michael Greger. Documentaries have their purpose and are great. However, I retain information in a different way when I read it. This book has many peer-reviewed scientific evidence studies that taught me about which foods to eat and which lifestyle changes to make to live longer. When faced with such a comprehensive amount of scientific and proven evidence, it's hard to ignore! From reading this book, I've learned that the biggest change I could make to my health is the food I eat. It's very easy to get caught up in the junk food vegan alternatives. They do have their place and taste AMAZING, but real health and nutrition lies in eating whole-foods that are plant-based.

WHAT ADVICE WOULD YOU GIVE A SMART AND DRIVEN 18-YEAR-OLD TODAY? WHAT ADVICE SHOULD THEY IGNORE?

Knowledge is key. The vegan movement is growing, which is incredible, but please take the time to go back to the basics and learn about food groups and nutrition. Everyone who goes vegan will have different experiences; however, ensure that you know how to look after yourself by fueling your body with the vitamins and minerals it requires.

One of the best apps I've found is Cronometer. I find it so useful to understand how nutrient-dense my food is and learn which plant foods provide you with higher levels of carbohydrates, calories, protein and fats.

With the world we live in, people naturally judge one another. Choosing an "alternative path" and going vegan may seem scary. You are choosing to live a lifestyle that is outside of the norm. Being different influences change. Veganism is a lifestyle that reduces both human and animal suffering as well as leaving a habitable planet for our future generations. Do it today, go vegan.

FREYA HALEY

CONNECT WITH FREYA:
INSTAGRAM: @FREYAHALEY
YOUTUBE: FREYA HALEY

"Sometimes the worst things only come back temporarily, to remind you of just how far you've come. I think when we embody our truest values and live accordingly, people will naturally want to follow or know more. This will "plant the seed" in some fashion. I believe that just by living out kindness, we may encourage others in a subtle way to do the same."

WHAT IS ONE OF THE BEST OR MOST WORTHWHILE HEALTH-RELATED INVESTMENTS THAT YOU HAVE MADE?

I can't just name one! I know it's not material, but investing time into myself and self-care. Really paying attention to where I'm at each day. Putting myself first. Putting everything into myself allows me to put everything into others.

AT WHAT POINT IN YOUR LIFE DID YOU DECIDE TO CHANGE YOUR DIET? HOW HAS THAT DECISION IMPACTED YOUR LIFE?

When I was around seven years old, I was living on a farm. I saw my brother and Dad kill a rabbit that was considered a pest. It absolutely broke my heart, and although I became vegan many years after that event, it really shaped my compassion towards loving animals and wanting to make a change.

WHO HAS BEEN THE BIGGEST VEGAN INFLUENCER IN YOUR LIFE AND HOW HAVE THEY HELPED YOU?

Probably Essena O'Neill back when she was on social media! Her posts and activism in regards to veganism triggered something within me. She helped me to form the connection between what I was eating and the reality of the industry.

HOW DO YOU THINK WE CAN ALL HAVE A BIGGER IMPACT ON INFLUENCING PEOPLE AND HELPING THEM MAKE THE CONNECTION TO HEALTH AND EATING A PLANT-BASED DIET?

I think when we embody our truest values and live accordingly, people will naturally see how much joy it brings us. This will spark the idea in others' minds; "plant the seed" in some fashion. I believe that just by living out of kindness, we may encourage others in a subtle way to do the same. Also, bringing this awareness into our "circle," whatever it may be. You don't need to be a celebrity or influencer to create change. Some of the largest changes happen to be a small ripple in the beginning. Gently educating our friends, peers, colleagues and family is vital.

WHAT WAS THE REACTION YOU RECEIVED FROM PEOPLE WHEN YOU ANNOUNCED THAT YOU WERE GOING VEGAN?

At first, it was rough. I was only about 16-years-old at the time and living with my parents. This meant getting my meals cooked by them too! My parents were shocked, to say the least! People from high school could be quite rude about it and make jokes and such. Even (and in particular) my friends. I had a few close girlfriends that went vegan at a similar time to me, and they were my rock. Nowadays it's chilled out a little more. Everyone accepts it, and my parents (who at first were mortified) now love the idea of having vegan food and treats too!

HOW HAS A FAILURE, OR APPARENT FAILURE, SET YOU UP FOR LATER SUCCESS? DO YOU HAVE A "FAVORITE FAILURE" OF YOURS?

Absolutely! Failure allows you to be grounded, wise and patient enough to follow through with deeper, larger goals. My "favorite failure" would be my ongoing struggle with depression and mental health. Coming from a traumatic childhood and being able to find the strength to not only empower myself but empower others is something I am truly proud of. It makes me really proud to look back on all the adversity I have experienced and know that I am now solid enough to move through any mountains.

WHAT ADVICE WOULD YOU GIVE A SMART AND DRIVEN 18-YEAR-OLD TODAY? WHAT ADVICE SHOULD THEY IGNORE?

1. Don't let other people tell you your dreams are too big. Life is too short to subscribe to the idea that you are "not ready" because you are "not old enough." Do your own thing, beat your own drum, make your own world.

2. Trust your intuition. If something doesn't feel right for you, you don't have to do it. Even if it feels like an amazing opportunity, know that amazing opportunities come and go. Don't feel pressured into one path just because it is the first option.

3. Surround yourself with like-minded friends. Seriously, the amount of time and wisdom I took from myself because I was too busy getting drunk is ridiculous! Women and men that are forward-thinking, wise, patient, kind, loving, understanding and driven are your key.

JASMINE BRIONES

CONNECT WITH JASMINE:
INSTAGRAM: @SWEETSIMPLEVEGAN
YOUTUBE: SWEET SIMPLE VEGAN
sweetsimplevegan.com

Jasmine Briones is the co-owner of the popular blog, Sweet Simple Vegan. Along with her partner Chris, Jasmine transformed the blog from a hobby website that she started in 2013 to one that helps share the vegan message to hundreds of thousands of followers/subscribers all over the world. The couple is passionate about sharing their love of animals, the environment and healthy food, through delicious recipes and resources that help their audience understand and experience the benefits of vegan food.

WHAT IS ONE OF THE BEST OR MOST WORTHWHILE HEALTH-RELATED INVESTMENTS THAT YOU HAVE MADE?

The most worthwhile investment for me was my nutrition education. I earned a bachelor's degree in nutritional science through CSULA as well as a certificate in plant-based nutrition through eCornell. Both have had a long-lasting impact on my lifestyle choices and perspectives on food and nutrition.

WHEN DID YOU DECIDE TO CHANGE YOUR DIET?

I went vegan when I was 18 and recovering from an eating disorder. At first, it was nothing more than a diet for me and the way I was going to gain back my health. After making the shift and eventually doing more research on the subject, my mind opened up to something much larger. I realized that I was focused so much on myself and the bubble of my own life, when there were so many other things happening in the world that I could focus my energy and attention towards. It was then I realized that I had found my passion in life, and it was then I dedicated myself to living a life full of compassion for not only myself, but for our planet and the animals. Veganism completely shifted my lifestyle and perspective for the better.

WHO HAS BEEN THE BIGGEST VEGAN INFLUENCER IN YOUR LIFE AND HOW HAVE THEY HELPED YOU?

My Mom has been the biggest influence for me. Although she was not vegan when I made the change, she always helped me stay positive and confident in my choices and beliefs, which helped so much with my transition.

393

HOW DO YOU THINK WE CAN ALL HAVE A BIGGER IMPACT ON INFLUENCING PEOPLE AND HELPING THEM MAKE THE CONNECTION TO HEALTH AND EATING A PLANT-BASED DIET?

By being compassionate and setting a positive example. From my experience, forcing my beliefs on others may be understood by them as more of criticism or an attack on their lifestyle choices rather than me trying to help them make an impactful change. I've learned that if I live out my life and my beliefs compassionately, others who are not vegan respond to it more positively and are then more open to discussion.

WHAT WAS THE REACTION YOU RECEIVED FROM PEOPLE WHEN YOU ANNOUNCED THAT YOU WERE GOING VEGAN?

When I went vegan in 2012, I was met with confusion and concern. My friends and family did not know any vegans, let alone vegetarians, so they could not fully grasp what the lifestyle change meant. They were convinced that all I could eat were things like carrots and lettuce, and they expressed concern in the "restriction" that I was putting upon myself.

My support at the time was the online vegan community as a whole, they helped me stay motivated, feel welcome and not alone. Since I did not know any other vegans in real life, turning to the online community really helped me flourish in the lifestyle and push through some of the hard times during the initial change.

HOW HAS A FAILURE, OR APPARENT FAILURE, SET YOU UP FOR LATER SUCCESS? DO YOU HAVE A "FAVORITE FAILURE" OF YOURS?

When I was in college, my goal was to become a nurse. I did not get into my first choice school when I applied, so I waited a year and applied a second time. I still did not get into the school, and I really felt like I had failed myself and my family. I did not realize it at the time, but that was a blessing in disguise. My heart was always in nutrition and this pushed my enrollment in the CSULA nutrition program. I realized that I was only pushing myself to pursue nursing because I felt like that was a stable and respected profession. Once I started the nutrition program, it was the first time in my life that I felt a true passion for something, and it brought me to where I am today.

WHAT ADVICE WOULD YOU GIVE A SMART AND DRIVEN 18-YEAR-OLD TODAY? WHAT ADVICE SHOULD THEY IGNORE?

To appreciate everything that happens to them in their life, the good and bad. I used to spend so much time trying to avoid negative experiences in my life, but as the years went by, I realized that negative experiences were just as important as the positive ones, if not more. Things happen in our lives so that we can learn and grow. As cliche as it sounds, everything happens for a reason.

SIX VEGAN SISTERS

CONNECT WITH THE SISTERS:
INSTAGRAM: @SIXVEGANSISTERS
YOUTUBE: SIX VEGAN SISTERS
FACEBOOK: SIX VEGAN SISTERS
sixvegansisters.com

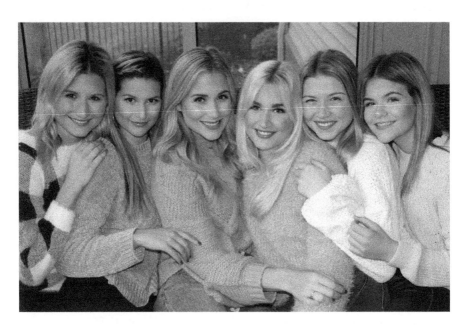

Molly, Emily, Carrie, Mary-Kate, Hannah and Shannon are the real-life sisters from Six Vegan Sisters, a popular website and social media platform advocating for animal rights and plant-based eating. By sharing mouthwatering and Instagram-worthy vegan meals, the Six Vegan Sisters have gained attention for their recipes that are all made from a plant base.

WHAT IS ONE OF THE BEST OR MOST WORTHWHILE HEALTH-RELATED INVESTMENTS THAT YOU HAVE MADE?

We can unanimously agree on this (which is surprising when there are six of us): an air fryer! Hello, perfectly crispy sweet potato fries.

AT WHAT POINT IN YOUR LIFE DID YOU DECIDE TO CHANGE YOUR DIET? HOW HAS THAT DECISION IMPACTED YOUR LIFE?

We all had different defining moments, and all became vegan at different times in our lives. For Emily, it began as a "diet," but for Molly and M-K it was after watching the "Dairy is Scary" video on YouTube. Hannah, Carrie, and Shannon switched from vegetarianism to veganism after realizing that vegetarian diets still cause harm to animals. Now, our end goal is the same, and it's to save animals, have a positive impact on the environment and live healthier, happier lives.

WHO HAS BEEN THE BIGGEST PLANT-BASED INFLUENCER IN YOUR LIFE AND HOW HAVE THEY HELPED YOU?

Hands down, our Mom. She was the first to go vegan (and has been a vegetarian since she was 15) and inspired all of us to follow in her footsteps. She always supported and educated us, but never forced her beliefs on us and let us make the decision all on our own, which in our opinion, is pretty darn amazing.

HOW DO YOU THINK WE CAN ALL HAVE A BIGGER IMPACT ON INFLUENCING PEOPLE AND HELPING THEM MAKE THE CONNECTION TO HEALTH AND EATING A PLANT-BASED DIET?

A huge reason we started Six Vegan Sisters was to inspire people and help make their transition to veganism a little bit easier. We aim to inspire and educate rather than belittle or put someone down for not being vegan – after all, we were all there at one point in our lives. We aim to create recipes that are super easy to make and that anyone will love - vegan or not vegan. We think that the best way to inspire others is to educate them, share easy and delicious vegan recipes, and show them the benefits that veganism can have not only on their health, but on the planet and the animals.

IF YOU COULD HAVE A GIGANTIC BILLBOARD ANYWHERE WITH ANYTHING ON IT, WHAT WOULD IT SAY?

You can't love animals and eat them too.

HOW HAS A FAILURE, OR APPARENT FAILURE, SET YOU UP FOR LATER SUCCESS? DO YOU HAVE A "FAVORITE FAILURE" OF YOURS?

When we first started our Six Vegan Sisters Instagram and blog, we honestly had no idea what we were doing. We had always been decent cooks, but we were new to veganism and had never taken a single food picture, let alone take pictures that would lead to successful social media accounts. We made lots of mistakes when it came to vegan cooking and photography. Continuing to make new recipes and take more pictures, all while researching how to get better, allowed us to learn how to find our photography style and create recipes that have kept our followers coming back for more.

WHAT VEGAN RESOURCE COULD YOU NOT LIVE WITHOUT AND WHY?

The first vegan cookbook that helped us get started with vegan cooking was the *Oh She Glows* Cookbook by Angela Liddon. We still make recipes from that cookbook to this day - our favorite is her tomato soup!

WHAT ADVICE WOULD YOU GIVE A SMART AND DRIVEN 18-YEAR-OLD TODAY? WHAT ADVICE SHOULD THEY IGNORE?

Our biggest piece of advice is to ignore negativity and stick to your beliefs. We have found that it can be hard to avoid people who don't agree with your lifestyle, but if you power through and find like-minded people to influence you and share your struggles with (social media is great for this!), you'll live a happier life.

ANY INSPIRING STORIES THAT HAVE HAPPENED TO YOU OR PEOPLE CLOSE TO YOU THAT HAVE NOT BEEN COVERED ABOVE. STORIES THAT CAN HELP OTHERS.

In September of 2017, our Aunt Colleen was diagnosed with stage four metastatic breast cancer that had spread to her spine. She had always been into living a healthy life, and she decided to focus on her diet in hopes of turning around her life-threatening diagnosis.

397

She began an organic plant-based diet consisting solely of fruits, vegetables, and limited grains. Her daily diet included about nine carrot juices, a big salad, oatmeal with fruit, green juice and freshly squeezed orange juice. A year and a half later, her cancer is "sleeping," and she feels that her recovery was greatly impacted by her diet. She has allowed small amounts of other foods, such as peanut butter, back into her diet because, as she says, "you can only eat so many carrots without going insane!" She has truly shown that food is medicine as long as you're eating the right food.

SNEHA ULLAL

CONNECT WITH SNEHA:
INSTAGRAM: @SNEHAULLAL
FACEBOOK: @SNEHAULLALOFFICIAL

Sneha Ullal is an Indian film actress known for her roles in Tollywood and Bollywood films, most notably for her roles in Telugu films, Ullasamga Utsahamga, Simha, and the Hindi film, Lucky: No Time for Love.

"Being vegan to me only means one thing: no animals harmed. To add to this, I must mention that along with my cruelty-free diet, I also maintain cruelty-free beauty and fashion choices. This means that I don't use real leather, fur or even cosmetics that are tested on animals. Being compassionate is my way of life now, and I'm proud of my choices. Animals deserve to live as much as children do."

AT WHAT POINT IN YOUR LIFE DID YOU DECIDE TO CHANGE YOUR DIET? HOW HAS THAT DECISION IMPACTED YOUR LIFE?

398

I decided that in order to live my life, I don't need anyone or anything harmed anymore. Yes, one might say that I harm plants, but we don't have any replacements for that.

I am always respected and looked highly upon when I express my vegan morals to someone. It feels amazing.

WHO HAS BEEN THE BIGGEST VEGAN INFLUENCER IN YOUR LIFE AND HOW HAVE THEY HELPED YOU?

No one, it's been me, my heart, my compassion and my will power.

HOW DO YOU THINK WE CAN ALL HAVE A BIGGER IMPACT ON INFLUENCING PEOPLE AND HELPING THEM MAKE THE CONNECTION TO HEALTH AND EATING A PLANT-BASED DIET?

I try to express and preach compassion as much as I can. When we are true to our heart and our cause, I am sure that it will make a huge difference some day. Obviously more education and support from our governments as well.

WHAT WAS THE REACTION YOU RECEIVED FROM PEOPLE WHEN YOU ANNOUNCED THAT YOU WERE GOING VEGAN? WHO WAS YOUR BEST AND WORST SUPPORTER?

Not many were great supporters. I would say it was more out of concern for the lack of vitamins and essential nutrients that one might get or not get from animal products. Also, a vegan diet in India is not very easy, so it's been tough. But it has been worth it obviously.

HOW HAS A FAILURE, OR APPARENT FAILURE, SET YOU UP FOR LATER SUCCESS? DO YOU HAVE A "FAVORITE FAILURE" OF YOURS?

Failure today means to succeed some other day. It's part of progress. I don't even think about that word.

WHAT ADVICE WOULD YOU GIVE A SMART AND DRIVEN 18-YEAR-OLD TODAY? WHAT ADVICE SHOULD THEY IGNORE?

Be compassionate towards all living beings. Believe in Karma. Avoid sugar. It's the root cause for any disease.

ANY INSPIRING STORIES THAT HAVE HAPPENED TO YOU OR PEOPLE CLOSE TO YOU THAT HAVE NOT BEEN COVERED ABOVE. STORIES THAT CAN HELP OTHERS.

I was born a non-vegetarian who loved meat like so many of you out there. Then I became a vegetarian, and then I became a vegan. You can do it. It feels amazing to be living a life where you harm no one. Start with avoiding animal products two days a week and increase it as you go.

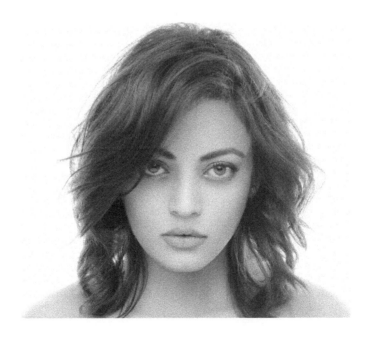

Chapter 7 | INFLUENCERS

THE VORA SISTERS (MEG)

CONNECT WITH MEG & KOMIE:
INSTAGRAM: @DELIKATERAYNE
delikaterayne.com

Komie and Meg Vora are sisters and co-founders behind the LA-based fashion label Delikate Rayne, a 100% cruelty-free, eco lux women's contemporary fashion line. Born and raised vegetarian, these sisters were taught to love animals. This love paired with a non-conformist attitude for traditional cultural and gender norms, they're fueled to create a brand that reflects strongly held beliefs in animal rights and freedom of self-expression.

With recent features in Forbes, NBC, WWD, and HuffPost, these sisters are disrupting the fashion industry with their cruelty-free women's label. They are redefining luxury fashion as sustainable, ethical and animal/cruelty-free. The Vora sisters take pride in educating others on the effects that the fashion industry also has on both humans and the planet, not just the animals. "Your choice of wardrobe can actually make a difference in the world. We want to make that choice easier for you."

400

WHAT IS ONE OF THE BEST OR MOST WORTHWHILE HEALTH-RELATED INVESTMENTS THAT YOU HAVE MADE?

Anything with Hyaluronic acid in it. It's a game-changer for achieving supple skin but has multiple beneficial properties to it as well. I'm really big on fresh, dewy skin without makeup and it's important to me to have that inside and out. Hyaluronic acid worked really well for me to do this topically, so I take vegan gummy glow supplements and make an effort to incorporate as many foods rich in it as possible when eating.

AT WHAT POINT IN YOUR LIFE DID YOU DECIDE TO CHANGE YOUR DIET? HOW HAS THAT DECISION IMPACTED YOUR LIFE?

With the conception of our company, Delikate Rayne, it made even more sense to become vegan and happened pretty organically. Around the same time, we were creating DR both my sister and I already had been actively looking into the effects of the dairy industry on the planet. When we discovered the link of cruelty to animals and the darkness of dairy farms, we started to question a lot of things.

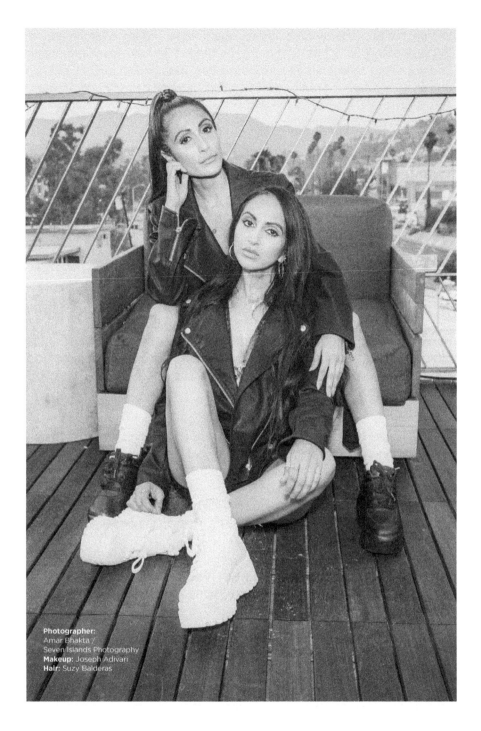

Photographer:
Amar Bhakta /
Seven Islands Photography
Makeup: Joseph Adivari
Hair: Suzy Balderas

Chapter 7 | INFLUENCERS

We wanted to do better for ourselves, the animals and the environment. Because of this, it did not feel right to be behind Delikate Rayne promoting and educating consumers about "cruelty-free" fashion and to not be vegan ourselves. I haven't looked back since. It's an integral part of our business and lifestyle, and it continues to encourage me to spread our growing knowledge about it to others.

WHO HAS BEEN THE BIGGEST VEGAN INFLUENCER IN YOUR LIFE AND HOW HAVE THEY HELPED YOU?

My parents and our upbringing. I grew up in a Jain and Hindu household where compassion thrived, and violence towards any living thing was unacceptable. My sister and I were raised vegetarian. Both sets of our grandparents were brought up the same way and raised both of our parents like that as well. This foundation helped set me up to see the world and feel differently from a young age. At first it made me an outcast, but with time it has gotten better, and I am thankful for it.

HOW DO YOU THINK WE CAN ALL HAVE A BIGGER IMPACT ON INFLUENCING PEOPLE AND HELPING THEM MAKE THE CONNECTION TO HEALTH AND EATING A PLANT-BASED DIET?

By being more compassionate in the way the vegan community spreads the knowledge about veganism. Everyone's heart is in the right place, but we all need to be kinder to one another, which includes respecting each other's ways of living even if we don't agree with it. Judgement and belittling doesn't influence change. We need to lead by example - bringing awareness to a lifestyle that is explicitly tied to compassion by forcing beliefs on someone is a complete turn off and is not going to result in the desired outcome. We can continue to present the facts and make sure we keep the conversation going; there is no expiration date on learning.

WHAT WAS THE REACTION YOU RECEIVED FROM PEOPLE WHEN YOU ANNOUNCED THAT YOU WERE GOING VEGAN? WHO WAS YOUR BEST AND WORST SUPPORTER?

Never having tasted meat before because I was raised a vegetarian and stuck with it, I don't think it surprised many when the transition into veganism was made. I still come across a lot of people who are foreign to the concept of veganism. Off the bat, they are genuinely surprised and usually think they can never do it. They feel its too daunting of a task. I like to walk them through it and answer however many questions they have. It's hard for them to support something they don't get yet, but once they know better, hopefully they too will do better.

HOW HAS A FAILURE, OR APPARENT FAILURE, SET YOU UP FOR LATER SUCCESS? DO YOU HAVE A "FAVORITE FAILURE" OF YOURS?

Every failure I endure has special elements that I hold onto for the betterment of myself. They remind me that obstacles, change and often times failure is inevitable...it's a part of the process. You need to go through failures in order to continue forward momentum in a positive way

WHAT VEGAN RESOURCE COULD YOU NOT LIVE WITHOUT AND WHY?

The Alchemist by Paulo Coelho and *In the Meantime,* by Iyanla Vanzant. Both books were instrumental in beginning my journey towards believing, self-love, realization and care. *The Celestine Prophecy* by James Redfield - an actual life analogy and manual in tangible form

WHAT ADVICE WOULD YOU GIVE A SMART AND DRIVEN 18-YEAR-OLD TODAY? WHAT ADVICE SHOULD THEY IGNORE?

Instead of giving up when something doesn't pan out, ask your yourself "what can I learn from this?" or "what is the universe trying to convey here?" By asking questions, you will more often than not uncover a hidden opportunity that will be more relevant than what originally did not work out. Times have changed and so have the so-called "rules"- so don't get caught up in thinking that there is only one path to success. The traditional model of achievement may not apply to you; don't fight it... success is fluid, we all attain it in our own way

ANY INSPIRING STORIES THAT HAVE HAPPENED TO YOU OR PEOPLE CLOSE TO YOU THAT HAVE NOT BEEN COVERED ABOVE. STORIES THAT CAN HELP OTHERS.

Try and not lose sight of the fact that we truly all have something to contribute. You may not know what it is yet, but that is a part of the journey. Trust it, enjoy it, believe in it and never stop learning

THE VORA SISTERS (KOMIE)

AT WHAT POINT IN YOUR LIFE DID YOU DECIDE TO CHANGE YOUR DIET? HOW HAS THAT DECISION IMPACTED YOUR LIFE?

We were raised vegetarian, so meat was already eliminated from our diet from the very beginning...we still have never tasted meat till this day. The transition into veganism slowly started happening even before I decided to purposely become vegan. Growing up, our mother would have plant-based alternatives in the house such as soy milk, flax seed and almond butter, etc. So I was exposed and aware of certain substitutes already. As I started getting older I stumbled upon gelatin, and once I learned about this active ingredient, I immediately cut that out from my diet.

Moreover, I was born with eczema, and many studies had proven that dairy was the cause of inflammations and I wondered if I stopped consuming dairy if that would help control the flare-ups...so I tested it out. It was all around the same time I was doing more research for Delikate Rayne and saw disturbing footage on how animals were being treated in the dairy industry, which I was not really aware of before. It opened up my eyes to a lot of things, and I decided from that day forward I would no longer ingest any dairy products.

WHO HAS BEEN THE BIGGEST VEGAN INFLUENCER IN YOUR LIFE AND HOW HAVE THEY HELPED YOU?

The concept of not harming any living beings stems from my upbringing. My mother was raised Hindu, and my father was raised Jain, so those principles of non-violence and compassion were taught to us at a very young age. However, the transition to veganism was really all me. It was a decision I made for myself and what I felt aligned best with my beliefs and purpose.

HOW DO YOU THINK WE CAN ALL HAVE A BIGGER IMPACT ON INFLUENCING PEOPLE AND HELPING THEM MAKE THE CONNECTION TO HEALTH AND EATING A PLANT-BASED DIET?

The best way to influence someone is through education. You cannot force or control anyone into doing anything, and that shouldn't be your job to do so either. Everyone is entitled to living a life they feel is best for them - we can only teach and share what we know based on our own experiences and knowledge. I have found having non-judgmental conversations and just simply sharing what you know is the best step to making an impactful connection. In order to make a difference, you need people to see why it matters so much and how they themselves can make a difference not only for themselves but the planet as a whole. I think once people register that into their minds and fully understand how dominant their decisions can be towards so many other factors, that is when you see the ultimate power of change.

WHAT WAS THE REACTION YOU RECEIVED FROM PEOPLE WHEN YOU ANNOUNCED THAT YOU WERE GOING VEGAN? WHO WAS YOUR BEST AND WORST SUPPORTER?

Most people thought I was crazy, because I was already raised vegetarian. They thought why would I take things a step further and eliminate even more things from my diet. It is interesting though, because the same people that would make fun of me are the same ones who are wanting suggestions on making the switch now.

HOW HAS A FAILURE, OR APPARENT FAILURE, SET YOU UP FOR LATER SUCCESS? DO YOU HAVE A "FAVORITE FAILURE" OF YOURS?

Failure is success. Without contrast, there is no want. In other words, if you always got what you wanted, you would never learn from the process... there would be no lesson learned. How do you grow if things always went as planned? Anytime we did not get that interview, sale, project, award, etc it is simply because in reality, it wasn't the time for us. People often associate "no" with failure or not being good enough. To me, I have redefined that word in my mind. I think of "No" as Not Over. You may not get that opportunity or desire fulfilled now, but it is Not Over...and that is what keeps driving me to get that yes.

WHAT VEGAN RESOURCE COULD YOU NOT LIVE WITHOUT AND WHY?

"Ask, and It Is Given" by Esther and Jerry Hicks

WHAT ADVICE WOULD YOU GIVE A SMART AND DRIVEN 18-YEAR-OLD TODAY? WHAT ADVICE SHOULD THEY IGNORE?

Ignore all the conditioning that you were taught when you were growing up. Create your own reality by the things you want to do. Think about how you can help the world and what impact you want to be remembered for when you leave your physical body. No one is you, and that is your superpower.

SARA HANSEN
(EDITOR OF THIS BOOK)

CONNECT WITH SARA:
INSTAGRAM: @SARAAAHANSENNN
rebelwritingco.com

Sara Hansen is a writer, editor (the one who edited the book you're reading right now!) and founder of Rebel Writing Company, where she writes and edits copy for a variety of health and wellness companies. After struggling with years of insomnia and digestive issues, Sara discovered the life-changing benefits of plant-based eating and has now made it a life mission to spread the message about the power of plants to as many people as possible.

WHAT IS ONE OF THE BEST OR MOST WORTHWHILE HEALTH-RELATED INVESTMENTS THAT YOU HAVE MADE?

406

The best health-related investment I've made recently was spending a few hundred dollars to attend a six-day yoga retreat in Thailand. It was an incredibly beautiful and heart-opening experience and so worth the money. It's part of the reason I've gotten much more into plant-based eating as well. Up until that point, I had never taken six days out of my life to really soak in self-care, self-awareness and stillness. I learned a lot about myself in that short period of time, and I really started to realize why avoiding animal products is so important to me.

AT WHAT POINT IN YOUR LIFE DID YOU DECIDE TO CHANGE YOUR DIET? HOW HAS THAT DECISION IMPACTED YOUR LIFE?

I decided to change my diet about two years ago after watching the documentaries *What the Health* and *Cowspiracy*. I had no idea how corrupt the animal agriculture and pharmaceutical companies in America were and it totally disillusioned me. I like to tell people that I became plant-based for the health aspect, but stayed plant-based once I learned about the environmental impacts of raising animals for consumption.

Choosing to go plant-based has impacted my life in so many positive ways! My overall health has improved drastically, and I no longer feel like I'm living in a fog. I have more energy even if I didn't sleep well the night before, but I generally sleep much better now overall anyways.

Going plant-based has also introduced me to a community of like-minded, high-vibe people who make me feel like I'm a part of this secret club where the entrance fee is only an open mind. When I meet other people who are plant-based or interested in this lifestyle, I instantly know that we will connect. It's really a community-building thing.

WHO HAS BEEN THE BIGGEST PLANT-BASED DIET INFLUENCER IN YOUR LIFE AND HOW HAVE THEY HELPED YOU?

This one is easy: Julie Piatt and Rich Roll. This is a husband and wife duo who are incredible plant-based advocates that are all about promoting compassion and authentic self-love practices. When I was struggling with my health a lot in the form of insomnia and digestive issues, I started to take daily walks to calm my mind and get some simple exercise into my day. On these walks, I started listening to the Rich Roll podcast, and I'm not exaggerating when I say that this changed my life. Rich is a plant-based ultra-endurance athlete who sits down with thought-leaders and change-makers who are at the top levels of their respective fields of study, and the discussions he has with these people are so insanely inspiring. Rich is the reason that I went plant-based in the first place, and I still listen to his podcast today.

HOW DO YOU THINK WE CAN ALL HAVE A BIGGER IMPACT ON INFLUENCING PEOPLE AND HELPING THEM MAKE THE CONNECTION TO HEALTH AND EATING A PLANT-BASED DIET?

I think living by example and discussing your diet choices when asked. I respect activists for animals/plant-based eating, but I don't think that approaching the issue in a combative or shaming way makes people listen. I think that makes people defensive.

Live your truth and express your reasoning as compassionately as possible if anyone asks you "why?"

IF YOU COULD HAVE A GIGANTIC BILLBOARD ANYWHERE WITH ANYTHING ON IT, WHAT WOULD IT SAY?

My favorite quote from the French writer/philosopher, Voltaire: "uncertainty is an uncomfortable position, but certainty is an absurd one." I think this is such an important sentiment because it speaks to how little any of us really know about anything, and that that's ok. I think if more people approached the world by embracing how much there is to life that we don't know/understand, we'd all be much kinder when it came to expressing an opinion/idea/belief about something.

HOW HAS A FAILURE, OR APPARENT FAILURE, SET YOU UP FOR LATER SUCCESS? DO YOU HAVE A "FAVORITE FAILURE" OF YOURS?

The greatest example I can think of is the real beginning of my journey to wellness. It started in 2016 when I was just out of college. I was lucky enough to land a full-time job right away, but a few months in I soon realized the toxic environment that I had gotten myself into. There was constant turnover with employees, making everything very unstable, the management team had a very "bow down to your superiors" attitude, and when I finally quit six months into the job, five other employees quit at or close to the same time (the office was only a team of twelve at full capacity).

Leaving this job felt like a huge failure to me because it was my very first full-time job out of college, and it was something I was initially so excited about. I honestly thought I was in the perfect place for me at the time, and quitting six months in made me have some serious self-doubt. I kept wondering if there was something wrong with me, if I was lazy, if I was incompetent, the list of negative self-talk goes on…

At this point though, I have really come to appreciate this experience because while it was happening, I was the most stressed out I have ever been in my life. The job was stressful, my boss was stressful, I was being called after hours and while on vacation so I didn't really feel like I had any sort of work-life balance, so it's no surprise that my health really started to suffer. It manifested most as a wicked case of insomnia, which I had never experienced before in my life. Up until that point I had always been a pretty good sleeper, but because of the stress I was feeling, I just about stopped sleeping completely.

This is when I really delved into researching health and discovered the effects of food on sleep. This, in turn, led me to discovering a community of plant-based eaters and advocates for vegan eating, and my world was changed for the better. If I had never experienced such a stressful point in my life, I may never have discovered the amazing benefits of plant-based eating.

WHAT VEGAN RESOURCE COULD YOU NOT LIVE WITHOUT AND WHY?

Definitely Rich Roll. He's one of those "influencers" who are influencing others in the most genuine way possible. You can just feel the authenticity oozing out of him because he really feels strongly about what he does and how it can help other people. I believe him when he talks, and I think he's incredibly credible because the people that he brings on his podcast are the real deal. They are high-level scientists, athletes, artists and business owners who have something important to share and who want to help other people, and that's what drives me too.

As a millennial having grown up with the internet for most of my life and steeped in this "influencer" culture, I think that I have a good feel for who is authentic and who is just trying to sell me something. Rich Roll is just trying to learn as much as possible and share what he learns in order to help raise the collective vibration of the planet.

WHAT ADVICE WOULD YOU GIVE A SMART AND DRIVEN 18-YEAR-OLD TODAY? WHAT ADVICE SHOULD THEY IGNORE?

I love this question because I think, as a 25-year-old, I'm still close enough to 18 to really remember what it was like and enough years past 18 to have some solid advice that I wish someone would have told me.

I have a few pieces of advice I wish I would have taken to heart as an 18-year-old:

Read as much as you can. It expands your brain and your imagination, and there is wisdom hidden within books that many cannot even fathom that will change you and expand your awareness. Read fiction, read non-fiction, read poetry, read memoirs; anything that interests you and even some things that don't because it will expand your brain in ways you never could have imagined otherwise.

Make a self-care practice a top priority. How you feel and specifically how you feel about yourself, affects every single other aspect of your life. If you are not prioritizing self-care, it will catch up to you fast.

409

Learn about meditation and start a daily practice. Your life will be better because of it, I promise you.

Practice non-judgement, starting with yourself. This is tied closely with number two and number three. Treat yourself the way that you want others to treat you and watch how your life turns into magic.

ANY INSPIRING STORIES THAT HAVE HAPPENED TO YOU OR PEOPLE CLOSE TO YOU THAT HAVE NOT BEEN COVERED ABOVE. STORIES THAT CAN HELP OTHERS.

I'm really into quotes, so I want to share this one from Brianna Wiest that inspires me every time I read it: "If you laid out your blood vessels, they'd circle the Earth four times. Your blood is iron running through you, filling your heart. Your entire body is bioluminescent, it glows and emits light that's invisible to the naked eye. There is more depth to you than you could ever realize, there is more potential within you than you've ever known, and there is a light to you that you will probably never see. But it is always there, burning, guiding you. You are a force more powerful than you could ever dream."

VEGAN &
PLANT-BASED
RECIPES

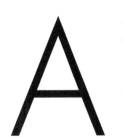

t this point, you may be feeling inspired, ready to make the change, motivated to do the thing that will have a positive impact on your mind, body, and overall wellbeing, but the hardest part is knowing where to begin.

I've compiled the following recipes per the recommendations of some of the women featured in Legends of Change. They are tried and tested for deliciousness, nutritiousness and in some cases, kid-friendliness.

I hope that these recipes will help ease you into those initial first steps towards creating the happiest, healthiest and best possible version of you.

Each one of these women or their recipes can be found on Instagram. Next to each recipe is their Instagram name: Please make sure if you try their recipes, share it with your friends, and make sure you connect with them and support their channels.

Happy eating :)

Rebecca Frith x

RECIPE INDEX:

VEGAN BUTTER THAT'S OIL FREE
RECIPE BY ANJA CASS
@cookingwithplants

INGREDIENTS:

1/2 cup plant milk, unsweetened
100-grams cauliflower, cooked (about 1 cup)
1/8 tsp turmeric powder
1 tsp coarse Celtic sea salt, or to taste
1 tsp psyllium husks

METHOD:

Place all ingredients in a food processor
or powerful blender and blend until smooth
and creamy.

LOW CARB, LOW FAT, PURE PROTEIN BREAD
RECIPE BY SAM SHORKEY
@samshorkey

INGREDIENTS:

2 cups vital wheat gluten
2 Tbsp ground flax
4 Tbsp chickpeas (garbanzo beans) flour
1 tsp baking powder
1 tsp sea salt
1.5 – 2 cups of water (Start with 1.5 cups
then add a little more if needed)

METHOD:

Preheat oven to 350 degrees F. In a medium-
sized bowl, mix all dry ingredients together.
Slowly add in water, starting with 1 cup, then
add the additional half cup. Knead into a dough
and add a little more water if necessary. You
should have yourself a big lump of dough.

Lay out two long pieces of aluminum foil and
spritz the bottom of each piece with a tiny
spray of avocado oil or extra virgin olive oil.

Cut dough in half then use your hands to roll
into two long-ish, somewhat thick-ish cylinders.

Lie each sausage shape of dough on top of the
tin foil. Twist the ends of the tin foil and roll
the sides around your dough but leave the top
open so the bread can rise and air can get out.

Bake for 45 minutes. Remove from heat and allow
to cool before cutting into your protein bread.

BANANA BREAD
RECIPE BY STELLA
@StellaTheLight

INGREDIENTS:

2 Tbsp flax
1/3 cup plant milk
1 Tbsp apple cider vinegar
2 Tbsp nut butter of choice
1 tsp vanilla
3-4 mashed ripe bananas
1/2 cup sweetener (I use maple syrup
or cane sugar!)
2 tsp of baking soda
1.5 cups flour (I usually do 1/2 cup oats + 1 cup
spelt or whole wheat! - feel free to mix/match
with your favorite flours!)
Add-ins: cinnamon, apple, blueberry, chocolate
chips, raisins etc! Any flavors you love!

METHOD:

Preheat oven to 350F and line your bread
pan with parchment paper or lightly oil.

Combine vinegar and milk in a bowl and
let sit for 1-2 min.

Add in the rest of the liquid ingredients
and combine.

In another bigger bowl sift together or
mix together dry ingredients and pour wet
ingredients in!

Transfer to the pan and bake for
about 40-45 minutes.

Cool for about 20 min before popping
out and slicing up!

Store in an airtight container for 1-2 days
at room temp, up to a week in the fridge
and up to 2 months in the freezer!

GINGER-PINEAPPLE CHIA PUDDING
RECIPE BY MARINA
@soulintheraw

INGREDIENTS (SERVES 1):

For the milk:
1 Tbsp raw, unroasted almond butter
1.5 cups water
1 medjool dates pitted
1/4 tsp turmeric powder
1 pinch black pepper
For the pudding:
1/3 cup raw chia seeds
1 cup mango fresh or frozen
1 cup pineapple fresh or frozen
For the topping:
1 Tbsp coconut flakes unsweetened
10 strawberries chopped

METHOD:

Blend all ingredients, except chia seeds,
until smooth.

Place in a bowl, and stir in the chia seeds.

Place in the fridge overnight to thicken
for the best results, but you can also eat after
about 1 hour.

Top with coconut and chopped strawberries.

VEGAN SPICE PUDDING
RECIPE BY CRISSI
@veganfitnessmodel

INGREDIENTS (SERVES 4-6):

4 cups of water
1.5 cups red rice uncooked
1 cup pumpkin puree
1 cup almond or oat milk
2 Tbsp blackstrap molasses or maple syrup
40gms Salted Caramel 'Prana On' Protein Powder* or Vanilla – Brown Rice Protein
1 tsp cinnamon
½ tsp nutmeg
½ tsp cloves
½ tsp ginger
Pinch sea salt
12 pcs pecans (for garnish)

METHOD:

In a medium saucepan, bring 3 cups water to a boil

Add rice, salt, and stir

Reduce heat, cover and simmer for a further 10 minutes

Add in pumpkin puree, molasses or syrup, and nut milk and stir thoroughly

Add all spices, sea salt and stir until cooked

Allow to slightly cool, slowly adding the remaining 1 cup of water, with plant-based protein powder or any vegan plant-based protein source like hemp protein, pea protein, sprouted brown rice protein

Add 2 x pecans to each serving (Optional)

MICROWAVE CAKE BOWL
RECIPE BY STELLA
@StellaTheLight

INGREDIENTS (SERVES 1):

1 cup whole wheat flour (can try other flours like oat flour, buckwheat, etc)
1 tsp baking powder
1 tsp vanilla
1-2 Tbsp peanut butter or nut butter of choice
1 cup plant milk
Sweetener to taste - I used two Tbsp raw sugar! Could also use agave, or maple syrup.
add-ins - choose whatever flavors, spices, you desire! Cinnamon, cacao, vanilla.

METHOD:

Mix everything together in a microwave safe dish.

I did 1/2 the batter in two small bowls

Microwave for roughly 2 min (if halved) or probably 3-3.5 minutes for the whole thing depending on microwave.

Top with warmed sliced apples and I drizzled a sauce of peanut butter, almond milk and raw sugar + cinnamon over top!

QUINOA SUMMER MANGO SALAD
RECIPE BY MRS JACKED ON PLANTS
@mrs.jackedonplants

INGREDIENTS (SERVES 4):

1 cup dry quinoa
1 small can low salt veg broth
3 Tbsp fresh lime juice
1/2 tsp ground cumin
2 tsp maple syrup
1/4 tsp ground ginger
1/4 tsp cayenne pepper (optional)
1 small can black beans, drained and rinsed
1 medium mango, peeled, cored and diced
1 red bell pepper, cored and chopped
1/2 cup sliced green onions
1/3 cup chopped cilantro
1 medium avocado (semi-firm but ripe),
cored and diced

METHOD:

Rinse quinoa well in a fine strainer. Transfer to a medium saucepan along with veg broth and 1/4 cup water. Bring to a boil then reduce heat to low and simmer until water has been absorbed, about 15 - 20 minutes. Allow to cool.

In a small mixing bowl whisk together lime juice, syrup, cumin, ginger and cayenne pepper. In a large bowl or salad bowl toss together quinoa, black beans, mango, bell pepper, green onions, cilantro, avocado and dressing.

Season with salt and pepper to taste and serve.

CREAMY CARROT AND APPLE OVERNIGHT OATS
RECIPE BY ROBYN
@robynchuter

INGREDIENTS (SERVES 1 TO 2):

1 cup rolled oats
1 cup plant milk
1/2 cup unsweetened plant milk yoghurt
1/2 cup grated carrots
2 Tbsp date syrup
2 Tbsp ground linseed/flaxseed
1 tsp cinnamon
1/2 tsp ground ginger
1/2 tsp allspice
1/2 tsp cardamom
1/4 cup sultanas
1/4 cup chopped walnuts
1 apple, grated or finely sliced

METHOD:

In a medium mixing bowl, stir together all ingredients except apple until well-combined. Cover and leave in the fridge overnight.

Just before serving, add grated or finely sliced apple.

*You can buy ready-made date syrup from specialty grocers, or make your own: just place pitted dates in a saucepan, cover with water, bring the water to the boil and simmer for 30-60 minutes, depending on how hard the dates are. When dates are mushy, remove from the heat, cool, then transfer to a food processor and blend until smooth. Store leftovers in the fridge.

CHOCOLATE PROTEIN SMOOTHIE BOWL
RECIPE BY MRS JACKED ON PLANTS
@mrs.jackedonplants

INGREDIENTS (SERVES 1):

2 medium frozen bananas
1/4 cup almond milk
1 Tbsp cacao nibs
1 Tbsp chia seeds
1tsp cocoa powder
1 Tbsp pea protein (or hemp)
1 tsp hemp seeds
strawberries (optional topping)
1 Tbsp chopped walnuts (optional topping)

METHOD:

Add frozen bananas to a blender and blend for 30 to 60 seconds

Add a bit of coconut or almond milk and protein powder and blend on low again, scraping down sides as needed, until the mixture reaches a soft serve consistency.

Scoop into 1-2 serving bowls and top with desired toppings. I prefer chia seeds, cacao nibs, hemp seeds or walnuts and strawberries

CANCER KNOCKOUT SMOOTHIE
RECIPE BY ROBYN
@robynchuter

INGREDIENTS (SERVES 1):

1 medium banana
1/2 cup fresh or frozen blueberries
1/2 cup fresh or frozen cherries
4 pitted dates or 2 medjool dates, pitted
1 Tbsp hemp hearts or ground flaxseed/linseed
1 Tbsp cacao (raw chocolate) powder
1/2 cup pomegranate juice
1/2 cup non-dairy milk
1 cup firmly packed baby spinach
1 cup firmly packed bok choy
1/4 cup chopped coriander, including stems
(optional – omit if you're not a coriander fan!)

METHOD:

Blend all ingredients at high speed until creamy and smooth.

417

SPROUTED AVOCADO SANDWICH
RECIPE BY MRS JACKED ON PLANTS
@mrs.jackedonplants

INGREDIENTS (SERVES 1):

2 slices sprouted whole grain bread or Ezekiel bread
½ cup sprouts (sunflower sprouts or any microgreens)
Romaine Lettuce
1 ripe tomato, thinly sliced
¼ avocado mashed
1 small cucumber thinly sliced
Pepper to taste

METHOD:

Mash or spread the avocado on both slices of bread

Layer the sprouts, lettuce, sliced tomato, and cucumber between the slices of bread

Season with pepper and enjoy.

WORLD'S GREATEST TOFU SCRAMBLE
RECIPE BY SAM SHORKEY
@samshorkey

INGREDIENTS (SERVES 2 T0 4):

1 Tbsp extra virgin olive oil
1 cup chopped onion
4 garlic cloves (minced)
½ cup chopped bell pepper
½ cup sliced white mushrooms
1 cup fresh or frozen spinach
300-gram package extra-firm tofu (cubed)
1 tsp smoked paprika
2 Tbsp nutritional yeast
1 Tbsp Bragg liquid aminos (healthy,
low-sodium soy sauce substitute)
1 tsp black pepper

METHOD:

Heat oil in a large frypan over medium-high heat. Add onion and garlic and sauté for 2 – 3 minutes until garlic is lightly browned.

Add tofu, vegetables & remaining ingredients and cook until veggies are tender.

LET'S GET SHREDDED WITH DR. ANGIE'S SALAD
RECIPE BY DR. ANGIE
@angie.sadeghi

INGREDIENTS (SERVES 1):

1 bag of spinach
1/2 a can of chickpeas
1 block of sprouted tofu from Trader Joe's
6 Tbsp of pre-cooked lentils
1 Persian cucumber
1 cup steamed broccoli
Handful of blueberries
Handful of cashews
Sprinkle nutritional yeast
Sprinkle pomegranate vinaigrette
Sprinkle balsamic glaze

METHOD:

Place all ingredients into a large bowl, Sprinkle with Nutritional Yeast, Vinaigrette and a touch of Balsamic Glaze. Enjoy

RAW PAD THAI
RECIPE BY CANDY MARX
@plantfedmama

INGREDIENTS (SERVES 3 TO 4):

For the noodles:
1 packet of kelp noodles
2 cups red cabbage (shredded)
1 red capsicum (thinly sliced)
1 large carrot (grated)
2 - 3 large handfuls of salad greens
1/2 cup cashews or peanuts
Handful chopped shallots
1/2 cup fresh mint (ripped, not chopped)

For the sauce:
1/2 cup almond butter
2 to 3 tbsp tamari
2 - 3 Medjool dates
1/4 cup apple cider vinegar
2 - 3 tsp fresh lemon or lime juice
1 tbsp ginger
1 garlic clove
1/8 cup olive oil (can replace with water if preferred)

METHOD:

Soak kelp noodles in filtered water for about 15 minutes. Add salad ingredients to a large bowl. Add all the sauce ingredients to a blender (or stick blender beaker) and blend until smooth and creamy. Adjust to suit tastes. Drain the noodles and toss with oil and add to salad. Pour sauce over the noodles and combine well, making sure all of the noodles are covered. Top with chopped nuts, shallots, and mint, then serve.

ISRAELI COUSCOUS & SWEET POTATO SALAD
RECIPE BY ROBYN
@robynchuter

INGREDIENTS (SERVES 1):

1 large sweet potato, peeled and diced
1 tbsp low sodium vegetable broth, or water saved from steaming vegetables
1 tsp cinnamon
1 tsp ground coriander
1 tsp ground cumin
1 cup wholemeal Israeli couscous
1 1/4 cups boiling water
1 head broccoli, cut into florets
2 cloves garlic, peeled
2 cm ginger, peeled
1 bunch coriander
2 tbsp tahini
Juice of 2 limes
Water to thin
2 tbsp walnuts

METHOD:

Preheat oven to 200°C. Line a baking sheet with a silicone baking mat or baking paper.

Toss sweet potato cubes with vegetable stock or steaming water, and spices. Spread on a prepared baking sheet in a single layer, and bake for 20 minutes or until tender, turning once during the baking process.

Steam broccoli florets for 5 minutes, or until just tender.

Add couscous to boiling water and simmer, covered, for 10 minutes. Allow to cool.

Combine garlic, ginger, fresh coriander stems and leaves, tahini and lime juice in a food processor or high powered blender. Blend until smooth, adding enough water to reach a pouring consistency.

Toss sweet potato, broccoli, couscous and dressing together in a serving bowl. May be served warm or cool.

PULLED BB-BBQ SANDWICH
RECIPE BY NARA
@naraschuler

INGREDIENTS:

Fake meat:
500 g banana blossom in brine, drained
and pulled in small parts
2 Tbsp fancy molasses
1 tsp smoked paprika
1 tsp garlic powder
½ tsp salt
½ tsp black pepper
½ tsp ground chili powder
¾ cup BBQ sauce of your choice

For one sandwich:
Ingredients:
1 round bread cut in half and toasted
100 g Pulled BB-BBQ MM
1 Tbs red cabbage shaved
1 Tbs grated carrots
1 Tbs red onions sliced
1 mashed avocado

METHOD:

Mix all ingredients, add to banana blossom
Heat on a skillet for about 2/3 minutes
Add water if needed, reduce heat and let it
cook for about 5 to 7 minutes
Remove from stove, store in the refrigerator.

For one sandwich:
Instructions:
Spread Pulled BB-BBQ on one side of the bread
Mix cabbage, carrots, onions and avocado
Place mixture on top of BB-BBQ
Top with the other side of bread

HEALTHY VEGAN TUSCAN RIBOLLITA
RECIPE BY AMBER
@mcammertime

INGREDIENTS (SERVES 4 TO 6):

2 large carrots
1 whole red onion
4 garlic cloves
1 bunch of kale
2 cans cannellini beans rinsed and drained
16 oz vegetable stock
3 cups of water
2 or 3 cans of diced tomatoes
1 Tbsp olive oil
1 Tbsp fennel seeds
Salt and pepper
Chili flakes (season to how spicy you want it)
Ciabatta bread or bread of choice

METHOD:

Prepare and wash all produce
Peel and dice carrots
Dice red onion
Mince or grate garlic cloves
Finely chop kale (stems and ribs removed)

In a large pot, add olive oil on low-medium
heat, add carrots, garlic, onions, fennel seeds,
and chili flakes. Stir on occasion and until
veggies are soft.

Once veggies are soft, add beans, tomatoes,
vegetable stock, 3 cups of water to the pot and
season with salt and pepper. Bring the heat to
medium-high until it boils. Once it boils, lower the
heat and let simmer 20 minutes. Stir occasionally.

Add the kale to the pot, stir and let simmer
3-10 minutes until soft.

Feel free to add ciabatta or bread to the soup.
Take off the heat and serve! But be careful it's
hot! Season with salt and pepper to taste!

ADUKI BEAN AND RICE BALLS
RECIPE BY ROBYN
@robynchuter

INGREDIENTS:

1/4 cup pumpkin seeds (pepitas)
1/4 cup sunflower seeds
1/2 cup polenta
1/3 cup savoury yeast flakes/nutritional yeast
1/2 tsp dried thyme
1 tsp dried oregano
2 tsp smoked paprika
2 tsp onion flakes
1 tbsp dulse flakes
2 cups cooked brown rice
2 cups cooked, drained aduki beans
2 tbsp no added salt tomato paste

Dipping sauce
2 Tbsp no added salt tomato paste
1 tsp dijon mustard
Juice of 1 lime

METHOD:

Preheat oven to 180°C. Line a baking sheet with baking paper.

In a food processor, combine all ingredients except for brown rice, beans and tomato paste. Pulse until combined into a coarse meal. Set aside.

Place rice, beans and tomato paste in a food processor and pulse until combined but still chunky.

Stir in seed, polenta and spice mix.

Form dessert spoons of mixture into balls and place on a prepared baking sheet. Bake for 20 minutes. Turn with a spatula or slotted spoon and bake for another 15 minutes.

Stir sauce ingredients together until well combined.

ETHIOPIAN LENTILS
RECIPE BY DR JOANNE
@drjoannekong

INGREDIENTS:

2 cups dried red split lentils
3 cups vegetable stock
½ teaspoon coconut oil
2 cloves garlic, minced
½ cup finely chopped, medium yellow onion
1 tsp peeled, grated ginger
½ tsp turmeric
¼ tsp ground cumin
½ - 1 tsp Berbere (Ethiopian spice mixture)
½ cup lacinato kale, coarsely chopped

METHOD:

Place lentils and vegetable stock in a saucepot. Bring to a boil, then simmer, uncovered, for about 8 minutes.

While lentils are cooking, cook the garlic, onions, and ginger in coconut oil over medium heat in a small saucepan, until slightly browned. Turn off the heat and stir in the turmeric and cumin.

Stir the onions and spices into the lentils, and add in the Berbere.

Stir in the kale, until wilted.

VEGAN & PLANT-BASED RECIPES

SPICY TOFU JERKY
RECIPE BY SAM SHORKEY
@Samshorkey

INGREDIENTS:

1 brick of extra-firm organic tofu (350 g)
2 Tbsp Bragg's liquid aminos (soy sauce alternative)
2 Tbsp sriracha hot chili sauce
1 Tbsp finely minced garlic (about 3 - 4 cloves)

METHOD:

Drain your tofu then wrap it in a paper towel and press out as much water as you can. Cut the tofu into thin slices (mine were about a 1/2" thick.)

Combine Braggs, sriracha & minced garlic in a small bowl and set aside.

Line a couple of dehydrator trays with parchment paper or actual dehydrator liners if you're cool enough to own them. Arrange tofu slices on dehydrator trays then brush each side with a bit of the sauce.

Dehydrated for a good 4 - 5 hours. Remove once "dry and tough"

NO-BAKE PEANUT BUTTER BARS
RECIPE BY MARINA
@soulintheraw

INGREDIENTS:

For the first layer:
1.5 cups rolled oats
1 cup raisins
1.5 cups medjool dates, pitted
0.25 cup raw almond butter

For the second layer:
2/3 cup peanut butter
3/4 cup medjool dates, pitted
2/3 cup soy milk
Topping (optional):
1 Tbsp cacao nibs

METHOD:

For the first layer:
Add rolled oats to a food processor, and process until slightly broken down.
Add raisins, dates, and almond butter, and process until the mixture starts to stick together.
If the mixture is still not sticking together well, add a few more dates.
Line a square 8-inch glass dish w/ parchment paper.
Press the mixture from the food processor into the baking dish. Set aside.

For the second layer:
Rinse the food processor - you don't have to rinse extremely well.
Add peanut butter, dates, and soy milk into a food processor.
Process until completely smooth - about 5 mins.
Add the second layer on the first, using a rubber spatula.
Sprinkle with cacao nibs (optional).
Set in the freezer for 1-2 hours.
Remove from freezer, and cut into bars.

VEGAN CAULIFLOWER LENTIL STEW W/ TZATZIKI
RECIPE BY MARINA
@soulintheraw

INGREDIENTS (SERVES 2):

For the cauliflower lentil stew:
¼ cup sprouted lentils
½ large cauliflower chopped very well
3 cups cherry tomatoes chopped in half
1 sweet onion chopped
3 Tbsp apple cider vinegar
2 Tbsp onion powder
1 Tbsp chipotle powder or smoked paprika
2 Tbsp chilli powder
1 Tbsp cumin powder

For the hemp tzatziki:
4 Tbsp of hemp seeds
2 cloves of garlic optional
Juice of ½ a lemon 2-3 Tbsp of lemon juice
2 Tbsp dried dill
2 Tbsp nutritional yeast
¼ cup of water
1 small zucchini about 1 cup, chopped
3 Persian cucumbers about 1.5 cups, chopped
½ teaspoon of sea salt

METHOD:

For the hemp tzatziki:
Blend all ingredients in a high-speed blender, besides the dill. Start by placing the zucchini and all liquid ingredients at the bottom, and then adding the rest and blending until smooth. Add dill, and pulse a few times in the blender to incorporate. Set aside.

For the cauliflower lentil stew:
Chop onions, and add them to a very hot nonstick skillet. Cook for 10 minutes until they start to brown.
Add finely chopped or processed cauliflower, halved cherry tomatoes, lentils, apple cider vinegar, and all spices.
Lower heat to simmer, and let cook for 30-40 minutes, or until the cauliflower is very soft and easily pierced with a fork.
Enjoy the stew with some spring mix, and a drizzle of the sauce.

VEGAN ALFREDO POTATO BAKE
RECIPE BY ANJA CAS
@cookingwithplants

INGREDIENTS (SERVES 4 TO 6):

Bake ingredients:
7 large boiled potatoes, peeled and cooled sliced thinly
1 medium to large white onion sliced thinly
nutmeg or paprika to sprinkle over the top

Alfredo sauce Ingredients:
(makes enough for 2 bakes or extra for over pasta)
1 1/2 cups filtered water
1/2 cups plant milk
1 large boiled potato, peeled
1 Tbsp miso paste (soy, chickpea or brown rice miso)
1/2 cups nutritional yeast flakes
1 tsp garlic powder
1 tsp onion powder
1/2 tsp coarse Celtic sea salt optional, to taste only
1/4 tsp white pepper
1 Tbsp tahini
750g steamed cauliflower (1 medium head)

METHOD:

Preheat oven to 200C/400F.

Layer potato and onion in a 2 litre size casserole dish (with lid). Finish with a layer of potato.

Next, place all of the alfredo sauce ingredients into a blender. Blend on high for a minute or two until smooth and creamy.

Pour the alfredo sauce evenly over the potatoes, making sure that the sauce runs down and around the sides of the potatoes. Lightly sprinkle with nutmeg or paprika, and cover with a lid. If you do not have a baking dish with a lid, use some aluminum foil to cover it tightly.

Bake in the oven for 15 minutes. Remove the lid and place back in the oven for another 15 to 20 minutes until the potatoes are cooked through and the top is browned to your liking.

Note: The alfredo sauce makes enough for 2 bakes or extra for over pasta. Will keep in the fridge for about 5 days.

LEMON BALLS
RECIPE BY PAM ROCCA
@prepwithpam

INGREDIENTS (MAKES 12 BALLS):

1 cup almonds, pulsed into flour
2/3 cup unsweetened coconut flakes
¼ cup vanilla protein powder
2 Tbsp of lemon juice
¼ cup agave or a little stevia to sweeten.
Optional 1 tsp poppy seeds

METHOD:

1. Pulse almonds in a food processor to make almond meal (flour like texture).

2. Add all ingredients in a bowl and mix with hands. If mixture is too dry add a little bit more agave or add a little almond butter. This makes approximately 12 balls.

Note - you can make these school safe (nut-free) by substituting almond flour for oat flour. Simply pulse 1 cup of gluten-free oats into flour instead - this recipe is delicious both ways.

CARAMEL TWIKS
RECIPE BY CANDY MARX
@plantfedmama

INGREDIENTS (MAKES 12 BARS):

For the biscuit base
1 cup cashews
1 cup macadamias
1 tbsp lucuma powder (optional)
2 tbsp pure maple syrup
Pinch pink himalayan salt

For the caramel
15 medjool dates (pitted)
3 - 3.5 tbsp almond butter
2 Tbsp coconut butter OR coconut oil (melted)
1 tsp vanilla powder
Tiny pinch pink Himalayan salt
4 - 6 Tbsp filtered water, added gradually

For the chocolate
1 cup cacao butter
2 Tbsp cacao powder
2 Tbsp pure maple syrup
1/2 tsp vanilla powder or extract
1/2 tsp ground cinnamon (optional)

METHOD:

Add all biscuit base ingredients to a food processor or blender, and blitz until the mixture comes together and resembles a crumbly dough.

Press the dough into a medium-sized rectangular tray (I use a bread baking tin) lined with parchment paper and place in the freezer. Prepare the caramel.

Add all caramel ingredients except for the coconut oil/butter to a food processor, and pulse until smooth. Add the coconut oil/butter and pulse until combined. Spread over the biscuit base and freeze for at least 2 hours, then cut into long, equal-sized sticks.

Prepare the chocolate when the caramel and base are frozen, or solid enough to cut up without it falling apart.

Melt cacao butter in a small saucepan or in a double boiler. Add remaining ingredients and stir until thick and velvety.

Dip and coat each stick with chocolate and place on a plate lined with parchment paper. I find this step is easiest working with frozen sticks, as a thick layer of chocolate hardens and sets immediately. Otherwise, only a thin layer of chocolate will cover the stick, and you will have to dip the stick in chocolate again.

Store in the fridge in an airtight container for up to a week, or store in the freezer for up to 6 weeks.

CHOC CHIP NICE CREAM
RECIPE BY REBECCA
@Legendsofchange

INGREDIENTS (SERVES 1 OR 2):

3 medium bananas, sliced and frozen
1/4 cup coconut milk
1–2 Tbsp pure maple syrup
(optional for sweetness)
1/2 tsp pure vanilla extract
2 Tbsp vegan chocolate
chips or cacao nibs.

METHOD:

Blend frozen bananas until crumbly.

Blend in coconut cream, maple syrup and vanilla, until smooth.

Pulse chocolate or nibs

MANGO & LIME SORBET
RECIPE BY REBECCA
@Legendsofchange

INGREDIENTS (SERVES 1 OR 2):

4 cups of chopped frozen mango chunks
2 Tbsp of fresh lime juice
2 Tbsp of fresh lemon juice
4 Tbsp of water
1 tsp of maple syrup (optional) it is sweet
enough without it.

METHOD:

Mix all the ingredients into a high-speed blender
Blend until smooth
Enjoy!

425

OIL-FREE GRANOLA BAR
RECIPE BY STELLA
@StellaTheLight

INGREDIENTS (8 BARS):

4 Tbsp peanut butter (or tahini!)
1 mashed banana or 3/4 medjool dates
1.5 cup oats
1/3 cup maple syrup
1/2 cup nuts /seeds/coconut etc
1/4 - 1/2 choco chips or cacao nibs (can omit!)
Feel free to add any other flavors

METHOD:

Preheat oven to 375F.

Pour oats + nuts + dates (or banana - but I would use dates if you can!) in your high-speed blender or food processor and pulse/blend until they are broken up (don't blend too long!!)

Add in nut butter + maple syrup and blend it up again! You might need to stop the blender and scrape down the sides.

Line an 8x8 baking sheet with parchment paper, scoop out the sticky mess and try your best to spread it evenly!!

Sprinkle dairy-free choc chips (or other toppings!) on top if you are using them.

Bake at 375F for 25-30 min

SIMPLE & DELICIOUS OIL-FREE DRESSINGS:
BY MRS JACKED ON PLANTS
@mrs.jackedonplants

BITTERSWEET DRESSING:

INGREDIENTS:

3 Tbsps balsamic vinegar
2 Tbsps Dijon mustard
1 Tbsp maple syrup

METHOD:

Mix all the ingredients together in a bowl
until combined.

Drizzle on your salad, buddha bowls
or rice and enjoy!

RANCH DRESSING

INGREDIENTS:

1/4 cup hemp seeds
1 tsp lemon juice
1/2 tsp salt
1 tsp dill
1/2 tsp garlic powder
4-6 Tbsp water

METHOD:

Mix all the ingredients together in a high-speed
blender and slowly add water until you have
reached the desired consistency.

Remember this will thicken much more once
refrigerated so a little runny is ok.

Drizzle on your salad use on your
veg burgers and enjoy!

TANGY TOMATO DRESSING

INGREDIENTS:

2/3 cup organic tomato ketchup
1/3 cup water
1/4 cup agave or another sweetener
1/4 cup vinegar
1/4 tsp black pepper
1/4 tsp garlic powder
1/4 tsp onion powder
pinch of cayenne
pinch of thyme
Pinch of paprika

METHOD:

Combine all ingredients in a small saucepan over
medium heat. Bring to a boil, stirring often.

Reduce heat and simmer for 5 minutes.

Cool and refrigerate.

USEFUL RESOURCES:

Our Recommended Books:

The China Study *by T. Colin Campbell*
Proteinaholic *by G Davis*
How Not to Die *by M Greger*
The Low Carb Fraud *by T. Colin Campbell*
The End of Diabetes *by Joel Fuhrman*
Prevent and Reverse Heart Disease
by Caldwell Esselstyn
Eat to Live *by Joel Fuhrman*
Power Foods for The Brain
by Neal D Barnard
The Starch Solution *by John A. McDougall*
Eating Animals *by Jonathan Safran Foer*
Animal Liberation *by Peter Singer*

Our Recommended Films:

Forks Over Knives
Dominion
Cowspiracy
What The Health
Food Matters
Plant Pure Nation
H.O.P.E What You Eat Matters
Veducated
The Cove
Eating You Alive
Land of Hope and Glory
Eating - by Mike Anderson
Game Changers

News:

www.plantbasednews.org
www.livekindly.co
www.veganlifemag.com
www.vegan.com
www.vegnews.com
www.vegansociety.com

Vegan Not for Profit Sites & Sanctuaries:

www.sanctuaryfederation.org
www.peta.org
www.veganuary.com
www.happycow.net
www.mercyforanimals.org
www.farmsanctuary.org
www.vegan.org
www.farmusa.org
www.foodispower.org
www.friendfarmanimalsanctuary.org
www.changeforanimals.org
www.ffacoalition.org

Podcasts:

www.thatvegancouple.com/podcasts
www.richroll.com/category/podcast
www.nomeatathlete.com/radio-archive
www.plantproof.com/category/podcast
www.player.fm/featured/vegan

Doctors:

www.plantbaseddoctors.org
www.veganaustralia.org.au/vegan_
health_practitioners
www.pcrm.org

Wellness & Healing Clinics:

www.thanyapura.com
www.drthomaslodi.com
www.balanceforlifeflorida.com

Restaurants/Food and Alcohol:

www.happycow.net
www.barnivore.com
www.isitvegan.net

Lightning Source UK Ltd.
Milton Keynes UK
UKHW012020051219
354856UK00004B/121/P

9 780648 672012